M000100524

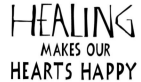

HEALING
MAKES OUR
HEARTS HAPPY

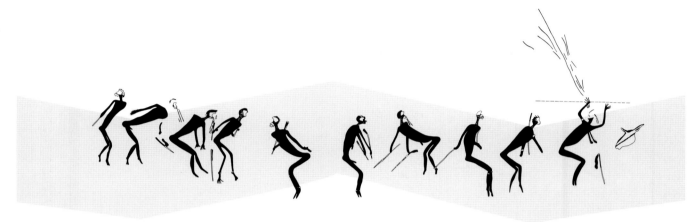

"The book is a compelling and sensitively written account of a people with a rich and vibrant culture. In many respects it's the parallel story of a culture which is shared by Indigenous people the world over. I am grateful to the Ju/'hoansi, as well as Dick, Verna and Megan, for the opportunity to experience a wonderful story of a people with whom I share a sense of kinship."

—Priscilla Settee, Indigenous Peoples Program, University of Saskatchewan

"I'm grateful for this sensitive and moving study of the contemporary Ju/'hoansi of the Kalahari. It must lead to a deeper appreciation of this people, the remarkable social technology they have developed, and the threats to their survival they now face. The acute account of the evolution of the healing dance at the core of Ju/'hoansi life is fascinating. If there is any justice, this exemplary essay in compassionate anthropology will bring critically needed help to these unique people."

—Norman Rush, author of *Whites* and *Mating*

"A moving and enlightening addition to humanity's healing paths."

—Daniel Goleman, author of *Emotional Intelligence*

"*Healing Makes Our Hearts Happy* is a breathtaking view of the Ju/'hoan culture; its practical and spiritual strength, its beauty and mystery, and the rapidity with which an ancient culture can be threatened by modern expansionism. The European ethic of bringing "civilization" to "primitive" peoples is not only challenged, but leaves the reader wondering how European culture might be enriched from a truly respectful exchange with Indigenous peoples worldwide. The researchers' sensitivity to the Ju/'hoansi, and their faithful commitment to the people's story for their own use as well as for Westerners, makes this book a rare treasure of integrity and knowledge preserved for all time."

—Joan Borysenko, Ph.D., author of *Minding the Body, Mending the Mind* and *A Woman's Book of Life*

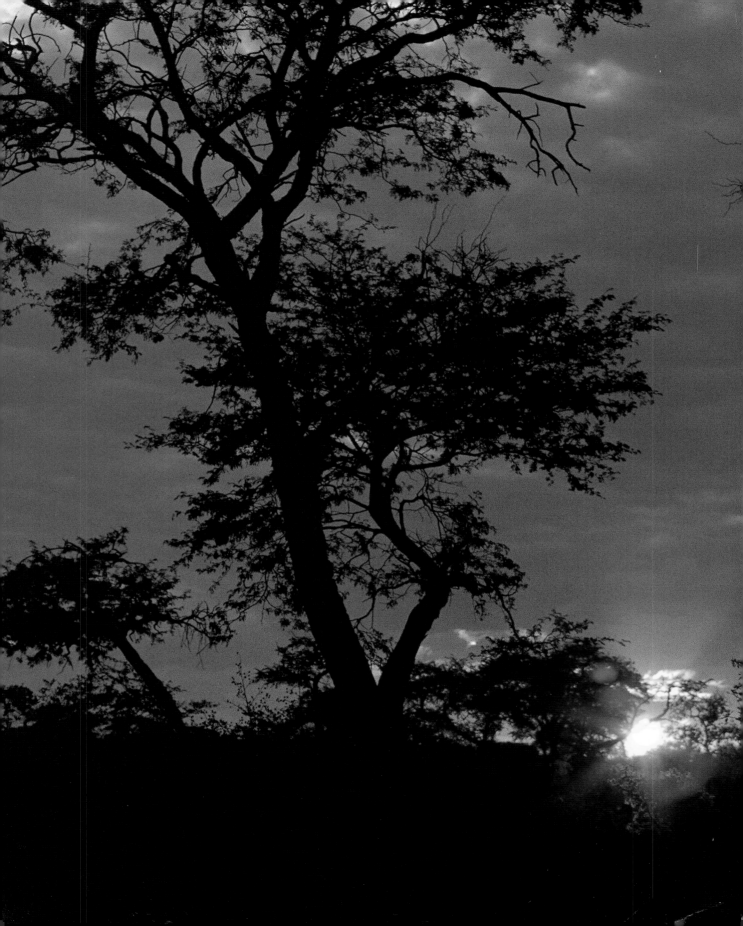

HEALING
MAKES OUR
HEARTS HAPPY

Spirituality & Cultural Transformation
among the Kalahari Ju|'hoansi

RICHARD KATZ • MEGAN BIESELE • VERNA ST. DENIS

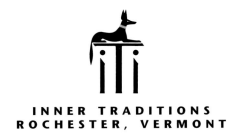

INNER TRADITIONS
ROCHESTER, VERMONT

Inner Traditions International
One Park Street
Rochester, Vermont 05767
www.gotoit.com

Library of Congress Cataloging-in-Publication Data
Katz, Richard, 1937–
    Healing makes our hearts happy : spirituality and cultural transformation among the Kalahari Jul'hoansi / Richard Katz, Megan Biesele, and Verna St. Denis.
        p.   cm.
    Includes bibliographical references and index.
    ISBN 0-89281-557-4
    1. !Kung (African people)—Medicine. 2. !Kung (African people)—Social conditions.
    I. Biesele, Megan. II. St. Denis, Verna. III. Title.
DT1058.K85K37   1996
306.4'61'089961—dc20   96-938
                                       CIP

The following publishers, journals, and people have given us permission to use material from their books, articles, and songs: Harvard University Press, Katz, *Boiling Energy*; *Ethos,* Katz, "Accepting 'Boiling Energy' "; Addison-Wesley, Katz, *The Straight Path;* University of Witwatersrand Press and Indiana University Press, Biesele, *Women Like Meat*; and Floyd Westerman and Jimmy Curtis, "Here Come the Anthros."

Cover photograph and all other photographs by Dick Katz (% Anthro Photo) except: Lesley Beake p. 154; Megan Biesele (% Anthro Photo) p. 34, p. 51 (bottom), p. 91, p. 152; Irven DeVore (% Anthro Photo) p. 9 and p. 14, p. 19, p. 52, p. 94, p. 146; Robert Hitchcock p. 157; Melvin Konner (% Anthro Photo) p. 18; Richard Lee (% Anthro Photo) p. ix; Verna St. Denis p. xix (bottom right), p. xx (top left), p. 82 (top), p. 148, p. 150, p. 155, p. 213 (top); Marjorie Shostak (% Anthro Photo) p. xii, p. 25, p. 111 (right); |Ukxa p. 176; Stan Washburn (% Anthro Photo) p. 64.

Printed in Hong Kong

10 9 8 7 6 5 4 3 2 1

Text design by Bonnie Atwater. Layout by Bonnie Atwater and Kristin Camp.
This book was typeset in Minion and Stone Sans with hand-lettered display type

Distributed to the book trade in Canada by Publishers Group West (PGW), Toronto, Ontario
Distributed to the book trade in the United Kingdom by Deep Books, London
Distributed to the book trade in Australia by Millennium Books, Newtown, N. S. W.
Distributed to the book trade in New Zealand by Tandem Press, Auckland
Distributed to the book trade in South Africa by Alternative Books, Ferndale

page ii: A Kalahari sunset.
page v: A young man decorates a drum that can be both used in the village drum dances and sold as a craft item.
page vi: Kinachau, a respected and experienced healer, at the end of an all night healing dance.
page 101: Totally blind, Kxao ≠Oah, a highly respected and powerful Jul'hoan healer, can "see" when in !aia during the healing dance.

The design element that appears on the chapter opening pages is a popular Jul'hoan beadwork motif called *g!acemhsi,* or "the little children of the rain," which refers to the blackbirds that swirl up into the sky when rain clouds gather.

DEDICATION

To the Jul'hoansi and their struggle to live as they choose

Nlang Jul'hoan ll'aea Ixoa

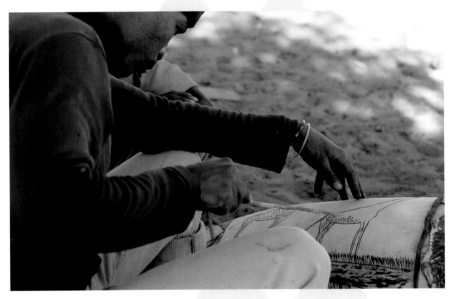

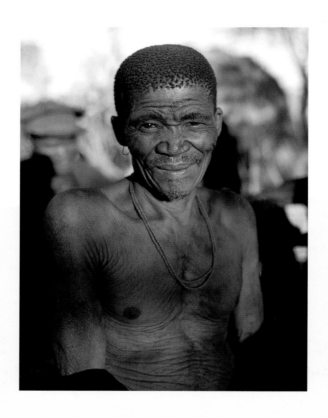

THE USE OF THE JU⏐'HOAN LANGUAGE

As a sign of respect and as an essential prerequisite to a true understanding
of the Jul'hoan people and their lives, we chose to use the orthography of
the Jul'hoan language that was developed under the auspices of their
people's organization and is now officially recognized in southern Africa as
well as internationally. Thus you will find Jul'hoan spellings, including four
click symbols (⏐, ≠, !, ⏐⏐), used for all Jul'hoan names and terms in the book.
These symbols remind us that the Jul'hoan language has specifics that
cannot be assimilated into English, but whose pronunciation can be
learned by English speakers. On p. xxii you will find detailed pronunciation
information.

CONTENTS

ACKNOWLEDGMENTS

WE ARE PRIVILEGED to be a part of an ongoing effort to work for Indigenous peoples throughout the world and, in particular, for the Jul'hoan people in the Kalahari Desert. Many people have offered resources that have made the book possible, and we hope that joining these resources together will further contribute to the struggles of all Indigenous peoples. In gratitude, we would like to acknowledge the following:

The Jul'hoansi of the Kalahari Desert, especially those living in the |Kae|kae area. They opened their homes and hearts to us and trusted us with the responsibility of becoming "paper people" for them.

The |Kae|kae research team, for guiding us toward the truths of Jul'hoan healing today even as they tolerated our foreign preconceptions and manners. The team included five healers and their wives: the healer ≠Oma Djo and his wife N≠aisa N!a'an, Tshao N!a'an and |Xoan, ≠Oma !'Homg!ausi and Ti!'ae, Tshao Matze and ||Uce N!a'an, and Kxao Tjimburu and N≠aisa; the Jul'hoan translators |Ukxa, Tshao Xumi, and Kxao Jonah |O|Oo (Royal); and the Tswana translator Florence Molebatsi. The translators' work was difficult—and indispensable. They translated far more than words.

Several Jul'hoan healers in Nyae Nyae, Namibia, who provided further understanding, including |Kunta Boo, |'Angn!ao |'Un, and ≠Oma Djo's son, G|aq'o ≠Oma.

The governments of Botswana and Namibia, for granting us permission to do research in their countries. In particular, we wish to thank the Ministry of Education, the Ministry of Health, and the Ministry of Local Government, Lands, and Housing, all in Botswana, and the Ministry of Basic Education and Culture in Namibia for their concerned support.

Colleagues whose work in the Kalahari has given us strength and insight, especially Robert Hitchcock, Melvin Konner, Richard Lee, Lorna Marshall, and Marjorie Shostak.

Colleagues who have provided specific historical and chronological material for chapter 2, including Robert Hitchcock, Polly Wiessner, Richard Lee, and Edwin Wilmsen.

David Lewis-Williams and Thomas Dowson, whose corpus of work on southern African rock art offered us fundamental understandings, and who, with the staff of the Rock Art Research Unit, Department of Archaeology, University of Witwatersrand, generously provided tracings of Bushman rock paintings.

Richard Lee, for the text of the "Haba-utwe Oration," which appears in chapter 8.

Robbie Davis-Floyd, Pat Draper, Richard Lee, and Renya Raimerez, who read an earlier draft of the book and provided exceptionally careful, perceptive, and caring critiques.

Students we have worked with over the years who, in the exchange of ideas and ideals, have helped us clarify our aim and strengthen our purpose. In particular, we wish to thank students at the Saskatchewan Indian Federated College, the University of Saskatchewan, Rice University, the University of Alaska at Fairbanks, the University of Toronto, and Harvard University.

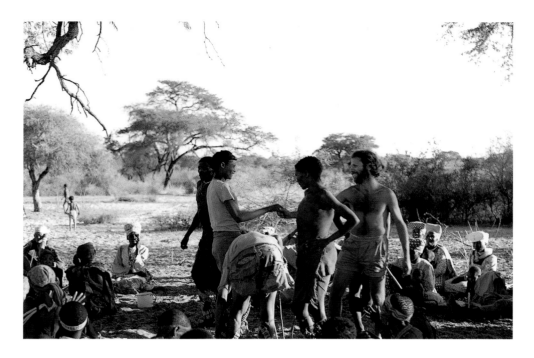

WITH ≠OMA DJO DANCING IN THE BACKGROUND, KXAO TJIMBURU AND DICK KATZ JOYOUSLY CLASP HANDS WHILE PARTICIPATING IN THE JUI'HOAN HEALING DANCE IN 1968.

Scholars and students who attended a talk given by Dick Katz and Verna St. Denis in February 1994 at the University of Puerto Rico at Mayaguez. Many participants offered enlightening perspectives on the issues of social change and spirituality.

The National Science Foundation (Grant #8804531) and the Mind Science Foundation of San Antonio, Texas (Grant #MH89001), for supplying the funds that enabled us to do our research at |Kae|kae in 1989.

The U.S. National Endowment for the Humanities, for providing funds under two translation grants (titled Jul'hoansi Kokxuisi I and II), some of which covered Megan Biesele's time in translating the interviews for this book.

Carl and Dr. Kathleen Brown of Chantilly, Virgina, and the Uniterra Foundation for providing funds to help in the production of the book.

The Saskatchewan Indian Federated College, for providing logistical support in the preparation of the manuscript.

Louis McCullum, whose dedicated typing helped make sense of the original Jul'hoan interviews as well as the manuscript, and Esther Eakin Biesele, who under time pressure transcribed the dialogue that is the basis for appendix A.

Margaret Eakin, for assistance with a computerized concordance to the manuscript for the glossary and names list.

Nancy DeVore of Anthro Photo File (of Cambridge, Massachusetts) and the photographers she represents, for their generous offer of Kalahari photographs.

Inner Traditions International and its president, Ehud Sperling, for their unconditional belief in the book and their pragmatic expression of that belief with the donation of a portion of the profits to the Kalahari Jul'hoansi.

Marie Cantlon, our agent and editorial guide, who understood the book and helped craft it.

Lee Wood, Larry Hamberlin, and especially Jeanie Levitan for their committed and sensitive editorial work on the book—and their patience.

John Matthews and DeAnna Satre for perceptive copy-editing.

E!a ui i!a waqnsi (We thank you all).

DOBE AREA
IN THE KALAHARI DESERT

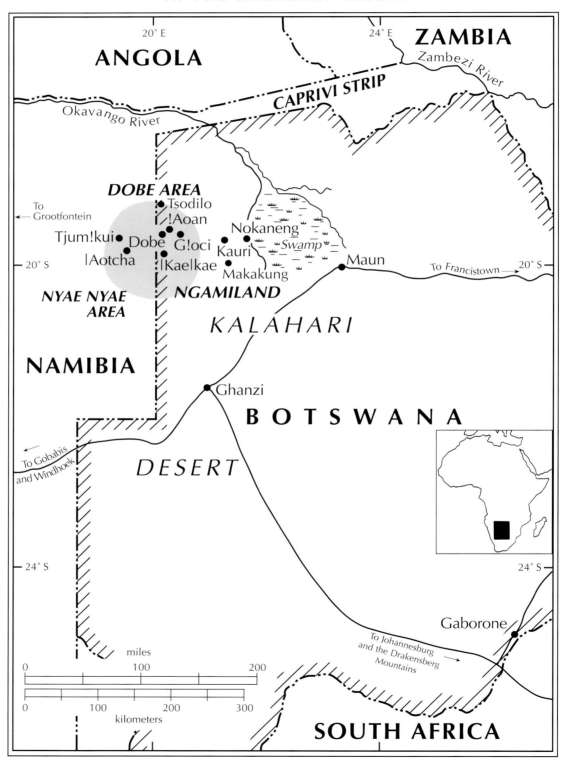

ZAMBIA

ANGOLA

20° E

24° E

Zambezi River

CAPRIVI STRIP

Okavango River

DOBE AREA

To
Grootfontein

Tsodilo

!Aoan

Nokaneng

Swamp

Tjum!kui

Dobe

G!oci

Kauri

Maun

|Aotcha

|Kae|kae

20° S

Makakung

To Francistown

20° S

NYAE NYAE
AREA

NGAMILAND

KALAHARI

NAMIBIA

BOTSWANA

Ghanzi

To Gobabis
and Windhoek

DESERT

24° S

24° S

Gaborone

To Johannesburg
and the Drakensberg
Mountains

miles

0   100   200

0   100   200   300

kilometers

SOUTH AFRICA

PREFACE

OUR OLDEST ANCESTORS were hunter-gatherers. They subsisted on the naturally occurring plants and animals around them, using a great fund of environmental knowledge and accumulating little in the way of possessions. Their often complex religious ideologies and social structures served their small groups' needs effectively. For countless millennia, hunting and gathering were the principal occupations of almost all human beings; only in the past few centuries has this way of life become something that most of us consider a part of an age long past.

The Jul'hoansi, a group of Bushmen of the western Kalahari Desert of southern Africa, are one of the few groups that still practice a hunting and gathering life at least part of the time. Though they are our contemporaries, they offer us profound insights into ancient human ways of relating as well as very useful information about efficient and low-technology systems.[1] *Bushman* has been used as a racist term by outsiders in the past. But today young Jul'hoan leaders, drawing on the word's original connotation of an "independent" people, suggest the term can be ennobled by the ways in which Jul'hoansi choose to use it.[2] We follow their lead in this book. The Jul'hoan people are one language group of Bushmen.[3] As they live in small groups, the Jul'hoansi enjoy a communal solidarity that goes far beyond Western rhetoric about sharing and healing. Their success at perpetuating fundamentally useful human social structures, such as extended families and ties to land and resources, has generated worldwide fascination with their culture. One of the most widely discussed peoples in anthropology, they also have captured the general public's interest through popular media, such as the widely seen but highly distorted *The Gods Must Be Crazy* films. Both popular and academic media have found it difficult not to romanticize the Bushmen.

Jul'hoan people themselves are much more pragmatic. Living in Botswana and Namibia, they once used a vast fund of information about Kalahari Desert ecology to produce a reliable and healthy, if spare, subsistence for themselves. Today they continue to use literally hundreds of plant, animal, and insect species on a rotational basis through the seasons. In general, men hunt—animals as large as giraffes and as small as tiny birds—and women gather the roots, berries, and nuts that make the Kalahari a bountiful environment to those with enough knowledge and skill. The men utilize spears, knives, and poisoned arrows,[4] and they rely on a great deal of tracking skill. Women often help men to track animals. The women also use digging sticks and antelope-skin cloaks, or *karosses,* to dig and carry home their wild vegetables and fruits. Traditionally, both men and women carried water to camp in the shells of ostrich eggs.

The isolation and independence of Jul'hoan and other Bushmen living in the western Kalahari have been compromised for a substantial period of time by the Herero and Tswana, cattle-keeping agricultural people who each speak one of the "Bantu" languages. Jul'hoansi call both Hereros and Tswana "Black" *(djo)* people, or "Blacks," as their skin is generally darker than that of Bushmen.

Herero and Tswana people began coming to the western Kalahari, including |Kae|kae, during the 1870s; thus their grazing activities have had time to make a significant impact on both the local sandveld ecology and on politics. In general, Tswana and Herero peoples have regarded themselves as superior to the Bushmen, and this attitude has had a measurable effect on intergroup relations.

In other areas of southern Africa, however, Bushman

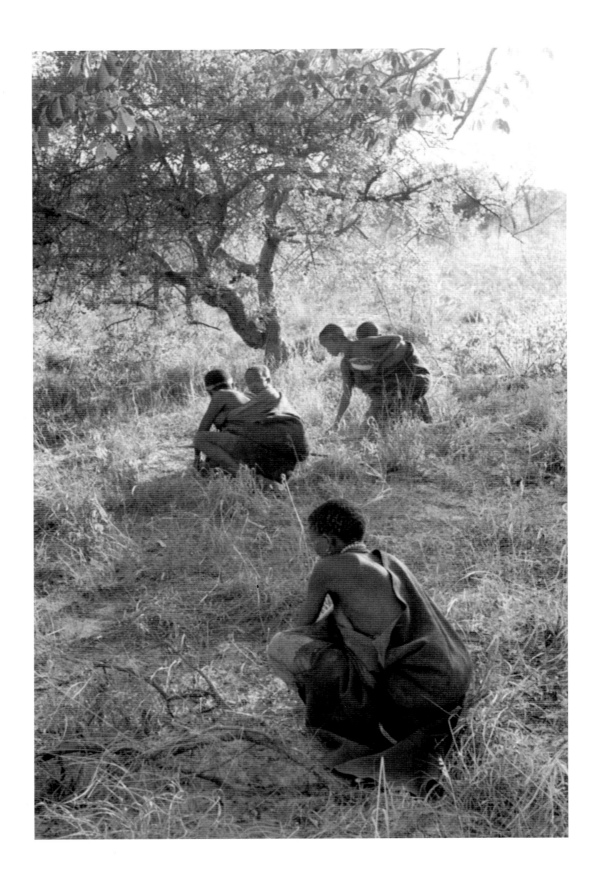

peoples live in different ecological situations and in both closer and more distant relationships with other peoples, including White Afrikaners, settlers of Dutch descent who first came to Botswana (then the British Protectorate of Bechuanaland) in 1897 from the South African Cape Colony.[5]

In recent years, the Jul'hoansi have begun to keep domestic stock and to grow agricultural produce on a small scale. They have found it increasingly necessary to replace their extensive economy of hunting and gathering, which requires a large land area, with more intensive economies so they can continue to live on a land-base that is dwindling. As is common throughout the world, Western-style products have become valued items, and school is viewed by some as a possible road to future improvement.

Many things about what is commonly referred to as "traditional" Jul'hoan life are changing, which is natural since the Jul'hoansi remain a vital people. The very concept of "traditional" Jul'hoan living must be questioned because it is misleading. The concept refers not to some abstract standard of living but most often is used to describe the way Jul'hoansi have lived during certain periods of their history when they were primarily engaged in hunting and gathering. Like all cultural traditions, Jul'hoan tradition is not a neatly bounded, static entity, but an evolving set of values and beliefs, permeable to outside influences.[6]

There are many important Jul'hoan values, beliefs, and ceremonies that persist from earlier times even as they change. For example, there is still substantial equality between the sexes in Jul'hoan society, with little difference in authority among individuals; each person is responsible for a set of personal tasks, and each person has a say in group decisions.

WOMEN GATHERING IN THE BUSH DURING

THE EARLY 1970S—TWO ARE CARRYING THEIR

BABIES ON THEIR BACKS.

One of the many ways in which harmony and consensus have long been maintained in Jul'hoan society is the community healing dance. Held on the average of four or five times a month on the basis of need or enthusiasm, the dance and its beautiful polyphonic music provide a highly social outlet for tensions, a spiritual vehicle for reinforcing the group's mutual reliance on one another, and a sense of place in their environment. The dance is celebratory, fun, solidifying, and deeply healing all at once, and everyone who is within earshot joins in. While people with specific sicknesses may be healed, all those participating can experience a sense of joy, renewed social commitment, and spiritual connectedness—a sense of healing.

Healing is based on *n/om*, a spiritual substance or energy residing in the bellies of the men and women who have been taught to activate it. N!om is said to "boil" when these people dance strenuously or sing the healing songs strongly; it leaves their stomachs and travels up their spines and out to their fingers, where it may be used to heal by the laying on of hands. The Jul'hoan people highly respect those who dare to feel the pain experienced when healing, and the synchronized presence of the whole community celebrates the healing power's existence. For the Jul'hoansi, the healing dance symbolizes an entire way of life, one in which their knowledge, strength, and willingness to help one another assert a secure sense of cultural identity.

Today, the traditional Jul'hoan way of life is especially threatened, and not just in the obvious sense of their ability to hunt and gather. In the more subtle and pervasive sense, their ability to maintain the spiritual and communal values that nourish and are nourished by that approach to subsistence are under stress. Jul'hoan attempts to forge new means for securing necessary resources meet obstacle upon obstacle. The threats and obstacles come from many factors, not least of which is a massive loss of land. More and more Jul'hoansi have to settle as landless and often unemployed squatters, either around other people's camps for grazing and watering cattle—the cattle posts—or around government centers.

The once self-reliant Jul'hoansi struggle to survive as a people.

In Botswana, powerful cattle syndicates, using modern machinery to drill for the water needed to feed their livestock, have almost squeezed the Jul'hoansi out of the land they once ranged as hunter-gatherers. And the government ideology of bringing Jul'hoan people into the "mainstream"—through a series of interventions it defines as acts of "progress"—has led to further attacks on Jul'hoan culture such as forcing Jul'hoan children to accept either schooling in a language not their own or no schooling at all. In Namibia, the South African apartheid system was in force until the country established its independence in 1990, sequestering the Jul'hoansi on a dwindling "homeland." It also lured them into militarized lives to fight against a Namibian liberation struggle they barely understood. In both countries Jul'hoan people and other Bushman groups stand at the very bottom of the social ladder and suffer bitterly from the economic dislocation of discrimination.

Many of their problems stem from misguided attempts to "civilize" them in African agriculturalist or Western styles. These colonizing forces, under the guise of "modernizing," seek to impose on the Jul'hoansi assumptions about what they should live for. Most of these assumptions arrive in the Jul'hoan world in the form of government strictures and "progressive" plans, many of which run counter to the Jul'hoansi's long-term successful use of their environment and to their own aspirations. Often well-intentioned efforts to help them "develop" tend to backfire when the Jul'hoan people themselves do not regard such changes as the next logical step in their own lives. Those who supposedly know best are bringing the fruits of modern education, medicine, and resource management to aid in what is justified as a "rescue" operation of the Jul'hoansi and other Third and Fourth World peoples.[7]

Yet these fruits do not always feed the recipients and can sometimes even poison them. An ancient, effective social system can change only at its own pace and through its own choice. The people best able to help the Jul'hoansi face changes substainably are the Jul'hoansi themselves. As this book sets out to demonstrate, the seeds of change and renewal lie within their own culture. Jul'hoansi have long known how to heal individuals and their communities. Their healing capacity could be a crucial ingredient in initiating and sustaining positive change.

As part of a colonial agenda, the West has too long imposed on Indigenous peoples its own definition of their problems, a definition that is largely self-serving. And we in the West are especially good at offering solutions but not so adept at recognizing and ennabling workable solutions that Indigenous peoples arrive at themselves. We must learn to ask the Jul'hoansi how we can best support them in their efforts to survive the upheavals that threaten their culture. But first, we cannot merely assume that they want our help.

As the Jul'hoansi find and follow their paths into renewed self-determination, they open a unique window of understanding into the future of humankind. Their attempts to solve conflicts force us to reexamine conventional approaches that seek social change through purely political or economic means. The Jul'hoansi remain intensely involved in their traditions of community healing and spirituality. "Healing," they tell us, "makes our hearts happy." The healing dance has supported the people in the past in their efforts to deal respectfully with problems within the community. In these times of accelerating social and political dislocation, can healing continue to energize changes that truly respect and restore people? That is not a question Jul'hoan people are explicitly asking; instead they are exploring its implications in their lives through the way they live. Yet in giving us permission to inquire into that question in this book, they make it possible to highlight some of the ways in which their healing tradition might have an impact on contemporary dilemmas.

Healing Makes Our Hearts Happy arose from a return, a kind of coming home. In 1989, more than twenty years after his first trip to the Kalahari, Dick Katz returned to

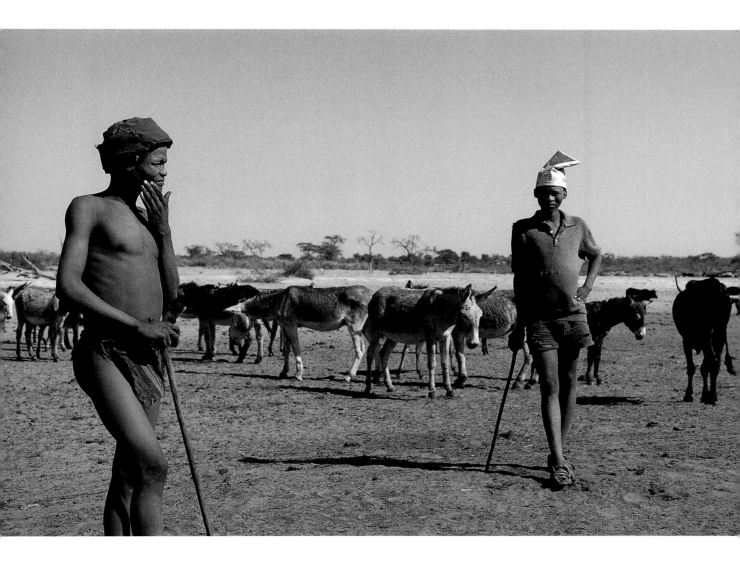

ǂKaeǂkae, the village that had become his spiritual home, and to the Juǀ'hoan healing dance and healers from whom he had learned so much. Accompanying him were two co-workers: his wife, Verna St. Denis, a Cree/Metis educator and researcher with special experience working with Indigenous people, and Megan Biesele, an anthropologist with almost twenty years of experience doing advocacy, development work, and anthropological research with the Juǀ'hoansi. But as the prologue explains, the trip was not a simple homecoming; instead, a new task presented itself. The Juǀ'hoansi asked the three of us to become "paper people," to use the power of the written word to make Juǀ'hoan needs and aspirations

TWO YOUNG JUǀ'HOAN MEN, ǀKAECE (LEFT) AND
KAQECE (RIGHT) IN 1968, TENDING LIVESTOCK FOR THE
TSWANA AND HEREROS WHO LIVE AT ǂKAEǂKAE.

known to those who were now controlling their lives. This book, emphasizing Juǀ'hoan voices rather than academic theorizing to better express the realities of their everyday lives, is one way we have tried to fulfill their request.

Part 1 describes the communal hunting-gathering lifestyle that has sustained the Juǀ'hoansi in the ǂKaeǂkae

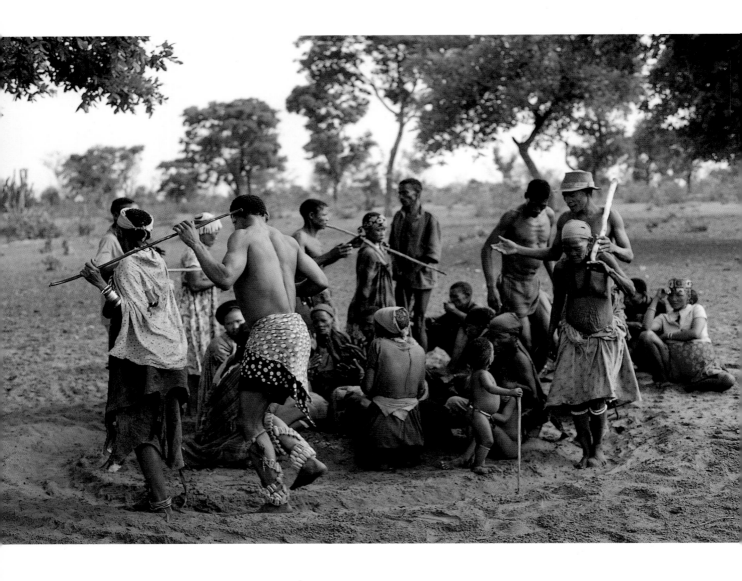

THE HEALING DANCE INCLUDES

THE ENTIRE COMMUNITY—

WOMEN AND MEN, YOUNG AND OLD.

area for many centuries and documents the dramatic and often traumatic changes that have disrupted their economic and political circumstances.[8] Despite these upheavals, the spiritual healing energy, the nǀom, continues to boil during their healing dance.

Part 2 looks at how "civilizing" efforts appear to be destroying the Juǀ'hoansi. Not only are the Juǀ'hoansi given an education that does not fully teach and a medicine that does not fully heal, but their own valuable traditions of teaching and healing are being cast aside by the government institutions of "progress." The healing dance, which makes the Juǀ'hoan people whole, is being ignored by these outside agencies.

We believe that neglect is ill-considered, for it is the still-vital Juǀ'hoan healing tradition that offers great hope of guiding the people toward more humanizing and liberating processes of social change. Yet the guidance remains subtle; at least for now the Juǀ'hoan do not talk about it directly. Nor are they committed to a strictly logical, outcome-oriented analysis of the dance, for example by describing the dance as "causing" an "effect" or by singling out its purpose. They dance for many different reasons and accept the ambiguity and paradox inherent in the dance and its functions. No matter how we ask about the relationship between healing and social change, the answer is the same: "The healing dance is one thing; these problems with our loss of land and resources are another thing." Whatever relationship now exists or might exist in the future will be unfolding in their actions and is not immediately obvious.

Part 3 explores this relationship by examining the dynamics and politics of nǀom. For example, we observed that a large number of healers, who practice their art during the dance, were becoming informal spokespersons about current land and resource issues, perhaps owing to the salience and moral authority they already held in their communities. Could this signal that the healing dance, and the nǀom it activates, might be evolving into a possible pathway for sociopolitical change?

This specific question raises more general questions about the relationship between spirituality and social transformation. Though there are many historical instances of a direct relationship—where, for example, a spiritual healer becomes a political leader or prophet—the Juǀ'hoansi offer another intriguing perspective: the very act of participating in the healing dance is a deeply affirming experience, giving the Juǀ'hoansi the strength to endure and adapt to disruptive social forces. The Juǀ'hoan struggle for self-preservation, only one expression of a global struggle among Indigenous peoples, demonstrates the essential role of spiritual traditions as a wellspring of cultural identity.

Part 4 and appendix A contain our thoughts on some troubling questions related to our research in the Kalahari and the responsibilities entailed. In critiquing our efforts, we try to highlight issues that permeate, too

often implicitly, the entire book. The question of power and control is central to our reflections. Is it possible to be fully aware of how disparities in power distort perceptions, allowing those in control, even when well intentioned, to pronounce half-truths as truths and claim the voice of others? Have we as researchers used the power inherent in our role so as to help, or at least not hinder, the Juǀ'hoansi? And can persons outside the Juǀ'hoan community offer genuine help? If so, how? What does it mean, for example, to say that we "want to help"?

Some Juǀ'hoansi have already taken actions that reveal likely future directions. In Namibia, a number of Juǀ'hoansi who are closely related to those in ǀKaeǀkae have formed the Nyae Nyae Residents' Council, a community-based organization that supports their efforts to drill water wells and purchase small herds of cattle to husband at their traditional hunting and gathering sites.[9] The successes of the Residents' Council have come slowly and setbacks remain frequent. But a viable future is being created by a people who have returned to their land, as is described in appendix E. This organization is only one example of the possibilities being unfolded by Bushman people in southern Africa; additional examples exist and others await birth.

In writing this book we hope to make a modest, practical contribution to these processes of birth and growth. Though we have worked according to standards of rigorous scholarship, we are trying to communicate beyond the academic community to a wider audience, especially the newly literate Juǀ'hoansi readership. As well, author royalties from the book will go toward establishing a fund for the Juǀ'hoansi, a fund that they will determine how to use. The publishers of this book have also agreed to contribute part of their share of the profits to this fund. It is time for us to demonstrate that we are struggling to hear the Juǀ'hoan story by a practical show of our support for their visions of their future.

MEETING AND TALKING WITH THE PEOPLE

Introducing people to each other puts the introducer in a mediating position. In the case of different cultures, languages, and social expectations, the "middleperson" position becomes particularly problematic. There are problems of representation, objectification, and unequal power. When people cannot meet each other directly, the erection of screens and distorting filters is likely. We have been acutely aware of this danger as we wrote the book, trying to navigate among various pitfalls such as romanticizing the Jul'hoansi and presenting our own assessments and judgments rather than those of the people themselves. We continued to ask how this could be a "book without authors." We have used this question as a spiritual exercise, an attempt to remind ourselves at every turn that this story is not ours to tell—we have merely been entrusted with the words of the Jul'hoan people, who have asked us to tell their story.

The Jul'hoan people live in the Kalahari Desert in southern Africa and this is their book. *Jul'hoan,* meaning "real," "genuine," or "ordinary" people, is their own name for themselves. They are members of a specific linguistic group within a larger group of Kalahari foraging people long called "Bushmen." In the past, Jul'hoansi have been referred to by outsiders as Bushmen, San, !Kung, and !Kung Bushmen. There are problems with all of these

names, which have been imposed from the outside. In this book, they reclaim their own name. At the same time, many Jul'hoan individuals who had been given Western names by outsiders are returning to the use of their own Jul'hoan names.[1]

MEETING SOME OF THE |KAE|KAE JU|'HOANSI

The Jul'hoansi who will speak to us are primarily from |Kae|kae and the Dobe area of Botswana (see p. x). In order for their words to convey more directly the lived realities they describe, we would like to introduce some of the |Kae|kae Jul'hoansi to you. Disembodied words cannot fully speak. Out of respect for the actual nature of their language, we have included various pronunciation markers to help you more accurately "hear" them (see The Use of the Jul'hoan Language on p. vi). Pseudonyms are not used—those who tell their stories here assured us they wish to engage openly in the Jul'hoan struggle for land and dignified living.

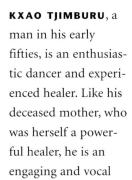

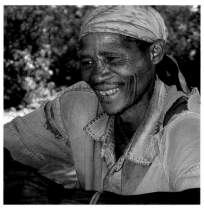

KXAO TJIMBURU, a man in his early fifties, is an enthusiastic dancer and experienced healer. Like his deceased mother, who was herself a powerful healer, he is an engaging and vocal conversationalist, yet he has a withdrawn, pensive side to his personality. Kxao Tjimburu and his family maintain a long-term and close economic relationship with a neighboring Herero family. Many in his extended family, especially his wife, N≠aisa, and other women and young girls, are actively involved in the healing dances. Having spent a brief time in an English-speaking mission school, Kxao Tjimburu can understand bits of English—sometimes during the interviews he captures the drift of our questions before they are translated, which becomes a source of mutual delight.

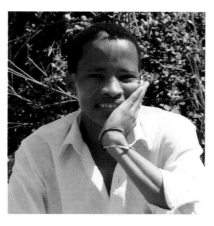

KXAO |O|OO is one of the few young Jul'hoansi in the Dobe and |Kae|kae region to advance in his formal schooling, having graduated with a Junior Certificate, the equivalent of a high school diploma. An outgoing and engaging person, he already has had an unusual amount of work experiences outside the region, although he is still in his early twenties. Having already developed a keen sense of the rhythms, demands, and assumptions of the Western-oriented work world as well as an excellent command of English, Kxao O|Oo is at the same time deeply rooted within his traditional Jul'hoan context. Just recently he has returned to using his Jul'hoan name instead of Royal, the name by which he was known. As a young person who walks in two worlds, Kxao O|Oo is an important person in the region and an important member of our research team.

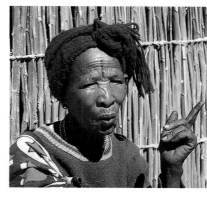

KXARU N!A'AN and her husband Kodinyau are one of the most active Jul'hoan families in establishing new means of subsistence. They own goats and cattle and plant a field behind their neat, mud-walled Tswana-style house. Surrounded by a solid, well-maintained reed fence, that house provides more substantial accommodations than most Jul'hoansi at |Kae|kae have. Though reluctant to discuss at length her involvement with healing, Kxaru N!a'an is acknowledged at |Kae|kae as having a strong connection with n|om, the Jul'hoan spiritual healing power—she is one of the strongest healing dance singers and one of the few women who regularly experience the healing trance (*!aia* or *tara*). Outspoken about the present situation and future possibilities of the Jul'hoansi, Kxaru N!a'an offers up her opinions with a sharp wit and a twinkle in her eye.

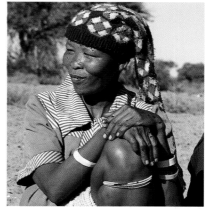

N≠AISA is one of the most animated, strong, and dedicated singers at the healing dances. Kxao Tjimburu is her husband. Though in her late thirties, she often laughs and jokes at the dance with enthusiasm and abandon, inviting others into her playful approach. Yet when healers are in need of support, she is there, working hard and risking her own sense of balance. Responsible for a large family, she at times seems overwhelmed; the joy then leaves her face and is taken over by weariness.

N≠AISA N!A'AN's energetic approach to life belies her nearly seventy years. Thoroughly engaged in village life and intimately connected to ≠Oma Djo, her husband of several years and a 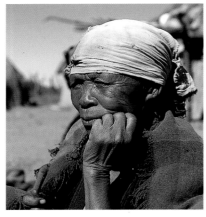 powerful healer, it seems that only her near-blindness slows her down. She works closely with ≠Oma Djo at the healing dances and is a source of reliably inspirational singing. At times N≠aisa N!a'an is preoccupied with her deteriorated sight, and she is a frequent focus of ≠Oma Djo's healing efforts. N≠aisa N!a'an speaks from her many years of experience in life and in the healing dance, and others listen to her with respect.

≠OMA DJO has become the "healers' healer" at |Kae|kae, the one other healers turn to for help. Though approaching eighty, he is a fervent healer and is unique at |Kae|kae in always being 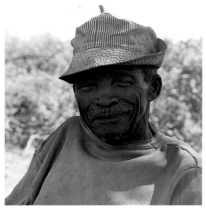 freely available for those who need healing. ≠Oma Djo and his wife, N≠aisa N!a'an, form a lively pair, teasing each other with joyful abandon and caring for each other with tenderness. ≠Oma Djo's long life has spanned many phases of Jul'hoan life, including the more traditional patterns of a hunting-gathering subsistence. Having experienced many intense pleasures and pains and fulfillments and losses, he has insight into a full picture of Jul'hoan life. His stories of his life are told with humor and captivating drama and are consid-

ered storehouses of Jul'hoan culture and knowledge. Most especially, ≠Oma Djo guides our work on Jul'hoan healing and does so with generosity, humor, and deep wisdom.

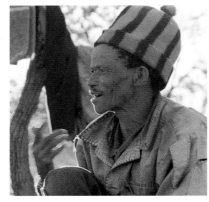

≠OMA !'HOMG!AUSI, an avid and respected hunter and healer, is an energetic man in his mid-fifties. His camp is noted for its strong singers and frequently hosts healing dances. ≠Oma !'Homg!ausi approaches activities, including his healing work, with a quickly generated intensity, entering into commitments without hesitation. One of the most consistent advocates of the bush as a continuing source of sustenance, ≠Oma !'Homg!ausi expresses his opinions with a quiet firmness.

TKAE||'AE N!A'AN (not pictured) is one of the oldest people living at |Kae|kae. When outside, she's usually reclining and wrapped in a blanket with her small, thin frame nearly hidden. But her spirit is alive, and her tiny voice conveys a wealth of knowledge about village life—and especially about healing. Though her frail condition prevents her from participating actively in the healing dances, everyone at |Kae|kae says the same thing: Tkae||'ae N!a'an is the one to talk to if you want to know about women and healing.

TSHAO MATZE's
quiet, even reserved,
demeanor belies his
articulate and force-
ful stance in regard
to the injustices suf-
fered by Jul'hoansi
and the urgent need
for change. An expe-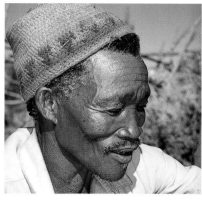
rienced and respected healer, he approaches the healing
dance carefully and earnestly, with little of the flamboy-
ance of some of the other dancers. He suffers from
tuberculosis, which is often manifested in his deep,
body-wrenching coughs. Tshao Matze is at times too
weak to carry on normal activities, let alone pursue
hunting and healing, activities in which he has been an
avid and skillful participant.

|UKXA is one of
the two students
who have graduat-
ed from the
|Kae|kae school
and gone on to
receive his Junior
Certificate (equiva-
lent to a high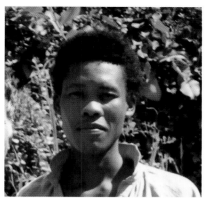
school diploma). A friendly, gentle young man in his
early twenties, he has yet to find regular employment
despite his educational achievement. With his firm
grasp of English, his ongoing involvement with his
|Kae|kae home, and his sensitive skills in communica-
tion and bringing people together, |Ukxa is an invalu-
able member of our research team. And his easygoing
humor is always a refreshing breeze in our sometimes
too serious work.

TSHAO N!A'AN
spent some time in
the 1960s living in
Ghanzi, an area that
lies a good distance
from |Kae|kae and is
dominated by the
large farms of White
Afrikaners.
Functioning there as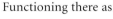
a healer, he developed a widespread reputation based as
much on his dancing ability as his healing power—he
often became something like a professional performer.
Now back in |Kae|kae and in his mid-sixties, Tshao
N!a'an is considered one of the two most powerful and
experienced healers in the village (the other is ≠Oma
Djo). Seeking a balanced approach in his views, Tshao
N!a'an is a reflective man who measures his words.

XUMI N!A'AN is an
articulate man,
committed to eras-
ing the injustices he
sees plaguing his
people. Though not
a healer, he is a ded-
icated participant in
the healing dances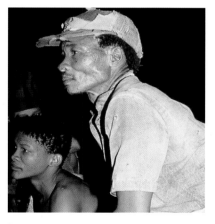
and a supporter of Jul'hoan healing traditions; he is
noted as an expert drum maker and player for the
drum healing dance. One of the most active Jul'hoansi
in |Kae|kae village politics, he is, for example, very
involved in how the school is being run, and his son,
Tshao Xumi, is one of only two |Kae|kae young people
to get a high school diploma. Now in his mid-fifties,
Xumi N!a'an's age and accumulated experience are
beginning to add extra weight to his already respected
opinions about Jul'hoan culture and the possibilities
for its future.

Learning about Jul'hoan people on their terms is not only a sign of respect but an essential prerequisite to any true understanding of their lives. Part of that respect entails the attempt to learn how to pronounce the words of their language used in this book. For a more detailed discussion of the political considerations in writing the Jul'hoan language see appendix C.

The Jul'hoan alphabet is very similar to the English one, except that it has four extra consonants for "clicking" sounds. Each of these clicks is as precise a tool for Jul'hoan speakers as, for example, our letter *b* is to us. The clicks are sounds produced with an ingressive air stream when the tongue is drawn sharply away from the roof of the mouth at four specific points of articulation described below.

The dental click ("|") sounds like "tsk, tsk," the English expression of irritation. It is made by putting the tongue just behind the front teeth.

The alveolar click ("≠") is a soft pop made by putting the tongue just behind the ridge located behind the front teeth.

The alveolo-palatal click ("!") is a sharp pop made by drawing the tongue down quickly from the roof of the mouth.

The lateral click ("||") is a clucking sound like that made in English to urge on a horse.

There are three other pronunciation features of the Jul'hoan language:

Nazalizations ("ng")

Glottal stops ("'"),

A "j," pronounced as the *j* in the French *jamais* or *je*

The word *Ju'hoan* has both a dental click consonant and a glottal stop; it sounds something like "Zhun-twa." *Jul'hoansi* sounds something like "Zhun-twasi." With all Jul'hoan words, you can get a first approximate of their pronunciation by saying them first without the distinctive Jul'hoan language features and then later adding those distinctive Jul'hoan features to be more accurate.

Until you master the less-familiar sounds of the Jul'hoan language, try substituting these pronunciations:

"|" and "≠" can be replaced by "t" as in "Toma" Djo

"!" and "||" can be replaced by "g" as in "gabesi"

"q" after a vowel indicates a low, exaggerated tone

"h" after a vowel indicates a low, breathy tone

Otherwise, most letters are pronounced as in English.

A WORD OF CAUTION

Healing Makes Our Hearts Happy exists within a complex context of social and economic power. As authors, we do not always acknowledge or even recognize all of these influences, especially when it comes to issues of power differentials between ourselves and the Jul'hoansi. "Control" of reality, especially another's reality, is an important issue. Hence this word of caution: we need diligent sensitivity to understand and deal with power's capacity to distort and transform truth. We want to suggest that certain dimensions of power—such as gender, wealth, and access to education—pervasively and often subtly influence this book. Therefore we encourage a general alertness to these dimensions in you, our readers. Perhaps, in reading the book, you will be able to highlight our shortcomings. We intend the words of caution in this section as a reader's guide, rather than an author's rationalization.

THE SPIRITUAL POWER OF NǀOM

At the core of *Healing Makes Our Hearts Happy* is the story of nǀom, a spiritual energy that is the foundation of Jul'hoan healing. Writing about such spiritual energy is difficult; that energy exists beyond words. But if we can follow the Zen teaching about never confusing the finger that points to the moon with the moon itself, writing about nǀom can indicate some of the dimensions, functions, and power of this energy. "We respect this nǀom," says ≠Oma Djo. "It can kill you." If we also respect Jul'hoan nǀom, we can begin to learn not only about the dangers of its power—one can die from its uninformed or unguided use—but also from its promise: in dying to oneself, one becomes able to heal others.

APPROACHES TO TRUTH

We have been asked by the Jul'hoansi to "tell our story to your people." As *Healing Makes Our Hearts Happy* unfolds, it will become clear how difficult a challenge that is. Jul'hoansi means "real" or "ordinary" people. How do we tell the story so that the reality of the Jul'hoansi comes through, so that they come alive as "real" people, as "ordinary" rather than exotic? How does anyone tell the story of another's truth, especially when the whole construction of truth is at question? The postmodernist anthropologist Michael Taussig described the subject of his ethnography as "not the truth of being, but the social being of truth, not whether facts are real but what the politics of their interpretation and representation are."[1] We cannot ignore such a perspective.

The fundamental principle that guides our work is that *we* cannot tell the *Jul'hoan* story. We try to provide a venue for the Jul'hoansi to tell their own story as much as possible. At the same time, we realize that this aim, as well as our own efforts to be accurate, truthful, and realistic, will never be fully met because of the context of power and power differentials within which we and the Jul'hoansi are situated.

For instance, the fact that we could choose to go to the Kalahari *and* choose to leave symbolizes a degree of power and entitlement that is both pervasive and ineffable. Our very attempt to provide a venue for the Jul'hoansi to tell their story, while expressing a sincere intention, also occurs because of our relative position of entitlement. The Jul'hoansi are not traveling to North America, nor trying to help North Americans tell the North American story—nor are they even interested in that task. They are unable to engage in such travels without external assistance. Since the relative power we possess is so pervasive, there are many times and ways in which we act from our positions of entitlement without recognizing it.

This problem of unacknowledged entitlement has historically plagued those who travel to the so-called far corners of the world. The classic pattern is for some Eurocentric White person to go to an "exotic" place and offer descriptions of the "strangers," descriptions that seek the "essential core" of that other culture, equating what is "real" or "authentic" in the culture with what is "traditional," "uncontaminated," or "isolated" from contact with "outside" influences. The apparently exotic is valued as the apparently authentic; tradition is viewed as an unchanging monolith of values, beliefs, and ceremonies.

Simultaneously, there is the evaluation of what is seen according to the traveler's own standards of correctness. And whether others are seen as "primitive" or the "true natural humans," both judgments are Eurocentric, denying the humanity of the persons being judged, turning them into the "other." This subversion of a people's true identity has been accomplished routinely by anthropologists, missionaries, soldiers, and traders.

Though we are aware of this legacy of stolen and misinterpreted identities and try to follow a different, more respectful path, we know we cannot be totally free of that past. It continues, sometimes in unconscious or subtle forms. It is imperative *Healing Makes Our Hearts Happy* be read while acknowledging both our intentions to respect the negotiated nature of truth and our inability to engage fully in that process of negotiation.

But the context of power within which we are working is infinitely more complex. One further element of complexity deserves mention. We three authors, though speaking for the most part in a single voice throughout the book, are each quite different from each other. For example, Verna, as a First Nations or Indigenous person, does not have the same struggle to overcome the tendency to romanticize or essentialize the Jul'hoansi. As the

three of us worked together, Verna's vision helped bring a new level of respect to our task.

In an effort to make *Healing Makes Our Hearts Happy* more accessible and to keep the emphasis as much as possible on the Jul'hoansi, we often merge our three authorial voices into one. There is a cost to that approach. The edges of difference between us are now smoothed over to make one combined, but hopefully more accessible and less intruding voice. The use of a single and relatively nonpersonal voice can introduce a false impression that we are detached from or neutral to the Jul'hoan situation; the opposite is the case.

Despite our realization that we must be concerned about Taussig's "social being of truth," we also still seek to understand the "truth of being"; we cautiously seek to understand in spite of our fears. As ≠Oma Djo says, "We still have our n!om. . . . N!om is just the same as long ago, even though it keeps on changing."

GEOPOLITICAL REALITIES

In *Healing Makes Our Hearts Happy,* contemporary Jul'hoan lives are seen as much as possible through the individuals' own eyes. The Jul'hoansi, a linguistic, ethnic, and economic minority whose once-remote hunting and gathering grounds are being engulfed by cattle and industrial interests, are living for the most part in independent Third World countries—but in a special category within those countries. Sometimes called "Fourth World peoples," Jul'hoansi and other Bushmen have been forced to occupy the bottom rung of every social ladder in southern Africa. This is true whether the Jul'hoansi dwell in Botswana or in neighboring Namibia—just as it has been true all over the world that foraging peoples have often been misunderstood by those who have cattle-based or industrial economies.

At the same time, we must always remember that though they have been disempowered in national or regional politics, the Jul'hoansi are anything but powerless; though they have been victimized, their lives are not adequately described by the experience of being victims. Part of the purpose of *Healing Makes Our Hearts Happy* is to present the actual and potential power of the Jul'hoan people.

The brunt of the Jul'hoansi's complaints about the devastating injustice of their situation is borne mostly by the neighboring Herero pastoralists and Tswana agriculturalist/patoralists.[2] If the Jul'hoansi seem to criticize the Tswana and Herero particularly, it is because their analysis of their situation is voiced in the idiom of regional specificity. Asked to render their voices as faithfully as possible, we could not avoid reporting on some of their specific grievances. But it must be remembered that the Tswana and Herero peoples have suffered their own history of being colonized. One way to put the Jul'hoan critique into perspective is to see them interacting with their pastoral neighbors as one people without much experience with formal state structures in communication with others, negotiating exchanges of most kinds in terms of mutual reciprocity, which they do not share with institutional governments. Only when economic abuse and/or violence become institutionalized in state structures do two-way negotiations cease and power positions become more static. We hope *Healing Makes Our Hearts Happy* can become a contribution to the effort of mutual respect that could help keep institutional abuse from happening in Botswana.

It may also seem as if the Botswana government is singled out for criticism. But Botswana's goal of uniting diverse ethnicities cannot easily result in a truly democratic government, and Botswana has struggled to achieve this for almost thirty years now—all the while coping as one of the vital "frontline nations" against the formerly apartheid-based South Africa.

Our work calls attention to *all* the Kalahari peoples who have tried to forge nations in southern Africa in the effort to dwell sustainably in the modern world. Our work is also a demonstration of the power and energy of a specific culture, a hope that its example may encourage recognition on national levels of the unique contributions made and to be made by regional minorities everywhere.

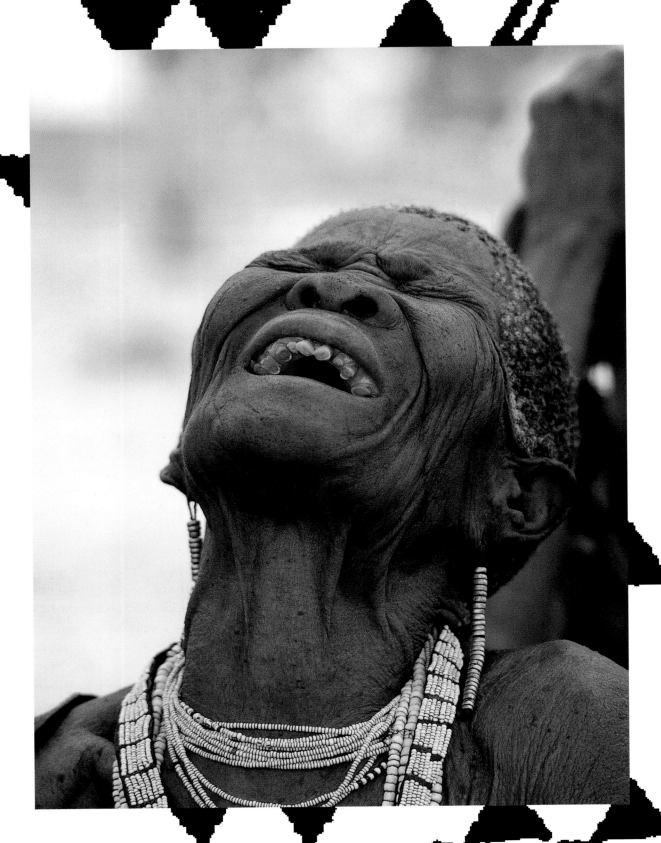

PROLOGUE

"TELL OUR STORY TO YOUR PEOPLE"

Twenty years have passed since I (Dick) first visited the village of ǀKaeǀkae in the Kalahari Desert in Botswana. This is the land of the Juǀ'hoansi, the "real" people.

In that initial visit, I had worked with Juǀ'hoan healers to learn about nǀom, the spiritual energy that boils inside them and brings on !aia, the enhanced state of consciousness that allows them to heal. And I had struggled to put that learning into practice by participating in their all-night healing dances.

Juǀ'hoan healing involves health and growth on physical, psychological, social, and spiritual levels; it affects the individual, the group, the surrounding environment, and the cosmos. Healing is an integrating and enhancing force, touching far more levels and forces than simply curing an individual's "illness."

The central event in the healing tradition is an all-night dance. It occurs on average four or five times in a

IXOAN NǃA'AN FROM GǃOCI, AN OLD WOMAN
GENERALLY REGARDED AS THE MOST
POWERFUL JUǀ'HOAN HEALER IN THE ǀKAEǀKAE
AREA DURING THE 1960S, EXPERIENCING A
STATE OF !AIA DURING A HEALING DANCE.

month. The women sit around the fire, singing and rhythmically clapping as night falls to signal the start of a healing dance. The entire camp participates. The men, sometimes joined by the women, dance around the singers. As the dance intensifies, nǀom is activated in those who are the healers and they experience !aia during which they heal everyone at the dance. The dance usually ends before the sun rises the next morning. Those at the dance confront the uncertainties of their experience and reaffirm the spiritual dimension of their daily lives. "Being at a dance makes our hearts happy," the Juǀhoansi say.

As Kinachau, a seasoned healer, says:

> You dance, dance, dance, dance. Then nǀom lifts you in your belly and lifts you in your back. . . . Nǀom makes you tremble, it's hot. . . . But when you get into !aia, you're looking around because you see everything, because you see what's troubling everybody.[1]

As healers learn to control their boiling nǀom, they can apply it to healing. They learn to heal, to "see the sickness and pull it out."

≠Oma Djo, a powerful healer, speaks of the feeling !aia gives—of becoming more essential, more oneself: "I want to have a dance soon so that I can feel myself again." A transcendent state of consciousness, !aia alters a Juǀ'hoan's sense of self, time, and space. !Aia makes healers feel they are "opening up" or "bursting open, like a ripe pod."

Through !aia, the Juǀ'hoansi transcend ordinary life and can contact the realm of the gods and the spirits of dead ancestors. Sickness is a process in which the spirits try to carry a person off into their realm. In !aia, the healer expresses the wishes of the living to keep the sick person with them and goes directly into the struggle with the spirits. The healer is the community's emissary in this confrontation. When a person is seriously ill, the struggle intensifies. If a healer's nǀom is strong and the great God wishes, the spirits will retreat and the sick one will live. This struggle is at the heart of the healers' art, skill, and power. In their search for contact with transcendent realms and in their struggle with illness, misfortune, and death, the healing dance and nǀom are the Juǀʼhoansi's most important allies.

My early experience in the Kalahari inspired my research and writing as well as my practice as a clinical psychologist. It also deepened a commitment to focus on healing, community, and culture. That experience changed me, increasing my openness to the potential and actuality of spiritual healing.

The struggle for that openness was hard fought. I can remember how my mind, nurtured for so many years by Western rationality, resisted the spiritual understanding my heart already knew. The conflict became crystallized around the experience of dying that Juǀʼhoan healers describe. "This nǀom kills us," they say. "We die in !aia," they warned me. When they saw me trying to "drink nǀom" at the healing dance, they were perplexed: "You want that nǀom!? Don't you know it is painful? Don't you know it can kill you?"

I went to Kxao ≠Oah, a powerful, respected healer, to speak about this death. In our exchange my Western notions of reality crumbled even further.

"Kxao ≠Oah," I asked, "you have told me that in !aia you must die. Does that mean really die?"

"Yes."

"I mean *really* die."

"Yes."

"You mean die like when you are buried beneath the ground?" I was already struggling with my words.

"Yes," Kxao ≠Oah replied with enthusiasm. "Yes, just like that!"

"They are the same?"

"Yes, the same. It is death I speak of," he affirmed.

"No difference?"

"It is death," he responded firmly but softly.

"The death where you never come back?" I was nearly at the end of my logical rope.

"Yes," he said simply, "it is that bad. It is the death that kills us all."

"But healers get up, and a dead person doesn't." My statement trailed off into a question.

"That is true," Kxao ≠Oah replied quietly, smiling.

"Healers may come alive again."[2]

I began to learn what those Juǀʼhoansi who become healers must know. To "kill" or to "die" is not just a metaphor, a statement about the overpowering strength of nǀom, a warning about the difficulty of getting it, or a test of one's desire to "drink" or receive it. The Juǀʼhoansi distinguish between a final death when the soul permanently leaves the body and the death of !aia when the soul goes out but then, they hope, returns, but there is only one *experience* of death, and that experience is what matters.

As my learning increased, I began hearing a request, first from one and then from other healers: "Tell our story to your people." Initially, I was not sure the Juǀʼhoansi knew what they were saying. Here was a people with no written language; did they know, for example, what it meant to publish a book, surely one of the ways I would use to tell that story? I kept reflecting on their request, and for a long while I wasn't clear about how to respond, even after I left the Kalahari. Finally, getting beyond the logistics of communication, I realized the deep simplicity of that Juǀʼhoan request. They felt I had learned enough about their healing to tell an accurate story—not *the* story, but *a* story. In fact, in their way, no one story is ever given total primacy; it is only a version of what happened. And it was not my story to tell. My responsibility was to put forth Juǀʼhoan words so their story could emerge.

The Juǀʼhoansi wanted others to hear about them, to learn about healing; they believed they had something to teach. And having given me permission to tell that story, they left it up to me to decide on the best form. That was my job; that was my area of expertise. I am grateful for their trust.

The Juǀʼhoan request to tell their story about healing resulted in *Boiling Energy: Community Healing among the Kalahari Kung* and a lifelong commitment to communicate about their tradition of healing in the context of a respectful exchange with their teachings.[3] Their request became a charge and with that a responsibility—an invitation and with that a challenge.

Since that time I have been asked by Indigenous Fijian people to "tell their story" and have been entrusted to select the proper vehicle. I have never taken such requests lightly. While the people are offering valuable techniques to my people and others, the story I communicate also deals with their own sense of self and history. But I always realize the limited significance of my work for them. Not only do I have only a small part of the story to tell, but the part I can tell is limited even further by my own historical circumstances, especially those stemming from my being from outside the culture. Nevertheless, I have been told by Indigenous elders that at certain points in a people's struggle toward self-determination, it may help to have available the view of an outsider who is deemed to have some understanding of the "inside." That outsider's view can offer a particular kind of argument or set of data in the people's larger discourse of liberation. I can only hope that in my telling I can bring a small measure of honor to my task.

A RETURNING

From the day I left the Kalahari, I always wanted to go back. My desire became a longing, and the idea of a return began to assume for me almost mythic proportions. I wanted to be with Jul'hoan healers again, to learn more from them, to share with them. And I know that there is more work to be done; the Jul'hoan story has moved beyond the healing dance to include a fervent call for political liberation. I strongly sense this new dimension in my obligation to "tell their story to my people." Whereas at the time of my first visit the Jul'hoansi were acting more as self-sufficient hunter-gatherers, now they have been pushed off their land by cattle-owning Tswana and Hereros, becoming a dispossessed people for the most part, increasingly dependent on government handouts. I already realize that I must go beyond the more descriptive focus of my earlier work and toward a stronger position of advocacy.

I know that within these currents of social destruction, the Jul'hoan healing dance, their central spiritual ceremony, has endured. But in what condition? And what role, if any, was it playing in the traumatic social changes that were surrounding the Jul'hoansi? What role might it play in the future?

Though many Indigenous peoples are suffering a similar destruction of their social fabric and cultural values, the Jul'hoan healing dance is an especially powerful and unquestioned resource for sustenance and renewal. Even Christianity, despite all its successes at undermining Indigenous spirituality and healing elsewhere, has yet to make an impact among the Jul'hoansi in the ǀKaeǀkae area. In the midst of the Jul'hoansi's negotiations of everyday life, there are important teachings for all of us about the relationship between spirituality and social change.

Twenty-odd years is a long time. So much energy spent reflecting on my experience with Jul'hoan healing. So much commitment built up to applying their teachings. And so many other experiences working with spiritual healing among other Indigenous peoples, which both were informed by the Jul'hoan teachings and shed light on them.

This myth of return springs from a soil rich in misunderstandings and full of unintended and less than desirable effects. But I would return with a more serious understanding of my *actual* relationship with the Jul'hoansi. For example, though I try to discourage the tendency of people in the West to treat me as an "expert" on Jul'hoan healing, only I know how little I actually know. Also, I realize that I am not anywhere near as important a part of their lives as they are of mine—in one sense, I am just another fieldworker who spent a brief time with them. And I understand more fully my position of entitlement that allowed me to make the first trip to the Kalahari and now allows me to choose to return. Yet I also appreciate that the telling of their story, energized by their ongoing presence felt within me, has inspired many others.

I know that my sincere desire to learn about their healing and my humility before their knowledge communicates a special respect to the Jul'hoansi. Through this respect, I struggle to go beyond the shadow of certain historical themes like the classic journey of the White traveler laden with the power and privilege of his culture who visits a far-off "exotic" people. I struggle to go beyond that shadow, all the while knowing that shadow is cast deep within me and will never be entirely erased.[4]

Within the limitations to what could be my contribution to the Ju/'hoan people, my hope, indeed my prayer, is that being respectfully *with* the people has provided a counterexample to the usual and classic pattern of the White visitor who abused his power—an abuse no less destructive to the people when it was unintentional. That hope, that prayer, makes the idea of a return possible.

I intensely wanted to return, but I was also ambivalent about returning. Is the Kalahari really a "home" for me in any way?

When I do go back to the Kalahari, the myth of "a return" begins to dissolve into countless, practical realities, and the actuality of the return assumes its own grounded dimensions. Most of the people I had worked with closely in 1968 have since died. As we enter |Kae|kae, the heart-beating excitement of a long-anticipated return is dulled by the anxiety of feeling like a stranger. Walking into the village, I see an old woman lying in the sand, resting. Her large overbite is unmistakable. Her face is familiar to me despite her aging body. I didn't know her well during my initial visit, but she is the first Ju/'hoan I recognize from that time. I greet her. She looks at me, a bit puzzled. I ask if she remembers me. And in an exquisitely polite manner, she responds, "Oh, I'm an old woman now, and my eyes are bad . . . but if I could see properly, I'm sure I'd remember you."

My heart sinks. I wonder: is it possible that her eyes can see—but not see and know me? Here I've come all this way to reconnect with people who have been such a deep part of my life, and they may not even remember who I am! I turn to my two co-workers—Verna St. Denis and Megan Biesele—and caution them: "We may be in for some disappointments."

Now, more eagerly, I seek out ≠Oma Djo, the one healer with whom I was closest in 1968 and who still lives at |Kae|kae. I have just learned that Kinachau, my other close healer friend, has recently died. "Is ≠Oma Djo here?" I ask, part of me afraid that maybe even he will not be around. "Out in the bush," comes the reply. We walk on and start setting up our camp. And then the commotion begins as people excitedly announce that ≠Oma Djo is coming. An old man walks toward me; his gait has a familiar, sprightly bounce. It is my old friend. He and I see each other, and the instant of recognition is overpowering. We embrace and cry and laugh . . . and cry some more. I feel at home, welcomed back.

Seeing ≠Oma Djo seems to open the gates of memory. Others I had worked with, though not known as well, come over, and we reintroduce ourselves and joyfully and instantly reconnect as we survey the passage of time on each other's faces.

The very next morning, ≠Oma Djo comes back to our camp to see "!Xam" again. !Xam is my Ju/'hoan name, given to me on my first visit to |Kae|kae. In Ju/'hoan culture there are a limited number of names, so there are a number of people called !Xam in the area.

"Yesterday," ≠Oma Djo says, "I was out in the bush, and someone told me that !Xam was here and was looking for me. 'What !Xam could be looking for me?' I wondered. So I came to see. When I saw you, I knew . . . but you've gotten old! I was surprised to see you, and I'm still surprised. It's such an amazing thing that someone who came so long ago would think to come back again.

"It's amazing that someone from so far away," he adds, "would continue to think about me. I myself thought about !Xam sometimes, and sometimes I forgot about him and just lived."

Yes, for most of these years we both "just lived." ≠Oma Djo's realism helps ground our meeting and my return and invites me to be the person I have become—more

THOUGH DANCERS AT THE HEALING DANCE ARE PRIMARILY MEN, WOMEN JOIN IN WITH A SPECIAL INTENSITY; HERE, IN 1968, TWO WOMEN—N!UNKA, WHO IS NURSING HER BABY, AND |XOAN N!A'AN FROM |KAE|KAE— DANCE WITH ≠OMA DJO (FAR RIGHT).

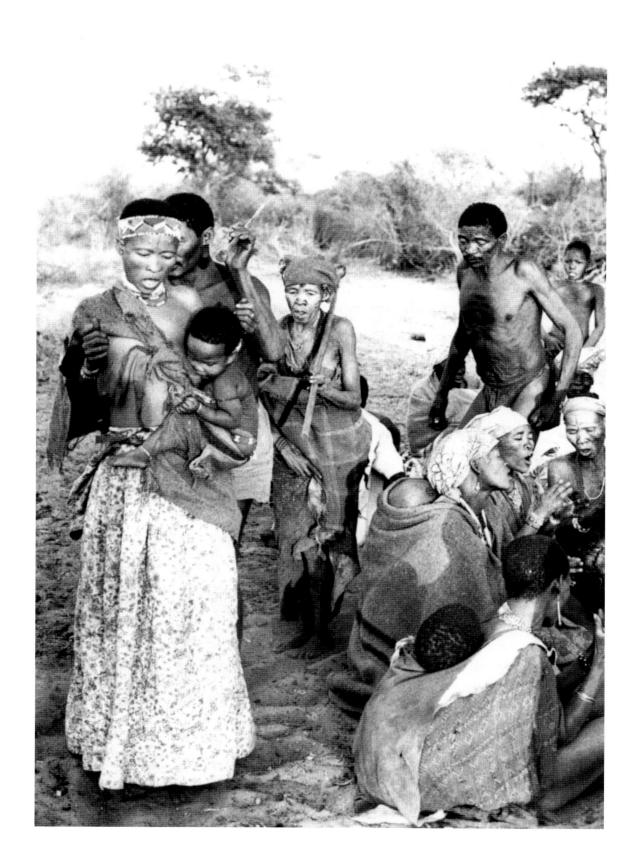

involved with everyday issues of the Jul'hoan community, more careful about working with nǀom than the young man of the first visit.

During my initial visit, I had focused almost exclusively on healing and the healing dance. Going to every dance that occurred at ǀKaeǀkae and trying to learn about "drinking" nǀom structured my stay in the Kalahari. ≠Oma Djo had then remarked, "!Xam, when I'm looking at you and watching you dance, I say, 'There's a guy that's concentrating on nǀom.'

"!Xam," he had continued, "I know you are a good dancer. I know you are a guy who is interested in dancing and nǀom. I've seen you in action. Someday, !Xam, you watch the dancing, and I'll dance and put nǀom in my dancing stick before I give it to you."

"≠Oma Djo, what if I came to you requesting that you teach me nǀom?"

"If you dance and get nǀom from me, don't you think the police will be after me for giving you nǀom?" ≠Oma Djo responded with mock surprise. "Some people might say, 'What sort of a business is it when a White man starts to !aia on Jul'hoan nǀom? Surely that can't be a good thing.' The word would get out that there's some crazy Jul'hoan upcountry who is pouring nǀom into a White man. I know you won't tell, but look, we do our nǀom training in public, and hundreds of people could see you !aia."

In his humorous and gently indirect way, ≠Oma Djo had been telling me I needed time to learn about nǀom, more time than I had allocated to spend in the Kalahari. There was no problem with the police—at that time there weren't any police in the area. The problem was with me. "Drinking" nǀom was a long, difficult, and painful process; ≠Oma Djo wanted me to know that with my heart not just my mind. I understood, but in my youthful exuberance so long ago I sometimes forgot what I knew.

Now, on my return, I do not focus so exclusively or literally on nǀom and healing. My fuller acceptance of the structural inequalities between myself and the Jul'hoansi, as well as my own growth in spiritual understanding, necessitates a more measured approach to nǀom. I am more involved in the requirements and responsibilities of the little camp that Verna, Megan, and I set up. In many ways, we are another ǀKaeǀkae family. The healing dance, though still a profound spiritual experience, is more a part of ongoing life events that constitute the days the three of us spend with the Jul'hoan community.

When dances are held, we go; I dance, Verna and Megan sing, and we visit—like Jul'hoansi do. But instead of trying to drink nǀom myself, I have a new aim: responding to the needs of those already engaged in the dance, and especially trying to calm down young healers overwhelmed with boiling nǀom. When healers are overwhelmed with the searing pain of boiling nǀom, their bodies often writhe in rigid, convulsing agony. Usually, I have to work with one or two other persons to muster enough strength just to hold such healers and prevent them from injuring themselves or running into the dance fire. Then we have to bring a sense of relative calm to the embattled healers so they can more effectively regulate—and cool down—the boiling nǀom and thence begin to heal. In that act of serving others, I begin to learn more about nǀom, and a different understanding emerges from when I had earlier tried to pursue nǀom more directly.

Another change comes about during this second stay in the Kalahari: hearing more about nǀom and healing, I also begin knowing less. During my first visit, the fundamentals of healing were presented, yielding a certain clarity; this was possible because the dance still had a relative integrity and coherence. Now, however, the dance is surrounded by the increasingly rapid currents of social change, and this integrity and coherence is under assault; a new degree of complexity and fluidity has entered into the dance.

As well, the questions we now ask as a team allow us to focus on more subtle and elusive aspects of healing. I am able to build upon my earlier fieldwork in the Kalahari and on subsequent experiences with traditional healers in other parts of the world. Verna and Megan, with their own well-developed areas of expertise, bring a many-layered richness to the interview process. Coupled with this maturational movement in our questions, the new level of inherent complexity in the dance keeps all of us in an ongoing dialogue of wonderment. Our assumptions and hypotheses are constantly being questioned, even dismissed.

Understanding that nǀom *can* "kill you," I came to respect more deeply the power of nǀom. Now, hearing healer after healer affirm, "We still have our nǀom," I became more optimistic about the power of nǀom to influence the course of social change among the Juǀ'hoansi. And it was to the forces of political and cultural destruction in their life that the Juǀ'hoansi directed us.

BECOMING PAPER PEOPLE

"We have lost our land so we cannot feed ourselves properly," ≠Oma Djo tells us. "We are barely alive anymore." With stark simplicity, ≠Oma Djo brings us up to date. With the loss of land undercutting their hunting-gathering, Juǀ'hoansi are turning more and more to other means of subsistence, including agriculture and cattle. But they are constantly obstructed in these efforts to create new means of survival. We hear the Juǀ'hoansi's pained frustration about their inability to halt the destruction surrounding them and their eloquent call for assistance.

Xumi Nǃa'an, for example, describes how Juǀ'hoan people must make demands on the Botswana government if they are to have access to agricultural and livestock resources. A respected elder and strong supporter of the healing dance, Xumi Nǃa'an sees meetings as one way of giving voice to Juǀ'hoan needs.

> All the Juǀ'hoansi here at ǀKaeǀkae are crying out for gardens, cows, and goats. Where will we get these things? The government says we should stay together, but how can it help us? Government people say we should lift up our hands and help the government. They say we should help in the field and get money that way to buy food and clothes. If I make a good garden and then ask them for money, when would I ever get it? Food now costs money.

> The government says I should lift myself up. But if I lift myself up, where will I get the money and food? Even seeds I don't have. My people aren't eating. So I say let's have meetings [with the government].

However, when meetings with the government are finally arranged, Juǀ'hoansi are not heard; their words, remaining in the oral mode, are dismissed. Describing a government meeting with rural people that includes the Juǀ'hoansi, Xumi Nǃa'an explains the dilemma:

> [At these meetings] we are like ostriches still closed up inside their eggs so they cannot see. [Those who run the meetings, the Tswana government people] can write, but I can't write. And they write down their own speech at these meetings, but they don't write down my speech. Even now I have papers from those meetings, but I haven't yet found anyone to read them to the ǀKaeǀkae people.

Xumi sees how words, to become powerful, must now also be written down. And this is where we, the "people who know about papers," become of particular value.

It is easy to take for granted the act of writing. But to the Juǀ'hoansi this use of pen and paper is a wondrous event, an expression of great skill, an opening toward great power. Except for their young people now attending school, the Juǀ'hoansi do not read or write. They realize that our pen-and-paper activity—our writing ability—surely could be of assistance.

Verna, Megan, and I are given a special task; we are to become "paper people."

> You [three] know about papers. You write on them. That is how you can help us. Send a letter to those government people. Tell them about how we are no longer a people. And tell them that we need our land back to become a people able to feed ourselves.

That is how Tshao Matze, a strong healer and a man who constantly struggles to regain the Juǀ'hoan land-base, speaks when we ask how we might help. He understands the new dynamics of authority, an authority exerted from a central government and conveyed by pieces of paper that unexpectedly keep telling him what he must do and not do—land-board papers about who owns wells and de facto the land around them; licenses to hunt, with restrictions on the number of game that can be killed; and lists of who receives food from special government assistance programs. These government papers threaten to submerge the traditional Jul'hoan modes of governance and authority, which are based on egalitarianism, consensus, and flexible oral exchange.

The need for this letter to the government—for many letters to various people in authority—is urgent. This book is an extension of one such letter. The ancient Jul'hoan land-base—the place of their hunting-gathering activities, the repository of their culture—is eroding rapidly. Cattle trample out their bush foods, entrepreneurs carve up their myths. Focusing on traditional Jul'hoan healing, this book hopes to epitomize the power, plight, and promise of Jul'hoan culture.

As authors of this book, we are messengers sent from the Jul'hoan people. Tshao Matze outlines our task:

> Bringing ideas to other people helps. Also, you take what we're doing to others, so they'll know. Those of you who have come over and over have each learned something and told other people. . . .
>
> I want us to call men and women together to hear what's really in everyone's hearts. Then we can tell it all to you who are our helpers.
>
> You people are "paper people." You can go speak to other people—big people—for us. We have "no hands" and don't know where we'll get water. There's water, but we don't get to drink it. You can contact the government for us—they now have the strength. And if we think of anything else later, we'll tell you.
>
> It's our thing [I speak of], not your thing. But what's important is to understand each other. If you're in pain about something, everyone should get together and come to an understanding.

It is the Jul'hoan "thing" that we write about, not ours. But to the degree we can "get together" with them, and "take what we're doing to others," we hope to carry the Jul'hoan message to those who can offer concrete help, aided if necessary by "moving" some papers.

We turn our pens and papers toward becoming scribes for the Jul'hoansi. Our task is to listen, to hear their words and the yearnings beneath them. And then, by providing with this book a place for their voices to speak, we could help to create the most powerful of advocacies possible. In this book, Verna, Megan, and I will be paper people, but always in the Jul'hoan way—with heart.

This emphasis on advocacy and action becomes a guiding principle of my return. Though nlom and healing remain the focus of the entire project, I now join in a more explicit and intensive manner others who have listened, described, and advocated—including Megan in her work with Jul'hoan people and Verna in her work with First Nations people in Canada.

Nlom and healing could be the linchpin to creating more constructive forces of social change for the Jul'hoansi. My prior experience with nlom in 1968, and my subsequent work over a twenty-year period with Indigenous spiritual healing traditions in other parts of the world, and with their relationships to Western therapies, encourage me to return to the Kalahari. I might have something to offer. In addition to wishing to join the Jul'hoansi in their journey to become n/omkxaosi (owners of nlom) or healers, I now wish to support them in remaining Jul'hoansi or "real people." Once again we are asked to "tell our story to your people"; and now the story encompasses new facts of life. In this enlargement of my earlier work in the Kalahari, I have found a way to return.

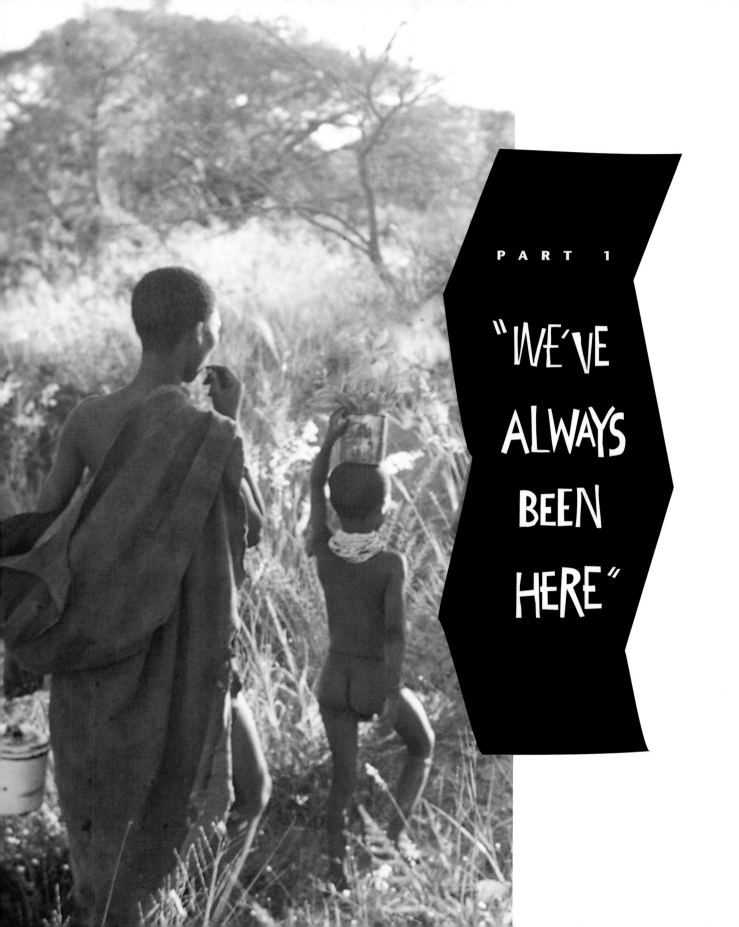

PART 1

"WE'VE
ALWAYS
BEEN
HERE"

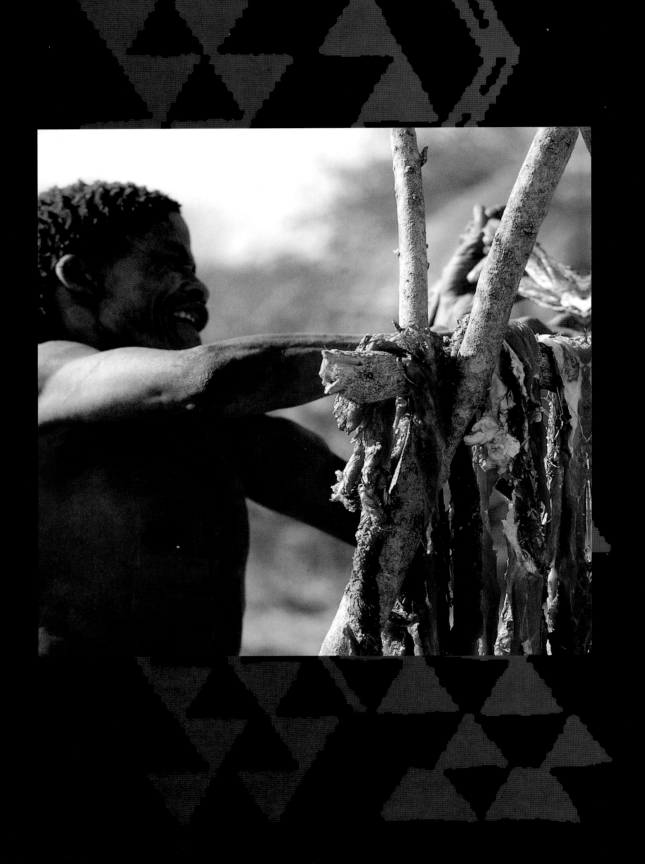

Jul'hoan people never lived in paradise. The ways of the past, though remembered fondly, were filled with their share of hunger, conflict, and tension. But the Jul'hoan people remember that in the past they lived with dignity, committed to each others' health and happiness. Through that commitment they supported their communities.

JUI'HOAN HUNTING AND GATHERING

The Jul'hoan hunting-gathering lifestyle, which predominated in the subsistence activities of the people at ǀKaeǀkae until the late 1960s, emphasized the sharing of resources, egalitarian relationships with each other, and a harmony of purposes between individuals and the community. The land provided sustenance and was used respectfully by Jul'hoan people.

≠Oma Djo, a powerful, highly respected Jul'hoan healer, reminisces with us in 1989 about his old hunting-gathering life.

> Long ago there was a lot of Bushman food we used to eat—wild potatoes, ca, and other things. Some of our food we dug out from the ground in the valleys, and some of it was in the dunes of sand. Bushman foods are very many. We lived here at ǀKaeǀkae and ate *mongongoes* and *gǃoan* berries and *nǀang* berries. And I'd shoot gemsbok and elands and we'd eat them. We drank from a small waterhole, which gave us "God's water." When I gave birth to my children and gave them food to eat, like things I'd killed, these were good times. In those days we didn't think of trouble.[1]

THE EQUITABLE DISTRIBUTION OF MEAT IS CENTRAL TO TRADITIONAL JUI'HOAN LIFE. HERE, IN 1968, A YOUNG ≠OMA ǃHOMGǃAUSI CUTS MEAT INTO STRIPS TO FACILITATE ITS DRYING AND DISTRIBUTION THROUGHOUT THE CAMP.

I

"WE USED TO DIRECT OURSELVES"

We can see that ≠Oma Djo is not just reminiscing; he is living those "good times" once more. The fertility of the land once allowed him as a hunter to "give birth," to give life to his children. And "God's water" guaranteed their survival. He also reaffirms what others long ago said about meat and sharing: "We Jul'hoansi always share our meat. We share so as to create good feelings among ourselves."

Implicit in this statement is a contrast with neighboring ways of life, such as those of the Bantu-speaking Tswana and Herero peoples. Both the Tswana ethnic majority of Botswana and the Hereros, who came from the west early in the twentieth century into Botswana (then Bechuanaland), are cattle-keeping agriculturalists. Their systems of labor and wealth distribution patterns are quite different from those of the Ju/'hoansi. Ju/'hoan sharing is a comprehensive means of social insurance in the context of their more variable, chancy, and immediate-return hunting-gathering means of production.

Their sharing ethic enabled the Ju/'hoansi to live in close quarters; individuals could spend their lives face-to-face with each other in relative harmony. The Ju/'hoansi typically lived in camps of between ten and thirty people closely related through kinship. Half a dozen or so woven-grass shelters supported by frames of sticks, usually forming a half- or quarter-circle, faced an open area and defined the camp. Remains of similar camps in areas immediately adjacent to |Kae|kae have been dated back many thousands of years. Some researchers see good evidence that, as many as forty thousand years ago, people made their living in the area much like today's Ju/'hoansi do.

That their lifestyle originated in the distant past is an understanding still conveyed today by both the Ju/'hoansi and their neighbors. Ju/'hoan and other Bushman people take pride in regarding themselves as the original inhabitants of a wide area encompassing the Kalahari Desert and beyond. The Herero and Tswana people are by and large respectful of these claims on a cognitive level, though they often disregard them on an economic one. These neighbors recognize that the hunting-gathering peoples possess special practical and spiritual powers associated with their longevity on this land. For instance, Ju/'hoan tracking ability and knowledge of animal behavior is seen as uncanny, and they have unquestioning awe for Ju/'hoan healing power. Ju/'hoan people thus occupy a moral high ground as cultural "seniors," although in practice they often are relegated to lower status in interethnic politics.

This ambivalence extends toward the Ju/'hoansi largely because of the special characteristics of their traditional way of making a living. Hunting-gathering is so different from the way most of Africa lives today that it causes distrust at the same time as it inspires wonder. Most Africans are agriculturalists, as were most Europeans and Americans until recently. Many African agriculturalists, like the Hereros and Tswana, specialize in "pastoralism," or the care of cattle and small stock.[2] The work ethics, distribution systems, storage patterns, and reward structures of agriculture have become so familiar to all of us who have inherited the agricultural mind-set that a different survival strategy can appear threatening.

Agricultural work ethics support repetitive, often drudging labor by rewarding it with delayed returns. Often agricultural social systems function by organizing the labor of younger or poorer people under an authority that controls wealth and distribution. The social stratification that occurs in such systems is often legitimized by religious and cultural ideologies. By its nature, agricultural wealth must be stored, whether on the hoof (as in animal husbandry), in granaries, or in other forms of long-term protection. Storage can quickly legitimize hoarding, and competitive ethics can arise and in turn become supported by ideology. Privatization of resources and encouragement of individual enterprise seem to go hand in hand in agricultural societies in ways that would be impossible in the hunting-gathering life, with its emphasis on egalitarian relationships and an immediate return from labor.

Ju/'hoan hunting-gathering is founded on social and economic premises that differ profoundly from those of agriculture. The economic system of the Ju/'hoansi is based on sharing collected wild food resources. Men mostly hunt, and women mostly gather; though women provide substantial help to the men in their hunting, with information about game and assistance in tracking, and men often gather when meat is unavailable. Between 60 and 70 percent of the diet by weight consists of wild vegetable foods gathered primarily by women.

Ju/'hoan local groups neither maintain exclusive rights to resources nor defend territories; reciprocal access prevails. Frequent visiting and sharing among the different groups mitigate the effect of localized shortages. Allied groups cooperate, coming together in a given area when there is sufficient food and water, living apart when sources of food and water are widely scattered. When food is brought into a camp, it is distributed for all to partake.

Resources of all kinds circulate among members of a camp and between camps, so that any one person draws upon the entire community's resources. Little effort is directed toward accumulating goods and property. Shelter, clothing, and tools are made easily, with ample leisure time to make them. Since individuals and groups must move to stay close to their food sources, personal property is kept to a minimum, usually less than twenty-five pounds per individual.[3] Frequent moves and the Jul'hoan emphasis on sharing also work to minimize food accumulation. The environment itself is their storehouse.

Accumulation of food would have distinct disadvantages in the hot Kalahari Desert. The Jul'hoansi only gather when they need food, and what they collect is immediately distributed and consumed fresh. There is also a marked absence of wealth disparity among the Jul'hoansi. No one is supposed to stand out from the rest of the group. If someone were to come back from a successful hunt showing excessive pride, he would be put firmly in his place, even if the kill were a large animal. With the freshly killed meat still over his shoulder, such an improperly proud hunter would hear the pointed teasing of his camp: "What is that you have there? What a scrawny little thing! You didn't kill that. It looks so sick and scrawny that it must have fallen dead into your arms."

Insulting the meat like this reinforces the rule of egalitarianism. The strong sexual egalitarianism of the Jul'hoansi is also reinforced by joking insults. For instance, there is a running joke in an oft-told folktale that pits male and female genitalia against each other in a

CHILDREN PLAY

AT GATHERING ACTIVITIES—

"DIGGING FOR ROOTS."

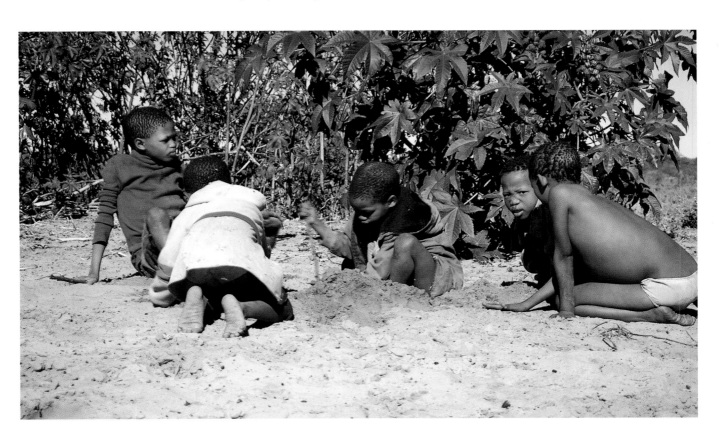

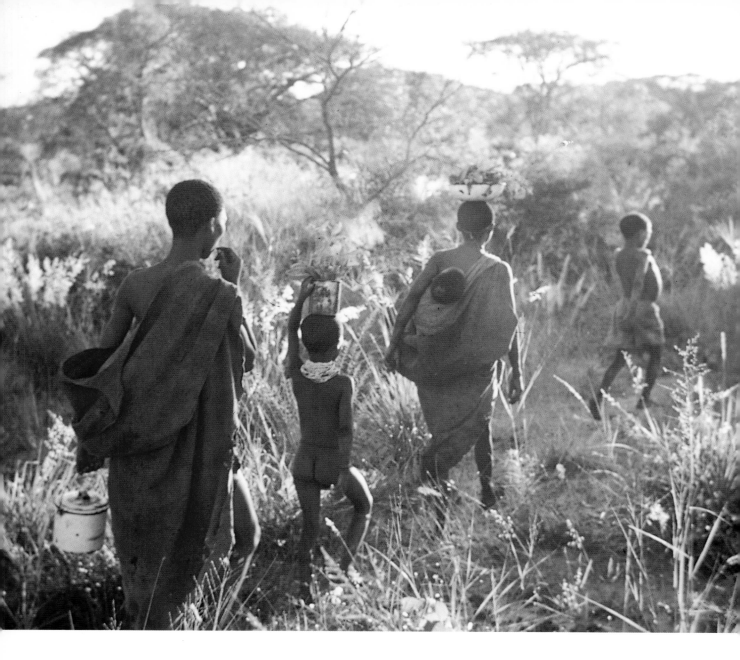

magical context. The tale is retold or alluded to with great delight by both sexes; in the end, neither side comes out ahead. Many social techniques like these combine to help their small groups work together in harmony. Since they live in a land that yields food and water only sparingly, they survive by joining in groups to share equally what they can hunt and gather.

Memories of Jul'hoan traditional life and self-sufficiency are vivid. Game was abundant, and the skills the hunters learned fitted them admirably to their work of providing meat. The huge, meaty eland, for example, was so important to the Jul'hoansi economically that it was considered spiritually important too. Eland symbolism marks many of the Jul'hoan rites of passage, including marriage, initiation as hunters, and the transformations of the healing dance. The simple technology of poisoned arrows made it necessary for hunters to be in superb physical shape to track and even chase down these animals on foot.

≠Oma Djo's relish for those old hunting days is expressed in his spirited account of an eland hunt when he was still a young man:

> I had come from ǀKaeǃkae and went this way. I stopped for water near a ≠'o tree. There I saw a steenbok and killed it. Then I saw an eland track and said, "What will I do with this steenbok?" So I stuck it up in the tree and stuck my quiver up there too. I tracked and tracked the eland until I came to where it was standing.
>
> I took the arrows themselves and the bow, leaving the quiver in the tree. I stalked the eland and stalked him and got close, took out one arrow and shot it, and it missed. Another arrow went past his stomach and fell. Then I shot it in the stomach and the eland ran. He went down a valley and climbed the dune on the other side. Up there it joined many other elands. So I went around the end of the dune and watched them. The others ran off, leaving the one I shot. So I cut him off from them. Then he went back down into the valley. He went under the shade of a big tree. So I went around the eland and shot at him again. He died there. I got my steenbok and quiver and went home, leaving the eland there.
>
> I went and got ǀAiǃae Nǃa'an and Glaq'o and we went to the eland, where we met Tshao, who had tracked my footsteps. I told ǀAiǃae Nǃa'an to go back and get more people while Glaq'o and I started to skin it. Rain beat down on us, and when the moon came out, it stopped. Then ǀAiǃae Nǃa'an came back with the people he had gone after. Glaq'o Nǃa'an (my mother's father) and my mother's younger brother and their wives came

and slept there. We all drank fat until the dawn broke.

> We sent Glaq'o Nǃa'an to get all the rest of the people because rain had brought water there so we all could drink. We lived there and drank the water the rain had brought. When the meat was gone we left there and went beyond the valley and lived.
>
> There I saw two more elands and tracked them. And when I got up to them, I ran between them and separated them. They ran off because they smelled me. I went after one and shot at it. It didn't die, so I left it. Then I went back to the camp, and by late afternoon I was telling them I had shot another eland. ǀUi's father was surprised and said, "Are you going to kill all the elands? There's still meat left and you've shot another."
>
> In the morning we packed up and went to the next eland, which had already died. It was raining again. We didn't stay there, but packed up the meat and went to live at ǀUihaba, where we ate the meat and drank from waterholes.

Concern for the environment is clear in this account, as is the highly social nature of hunting and sharing. What is most clear, however, is the sense of joyful mastery ≠Oma Djo describes, from the days when he felt his own skills and strengths were sufficient to the tasks of his life.

Since Dick initially worked closely with the Juǀ'hoansi in the 1960s, in this area of what is now Botswana, profound changes have come in the degree of self-reliance possible for the people. Once their isolated situation in far northwest Botswana protected them from very much outside contact. Before then, the Juǀ'hoansi of this area, with their close relatives to the west in adjacent Namibia, were among the last relatively independent hunter-gatherers in southern Africa. Living from foraging wild foods in this area required approximately 23 square miles (37 square kilometers) per person in order to support a stable population. It also required that people live in small, widely scattered groups in order not to put too much pressure on local resources.

Women were honored for providing the reliable majority of the diet. Men were honored for providing the chancy but coveted wild animal meat. A few staple vegetable foods, like the *morama* bean and the mongongo nut, were augmented by over a hundred edible plant foods.[4] More than fifty kinds of mammals, along with birds and reptiles, provided a solid subsistence base.[5] The Jul'hoansi prized most the meat of giraffes, warthogs, and the antelopes: eland antelopes, kudu, wildebeest, gemsbok, Cape buffalo, hartebeest, impala, roan, and the smaller bucks like duiker and steenbok.

Wild honey, though rarely found, was a delicacy. Especially delicious fruits like the *n!oh* orange were enjoyed in their season. Areas where different prized foods were to be found were fondly remembered. For instance, the morama bean fields between the Aha Mountains, northwest of |Kae|kae, were thought of as a kind of fertile heartland for gathering. The Ahas themselves reminded people of the satisfying *marula* nuts that grow in abundance there.[6]

To find such foods requires that the Jul'hoansi have intimate knowledge of their area. Food is abundant in season but ultimately limited, so one of the most important pieces of information is how local resources should be shared. In general, a band of related people makes use of the resources of its own *n!ore,* a roughly circular area of land with undefended borders that provides sufficient food and water to maintain a band over the course of a year of seasons.

One reason a n!ore can sustain a band of people is because a group of n!oresi function as an interlocking, co-operating entity. Those living in different n!oresi and linked to each other by marriage alliances have sharing arrangements based on visiting back and forth. Sometimes the rain may be spotty, causing bush foods to sprout or ripen faster in one n!ore than another. People often go to visit their relatives at the favored n!ore at this time, expecting in turn that they will receive a return visit when their relatives need something they can provide. Also, some n!oresi have bush foods or animal resources not found in others. Reciprocal access by kin and other

sorts of extended land-use rights are necessary to ensure a well-rounded and adequate food supply.

Leadership of n!oresi is not hierarchical. Each n!ore has as stewards a core group of brothers and sisters who share primary access to its resources and have the responsibility to share these resources with others. The n!ore system regulates the ratio of the numbers of people to the land and available resources, ensuring that local areas have stewards to keep foods from being hunted or gathered out. Because the system is based on well-known kinship rules, there is clear social agreement as to which people have rights to which areas.

Within these known areas, the boundaries of allied bands' territories are not precise. A hunting territory is a vague area extending, for example, south and west of a certain line of hills or a pan.[7] But animals within these territories belong to no one until they are shot, and they may even be shot by visiting bands. This flexibility is important in alleviating local food shortages in times of mild or scattered drought.

In years of severe drought, however, food scarcity is universal, so there is no point in visiting an allied band's territory. This practical fact is what has kept explosive situations of conflict over scarce resources from occurring. The flexible use of territories belonging to allied bands is an example of what might be called the "controlled opportunism" with which Jul'hoan hunter-gatherers successfully utilized their Kalahari environment. This pattern of flexible land usage is one "social technology" used to maximize the benefits of a chancy environment.

An important way that opportunism is monitored and kept social rather than individual or exploitative is through the Jul'hoan concept of *kxaosi* or "owners." Ownership for the Jul'hoansi is actually a form of responsible stewardship. A kxao or owner is also a "master," in the sense of "knowing fully." A *g!ukxao* (literally "owner of water") is more an informed person who cares for a water resource so it can be shared than an exclusive holder of rights to that water. This concept of ownership extends to many commodities and activities in Jul'hoan life that benefit from stewardship. As we shall soon see,

Juǀʼhoan healers are such stewards and masters.

The meat of animals is another essential commodity to which kxaosi is applied. In the 1960s, the Juǀʼhoansi who lived just across the border from ǀKaeǀkae (in what was then South West Africa) usually hunted down between fifteen and eighteen large mammals per year for a single band (averaging twenty-five people per band).[8] When the animal was killed, its kxao or "owner" (who might not necessarily be the hunter but sometimes the maker of the decisive arrow) had the right to distribute the meat. Almost without fail, meat was shared with all members of the local groups—along rather definite lines of division. This rigorous sharing of meat may have evolved in response to the universal human need for protein. Even those who might never have primary access to meat with which to reciprocate at a later date—such as women, crippled individuals, or those who for some reason just could not manage the discipline of hunting—would be given shares. The distribution of meat continues to be a high point of tension in Juǀʼhoan culture, and if anyone is left out, intense negative feelings can occur.

Vegetable foods are not shared as rigorously as meat. Though far outweighing meat in importance in the total diet, bush foods are shared by the woman who gathers them within her nuclear family, and the sharing is done much more casually than is the case with meat. What is *not* casual about the bush foods, however, is their ownership by different bands while these foods are still in the ground. Because ownership of groves and gathering places is clear, the kxaosi can do their work of regulating the pressure on these resources.[9]

Though nuclear families are the units within which gathered foods are shared, one nuclear family alone is not enough to sustain the arduous hunting and gathering life. So families are organized into extended-family bands. These bands provide enough men for reliable hunting and enough women to guarantee companionship on gathering trips. Subsistence activities are also social activities, with a great deal of daily business and satisfying talk and play interwoven.

The great equalizer in Juǀʼhoan social life is the need to share. If people live as they should, the Juǀʼhoansi say, the sharing of today will be paid off at a future date, sure to arrive, when those who have given come home empty-handed. Ownership, then, is essentially the ownership of the ability to share. Sharing itself, which minimizes risk, is a resource to be reckoned with in the marginal environment where the Juǀʼhoansi live.

One of the major ways the sharing ethic is promoted among the Juǀʼhoansi is through *xaro*, the giving of gifts. Gift-giving is more a way to stay in long, friendly relationships than it is a means to circulate goods. A man named !Xuma from Bate, north of ǀKaeǀkae, put it this way: "Xaro is when I take a thing of value and give it to you. Later, much later, when you find some good thing, you give it back to me. When I find something good I will give it to you, and so we will pass the years together."[10]

THE JUǀʼHOAN HEALING DANCE

As harmonious as these descriptions of their ideal life may sound, we should not assume that the Juǀʼhoansi have lived without conflict.[11] In fact, the detailed nature of their social technology for getting along with each other is evidence that conflict always has been a fact of their lives. One reason healing and the healing dance are so important to the Juǀʼhoansi is to help keep peace between people. Individuals might well become exasperated with each other under the sometimes harsh conditions of their life. Since they depend so much on each other, conflict could actually keep them from having shelter or enough to eat. Basic necessities depend on the continuation of goodwill.

But the Juǀʼhoansi's everyday life goes beyond survival in a harsh land; their healing is but one reflection of a profound spiritual dimension that pervades their lives. This spirituality is highlighted by intense and exhilarating all-night healing dances, dances that in the late 1960s remained at the very center of Juǀʼhoan ceremonial life, expressing the deepest Juǀʼhoan spiritual yearnings.[12] In these dances they share a spiritual power that heals, protects, and gives well-being to them all. Their approach to healing leads them to include everyone in the dance,

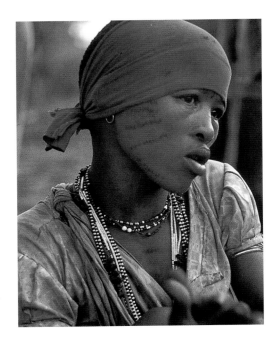

whether obviously ill or not; for in healing, the Jul'hoansi make no distinction among their physical, emotional, and spiritual needs.

The healing dance is their main method for treating sickness, though the Jul'hoansi also use medicinal herbs and salves for minor injuries and infections. Through recently introduced government clinics, the Jul'hoansi also have access to antibiotics, which they sometimes use against infections, for example, but they rely on the healing dance for the treatment of virtually every illness. However, dances are not held primarily to treat sickness; instead, they are opportunities for people to join together in a spiritual journey, occasions during which community is healed and reformed.

The Jul'hoansi bring more than just their medical and psychological problems to the dance; rips in the social fabric, such as arguments between villages or disagreements about the distribution of meat, are illnesses that often are mended in the dance. If someone's illness takes a serious turn, a regular dance involving the entire community may be convened. More often, however, there will be a smaller healing ceremony in which one or two healers, with several singers, work exclusively on the sick person. The healing dance, since it speaks to so many differ-

ent levels, is not strictly tied to any specific illness. And since the healing energy originates from the gods, the dance is itself a spiritual exercise.

In the healing dance of the Jul'hoansi, everyone shares a spiritual power called nlom. Some anthropologists have translated *n/om* as "medicine," but it is more than just medicine. Nlom is energy, spiritual energy. There are many referents for nlom, and the limits to these referents are purposely ambiguous.[13] Things of power, including things out of the ordinary, such as herbal medicines, African sorcery, menstrual blood, and the vapor trail of a jet, are among the contexts in which the word *n/om* is used. Therefore the phenomenon of nlom does not yield to a Western-oriented logical analysis, and we were constantly frustrated in any attempt to pin down its "meaning." Jul'hoan people say that nlom is a thing unto itself. But in whatever form or function, nlom is felt as strong—and the word *n/om* itself carries the power of nlom.

Nlom is "invisible," though it can be seen and picked up by experienced healers during a state of enhanced awareness. Otherwise nlom is known only by its action and effects. It is located only by its existence in a particular form, whether it be a person, a song, or a bee. Nlom is not personalized nor personified. No one can possess it exclusively nor control it completely.

Nlom, this primary force in the Jul'hoan universe of experience, is at its strongest in the healing dance. It resides in the dance fire, in the healing songs, and most of all in the healers, concentrated in the pit of their stomachs and the base of their spines. The dance activates the n!om in the healers; their singing and their dance movements, they say, "heat up" the n!om. When n!om boils, it vaporizes and rises up the spine. Kxao ≠Oah, one of the strongest healers in the !Kae!kae area, describes the feeling of n!om:

> In your backbone you feel a pointed something and it works its way up. The base of your spine is tingling, tingling, tingling, tingling. Then n!om makes your thoughts nothing in your head.[14]

Kxao ≠Oah goes on to describe how painful the boiling n!om is: "It hurts," he says. "It is like fire—it burns you."

As n!om reaches the base of the healers' skull, they enter a state of transcendence called !aia. Once in this state, the dancer can heal. !Aia, often translated as "trance," is actually a state of enhanced awareness in which the healer claims, among other things, to travel physically and psychically over great distances, to see inside other people's bodies, and to contact the gods—all in the effort to heal.

The healing dance often goes on from dusk to dawn, usually four or five times a month. Most of the community members come to the open center space of the camp where the dance revolves around a fire. The women sit around the flames, shoulder to shoulder, legs intertwined, and sing the healing songs to the beat of their rhythmic clapping. The dancers circle around them; they are mostly men, who do most of the healing, although singers sometimes heal as well. Toward the edges of the open area around several smaller fires, others sit, talk,

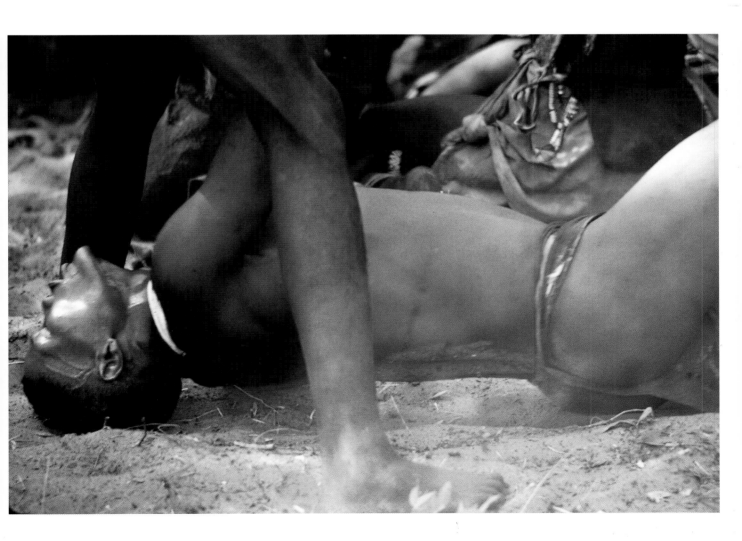

and rest, supporting the dance with their presence and at times singing and dancing.

At the start, the singers and dancers warm up, and the mood is casual and jovial. At first, there may be only a few women singing softly, and many of the dancers are adolescents, showing off new dance steps. Laughter and banter fill the air. Then, almost imperceptibly, the mood grows intense; many women have joined the circle of singers, and experienced healers begin to dance. The singing and clapping become spirited, the dancing focused.

But laughter is never far away. The same strict Western distinction between the sacred and profane does not exist for the Jul'hoansi. The dance is their most intensely spiritual event, but during it they exchange some of their spiciest jokes and tease each other with friendly vigor about their dancing. The dance does not have an atmosphere of solemn piety, though the sense of awe is profound. As nǀom boils and the mood of the dance intensifies, laughter recedes, but only because working with those in !aia requires great concentration and care. Even when the mood is most tense and all are filled with concern for a dancer overwhelmed with boiling nǀom, someone may joke, lightening the atmosphere and giving reassuring support.

The dance usually culminates for the first time toward late evening, while in the darkness of the desert the fire flickers a captivating, pulsating light on the singers and dancers. Accentuating the intensity of the singing, the women rise up on their knees as they clap. "We do this," says N≠aisa, "when our hearts are happy." Feelings run high; the dancers sweat profusely. Transcendence is at hand. Soon one or two healers begin to stagger, then one falls. A healer may shudder and shake violently, convulsing in pain and anguish. Others may walk about stiff-legged, their eyes glazed. The state of !aia has come and the healing begins.

Healing for the Jul'hoansi is much more than curing

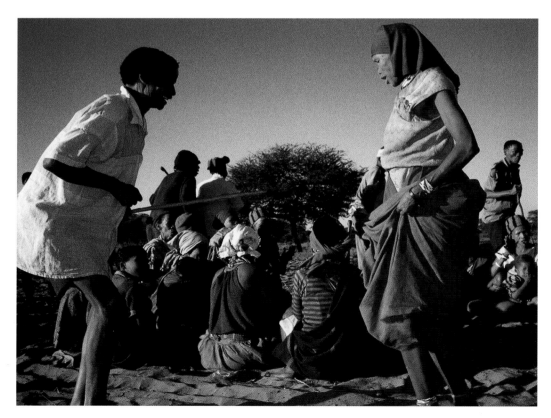

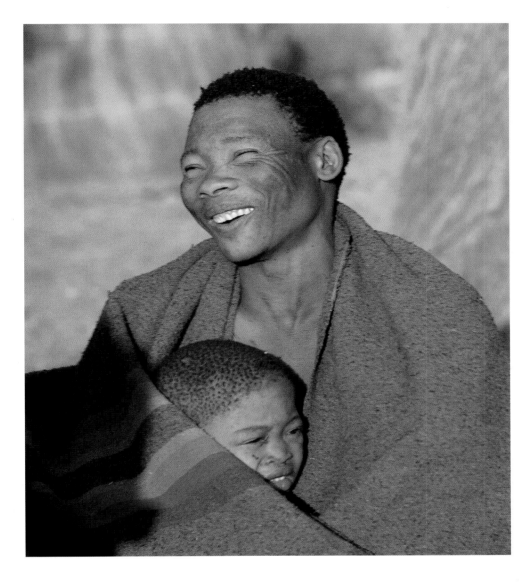

physical or psychological ailments, although it includes that. Healing nurtures each person's emotional and spiritual growth as well. The healer who is in !aia goes to each person at the dance, whether showing symptoms of illness or not. All receive the protection of healing. Healers plead and argue with the gods to save the person from illness. They lay their hands on each person and as they "pull out the sickness" (≠hoe) they usually utter their cries of healing, earth-shattering screams and howls that show the pain and difficulty of the healing work, which may go on for several hours.[15]

As the dance moves into the early morning hours, a calm sets in. Some dancers doze off outside the dance circle. The talk is quiet, the singing soft. The dance is resting. Before dawn comes, the dance awakes again as sleeping forms rise and move toward the dance circle. The singing again becomes strong, the dancing active. There is usually another period of healing as the sun begins to throw its golden light and warmth on the group now huddled around the dance fire. Before the sun becomes too hot, the healing usually subsides, the singing slowly softens, then stops. The dance is over.

To the Western eye, it may seem that the men, most involved in the dramatic role of dancing, are more im-

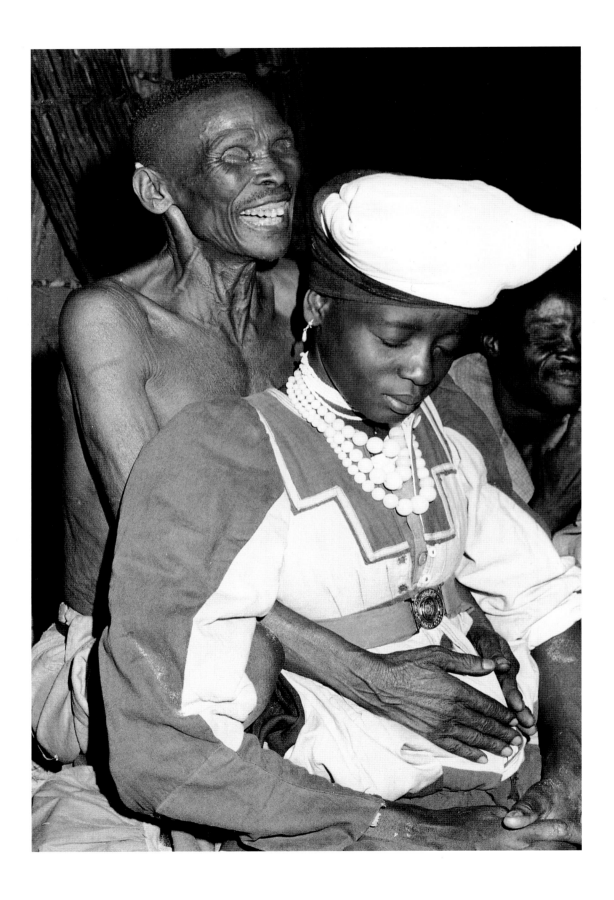

portant to the dance than the women. This is not so, say the Jul'hoansi. Men and women make different but equally valued contributions. The singers and dancers need each others' help to activate the healing energy. Though the actions of the men and women at the dance differ, the nǀom that boils in them is considered the "same nǀom" and their experiences of transcendence—the heart of the dance—are of the same dimension. Men and women are bound together in the dance by their shared, enhanced consciousness as tightly as they are bound together in their efforts at subsistence through their communal approach to hunting and gathering.

The Jul'hoansi enter !aia in order to heal—anyone who seeks to use the !aia experience routinely for other purposes is not supported. Healing has three main aspects: "seeing properly," pulling out the sickness, and arguing with the gods. Seeing properly allows the healer to locate and diagnose the sickness as well as to begin the actual healing with the healer's "absolutely steady" looking.

Seeing properly enables the healer to see beyond mere appearances to other realities. Kxao ≠Oah, an old, blind healer, tells the story of his seeing:

> God keeps my eyeballs in a little cloth bag. When
> he first collected them, he got a little cloth bag and
> plucked my eyeballs out and put them into the
> bag, and then he tied the eyeballs to his belt and
> went up to heaven. And now when I dance, on the
> nights that I dance and when the singing rises up,
> God comes down from heaven, swinging the bag
> with the eyeballs above my head, and he lowers
> the eyeballs to my eye level, and as the singing
> gets strong, he puts the eyeballs into my sockets
> and they stay there and I heal. And when the
> women stop singing and separate out, he removes
> the eyeballs, puts them back in the cloth bag, and
> takes them up to heaven.[16]

Whereas in ordinary everyday life, Kxao ≠Oah needs his wife to lead him as he walks falteringly about, during the dance he moves gracefully, finding all he needs to touch with his healing hands. In the dance, he sees properly.

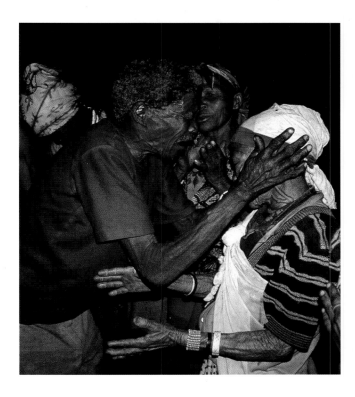

During !aia the reality of the unseen dominates. ≠Oma Djo puts it this way: "In !aia you see everybody. You see that the insides of well people are fine. And you see the insides of the one the ghosts [the spirits of the dead] are trying to kill."

Like healers in most other parts of the world, the Jul'hoansi lay on hands to pull out the sickness. They place their fluttering hands on either side of the person's chest or wherever the sickness is located. They touch the person lightly, or more often vibrate their hands close to the skin's surface. At times healers wrap their bodies around the person being healed, rubbing their sweat—believed to carry healing properties—on the person. The sickness is drawn into the healers, who then expel the sickness from their own bodies, shaking it from their hands out into space, their bodies shuddering with pain.

Ordinarily, the Jul'hoansi do not speak of the gods. But as the healers work, they not only talk directly to the gods, they may also bargain, insult, or even do battle with them. Healers struggle with the ghosts—the spirits of the dead—whom the gods send to carry the sick person away. If a healer's nǀom is strong, the ghosts will retreat and the sick one will live. This struggle is at the center of the healer's skill, art, and power.

Information on the Jul'hoan gods is neither codified nor logically consistent. The gods and one's relationship to them remain a very individual matter. This can create a predicament for an interviewer looking for such consistency, as Lorna Marshall so openly shares:

> I could discover no formulated myth of [the great God's] creation which . . . [all the Jul'hoansi] knew or anything which told how he created himself. People simply said they did not know. . . . [One Jul'hoan woman] turned on me and asked me if I knew. When I said I did not, she snapped, "How then did I expect her to know?"[17]

But generally Jul'hoansi have in their tradition a great God, who is known by several names. One prominent name used in ǀKaeǀkae is !Xu.[18] It is from !Xu that nǀom is said to have originally come to humans, and in special cases, still does. And it is to !Xu's home or village that healers travel to rescue the souls of the sick. The great God, a lesser god, who generally is associated with evil and sickness, and the spirits of the dead (or ghosts), who are more directly linked to sickness as they try to carry the sick one off into their own realm, are all referred to as *gǁaoansi*.

To meet the gods and thereby rescue the sick, healers must travel to God's village. They "slip out of their skins" and leave their bodies. ≠Omo Djo describes leaving his body as "breathing, like your breath leaving your mouth."

Outside their bodies, they climb the tortuously thin and fragile "threads" or "wires to the sky" that lead them to God's village. These threads can break—and the fall to earth is frightening.

Sometimes healers become lions or other animals in order to travel more rapidly. "You feel like wind. Your breath turns into an animal, and your soul *(moa)* changes," is how ≠Oma !'Homgǃausi describes the transformation. As lions, healers can travel especially fast and more widely, allowing them to check up on relatives in faraway places and bring healing when necessary. They *are* lions. Tshao Matze expresses the transformation this way:

> When I turn into a lion, I can feel my lion-hair growing and my lion-teeth forming. I'm inside that lion, no longer a person. Others to whom I appear see me as just another lion.

As healers leave their bodies, they fly off to do their healing work. ≠Oma Djo describes it this way:

> It's like the way a vulture travels—fly and then sit and look around, fly and then sit and look around. You're like a plane—you run and then sail up into the sky. When you come back, you press your feet into the sand.

The humor that pervades Jul'hoan life does not stop when healers are traveling outside their bodies. At times, for example, when they have become lions, healers will tease and joke with each other about the fear the lions induce. Kxao Tjimburu talks about this mutual joking and laughs at himself and ≠Oma Djo as he describes the fear they experienced:

> One night I was walking around at the cattle post during the rainy season. ≠Oma Djo, who had turned into a lion, came to frighten me. I had to run off with the women. At the cattle post we always joke. And sometimes I turn into a lion and frighten ≠Oma Djo. I softly came to him one night and he grabbed his wife, and they ran into a small hut, trembling!

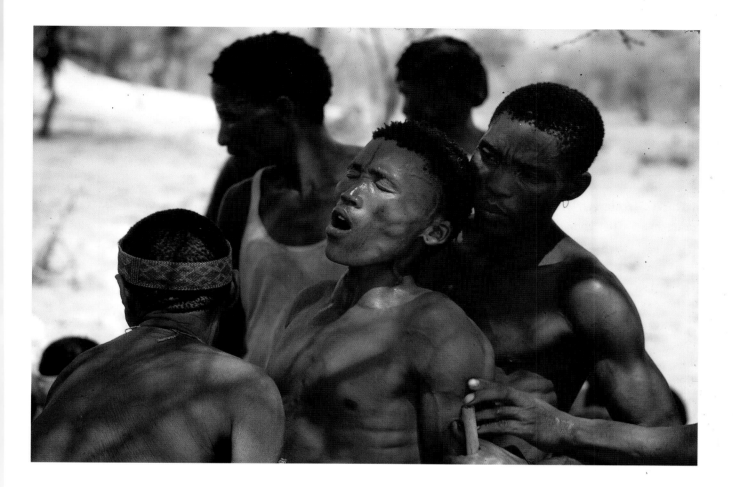

≠Oma Djo is sitting with us as Kxao Tjimburu tells this story. "How was your sleep last night?" he asks Kxao Tjimburu. "Not too good," replies Kxao Tjimburu, somewhat sheepishly. "Really?" asks ≠Oma Djo, a smile beginning to form. "Did something bother you?" he continues on. After some hesitation, Kxao Tjimburu answers: "Yes, something scared me." "A lion. Was it a lion?" ≠Oma Djo asks, now bursting out in laughter. Then Kxao Tjimburu realizes that ≠Oma Djo had visited him last night, mischievously disturbing his sleep. The two healers enjoy a full laugh together.

The healers' vocation is open to all, and most of the young men and many of the women seek to become healers. About half the men and a third of the women succeed; but there is no stigma attached to those who do not. The training is difficult. Not everyone can stand the

BOO "TIBET" STRUGGLING TO LEARN HOW TO REGULATE HIS PAINFULLY BOILING N|OM, IS SUPPORTED BY OTHERS WHO HOLD AND RUB HIM.

excruciating pain of the boiling n|om, which is said to be "hot and painful, just like fire." It makes one cry and writhe in agony.

The ultimate part of the pain comes from facing one's own death. To heal, one must die and be reborn into the !aia state. This is no allegorical rite of passage, but a terror-filled experience of death. |Ui, a powerful healer, says that

[in !aia] your heart stops. You're dead; your
thoughts are nothing. You breathe with difficulty.
. . . You see spirits killing people. You smell burn-

ing, rotten flesh. Then you heal, you pull sickness out. You heal, heal, heal. Then you live.[19]

The terror of !aia remains despite years of healing, and learning to accept this recurrent death is at the core of the healer's training.

The singers, dancers, and anyone else at the dance who chooses may help those seeking the enhanced state of !aia. With emotional and physical support, they may help the seekers regulate the intensity and speed with which nlom boils up inside them so as to keep a balance between the fear of !aia and the intensity of the boiling nlom. If !aia is coming on so rapidly that a dancer's fear is out of control, supporters may urge the dancer to stop dancing or lie down and drink some water to cool down the too-fiercely boiling nlom. But when the nlom is too cool, it cannot be activated for healing. If the fear can be contained or, even better, accepted, the dancer will want the nlom to boil more strongly, to become hotter. The stronger the nlom, the stronger the healing power. And though nlom is at its peak when the songs are sung with the most abandon and enthusiasm and the healers are doing their work with the most intensity and depth, the regulation of nlom remains critical, especially with inexperienced healers.

In one dance, for example, a young man new to !aia was on the brink of being overwhelmed by his boiling nlom. His fear was out of control, and he raced away from the dance. Immediately, two men brought him back to the dance and "danced him," one holding him from the back, the other supporting him from the front. The three danced as one, and the singing reached new levels of commitment. The young dancer now faced what he feared most—and in an even more intense form. But with the support he was receiving, he overcame his fear, experienced !aia, and began to heal.

As demonstrated by research conducted in 1968 by Dick, healers have richer fantasy lives than those who do not heal.[20] They also have a more inner directed functioning, are more able to cope with unfamiliar visual images, and are more easily aroused emotionally. All of

these qualities prepare a person to accept an enhanced state like !aia; these characteristics are both predispositions that may lead one to become a healer and attributes of the healer that intensify and are intensified by !aia. The older healers have experienced !aia perhaps a thousand times. Having so many profound experiences begins to affect the nature of the healer's inner life.

Even though healers have special psychological characteristics, they enjoy no privileges. Healers, like all Jul'hoansi, are first hunters and gatherers—only secondarily are they healers. Yet for a few of the most powerful healers things are somewhat different. With these few, a spiritual dimension seems to pervade their daily lives in a special way. They, for example, dance frequently, sometimes every day. They can heal themselves and others without the support of a full dance. Unlike ordinary healers, these powerful healers routinely travel to God's village during !aia. Their healing abilities and general wisdom are widely acknowledged, but they neither accumulate marks of prestige nor hoard their power.

Healing and spiritual powers are held in great respect, but just as the Jul'hoansi freely share their food and water, they share their healing energy. Healers or nlomkxaosi are "owners or masters of nlom"—stewards of that energy who guide it toward the service of others. Nlom cannot be hoarded; the more it is aroused in one person, the easier it is for someone else to share it. As one healer enters !aia, it becomes more likely that another will also. Nlom expands as it boils; and the more it is used for healing, the more that then becomes available for more healing. Boiling nlom is likened by the Jul'hoansi to the sparks that break out into the dark night in all directions when the burning coals in a fire are stirred roughly with a stick. The sparks reach into the far corners of the night, touching all in the area with their special glow. Through the healing dance, members of the group stimulate each other's well-being. Through the dance, each person receives more healing than would be derived through individual efforts. A synergy prevails in which the group's healing effort becomes more than the sum of the individual efforts.

Although many other cultures usually have only a few people devoted to healing work, the percentage of Jul'hoansi who become healers is large. Since most of them must also hunt and gather to survive, only a few of the most powerful healers can put hunting and gathering aside for a more total involvement with healing and the spirit—and those few are usually older persons whose contribution to hunting and gathering would be minimal anyway. The Jul'hoansi see the need for feeding the body and the spirit as equally important tasks.

It is tempting to draw inferences from archaeological evidence about the longevity of the healing dance among the Jul'hoansi's ancestors. Not only are there characteristic hunter-gatherer camp remains in the Dobe area, which includes ǀKaeǀkae, but rock paintings on stone surfaces not far from ǀKaeǀkae at Tsodilo—and all over southern Africa—show scenes and metaphors of healing dances strikingly similar to those of the Jul'hoansi today (also see pp. 53–54). There appears to be a strong cultural tradition linking the ideas by which Jul'hoansi now live with ancient spiritual traditions and practices.

Richard Lee and Irven DeVore carried out a survey to begin anthropological work in the Dobe area of what is now Botswana in 1963, and Lee stayed at this work through January 1965. One of his co-workers on a field trip three years later was Dick Katz, who had come to study the Jul'hoan healing dance. At that time three-quarters of the Dobe area people were hunting and gathering and the rest worked for Tswana and Herero cattle

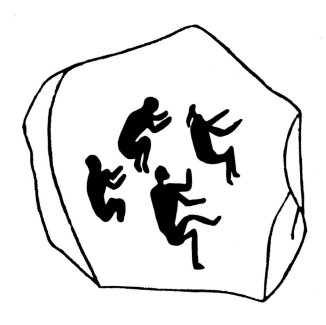

IMAGES OF DANCE POSTURES ADORN ROCK SHELTERS IN MOUNTAINOUS AREAS AND ROCKY OUTCROPS AROUND THE FRINGES OF THE KALAHARI DESERT.

owners. Independence and self-sufficiency still characterized much of Jul'hoan life. In fact, up to the mid-1960s there was a history of only *gradual* encroachment on Jul'hoan land and livelihoods in the Dobe area. The time of more rapid and rapidly dislocating change lay immediately ahead.

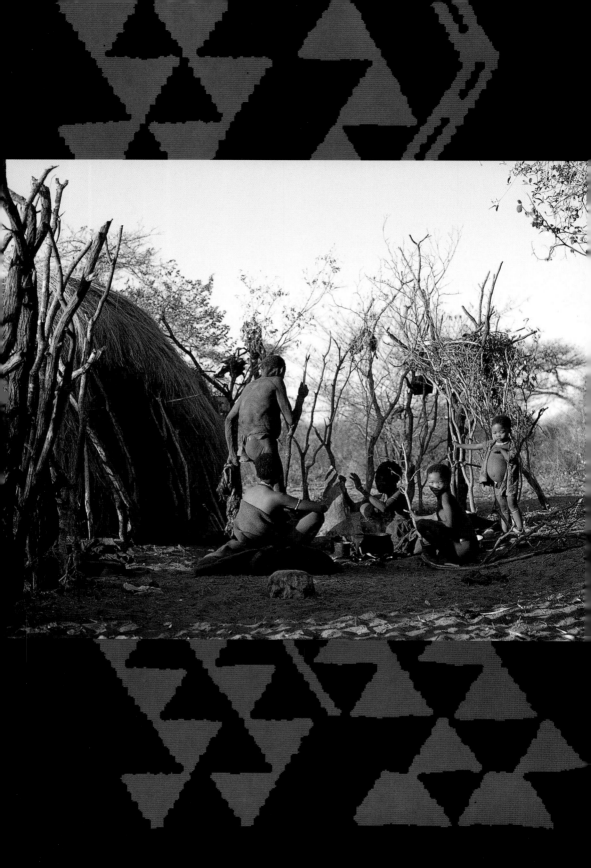

The social relationships of the Jul'hoan hunting-gathering lifestyle run very deep. Yet the Jul'hoansi are caught now in a mixed economy combining the tried-and-true of hunting-gathering with what are, for them, risky new options such as agriculture, herding, and wage labor. Further, not all groups, nor all individuals within a particular group, are equally enmeshed in one or the other economic alternative. Consequently, their old way of sharing no longer provides the mutual insurance they have relied on.

Their economic predicament is a result of environmental and political forces; however, their spiritual lives also face increasing social pressures from outside their communities. Government presence—in the form of local administration, land allocating boards, clinics, schools, and drought relief schemes—has brought many changes to the Jul'hoansi at |Kae|kae. "We used to direct ourselves, but now the government directs us," says Kodinyau, a respected older man who, with his wife, Kxaru N!a'an, is one of the most economically progressive |Kae|kae families. Outsiders, especially settlers with large herds of cattle, have challenged the Jul'hoan people's reliable spiritual and practical relationship to their land and resources.[1] As he considers the present situation at |Kae|kae with the Hereros and Tswana living there, !Xam, a somewhat carefree young man approaching late adolescence, becomes wistful, even pessimistic: "I don't know how everyone will manage to live together. What will they eat?"

Talking with Jul'hoansi in 1989, we sense anxiety over whether Jul'hoan social strengths, including their shared

2

"NOW THE GOVERNMENT DIRECTS US"

spiritual healing dance, will be able to persist as things change. Young people, of course, have been particularly affected by the alternative models posed by government workers in the form of clinic and school employees. Many young people cannot help but feel that, in comparison with the lifestyles of these government workers, their own elders' lives seem impoverished. The orientation of these younger Jul'hoansi is now more toward wage labor and purchased food and clothing than it is toward living from their skills on the modest support the land could once provide.

It is clear that younger people increasingly find something socially problematic about following their elders' examples, whereas in the 1960s such ambivalence was largely absent. Generational splits have surfaced in areas like education, attitudes toward gainful employment, traditional economic pursuits versus more "modern" options, popular culture, and adornment. These splits are minor compared with those experienced by urban people, but they are recognizable nonetheless. A restlessness exists among young people who, as they watch the newcomers to their area, seem to be caught between heightened expectations and renewed awareness of their remoteness from new kinds of opportunity.

This growing sense of desperation is more palpable among Botswana Jul'hoansi in 1989 than among their relatives just across the border. In Namibia (then South West Africa), a movement began in 1986 that evolved into the Nyae Nyae Farmers' Cooperative (see appendix E). That movement helped people explore new and viable economic and political options that, in some cases, involved a creative blend of old and new. But in Botswana the combined lack of economic opportunity and real educational advancement was making young people feel less hopeful.

The older Jul'hoansi observe the existential bind felt so poignantly by some of the young people, but in a matter-of-fact manner; there is no blame in their descriptions or assessments. In general the view is that the only future for young people lies in formal education and the jobs assumed to follow on its heels. Loss of land and resources due to the encroachment of cattle-owning people on the Jul'hoansi's former n!oresi, or foraging territories, has made the traditional hunting-gathering life, despite its continued attractiveness for many, a disappearing option.

Quite a few of the people we speak with—even adults—point to employment with non-Jul'hoansi as the only way for them to now keep from starving. Tshao N!a'an, a well-respected healer in his fifties, had at one time in his life been paid by White and Black Ghanzi farmers to put on dances and heal their sick. He tells us about employment in some dismay.

In the future I don't know what will help me. I have no work. I'm just sitting here not knowing what will help. If White people were here, they'd give you farm work and you'd stay alive. But I have no work here. . . . I still don't think of any work I could do, but if they give me some, I'll do it.

We talk to Kxao Tjimburu and Tshao Matze about employment, schooling, and the livelihoods of Jul'hoan people at IKaeIkae. We wonder what the young people who have gone to school but not found work will eat in the future—especially if they have not learned to hunt and gather.[2] Tshao Matze responds with sadness:

This is a good question. Many kids from IKaeIkae have been to school but not one of them has got a job. We see that the land of the Tswana has no help for us.

Little Tswana get work but our kids don't. Our kids just have to go around with their mothers. Even if they go to Maun [about 153 miles or 274 kilometers away] they don't find work.

We Jul'hoan parents won't be able to feed our children anything. Because our bush foods, like g!oan, and kaq'amakoq, mongongoes, ca, and dcaa—if it doesn't rain, these foods won't come up. And the food that is here today is food that comes from work. You work and you work and you work and you get money to feed your children, and you buy blankets to cover them from the cold! You buy clothes to wear. If you have no work and no n!ore, you die.

We today think we have a n!ore but it isn't ours: they've taken it from us and we have no other n!ore to which to go. If it were a place like N≠aqmtjoha, or N≠oa, or IAotcha [all now in Namibia, see map on p. 33], which all have water from a well, we'd move to them. Or if places like Glam and ≠Ogllaqna . . . were still open to us, we'd go there, but they are beyond [the border fence] now. If there were no fence we would long ago be there. If we were still alone at ≠Ogllaqna instead of

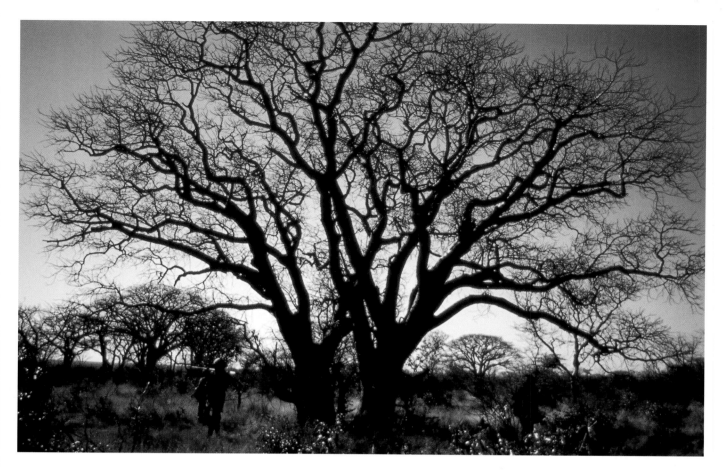

living here [at |Kae|kae] with the Hereros, who per-
secute us, maybe our kids would see some life.

The big thing, the hard thing, is that we can't
kill meat now. If we take up our bows and arrows
to try to kill an animal, they [the government] give
us a "pass" for only one animal, just like that. They
say we mustn't kill two animals [of the same kind
in one year]. It's a crime. Today we are in pain. So
that's why we say we have no n!ore, and no food
unless we have work and can buy it—a little sugar
to drink with tea.

Contrasting the sense of hopelessness and hunger of
today with the relative plenty in which the Jul'hoansi
once lived, ≠Oma Djo always describes the world around
|Kae|kae in which he had grown up in vivid terms. But
his criticism of the present situation is stark.

The Tswana have changed things for us. Today
people are insulting each other and fighting.

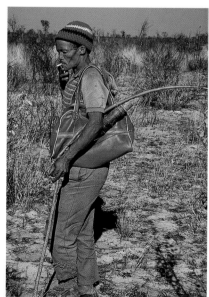

ABOVE: THE MONGONGO
NUT TREE PROVIDES A
STAPLE FOOD FOR THE
JUl'HOANSI. HERE
WOMEN GATHER THE
NUTS AFTER THEY HAVE
DROPPED FROM THE TREE.

A RED PLASTIC AIRLINE CARRIER BAG IS ONE OF THE

NEWER TOOLS |KAECE USES AS HE HUNTS TODAY.

ǀKaeǀkae has become a bad place. Juǀ'hoansi fuss with each other.

Beer is stuff that comes from the land of the Tswana, and that's why I say that Tswana have changed things so much. . . . Many Herero people [also brew beer here.] . . . Things have changed, and are different now. The Tswana are killing us. . . . We are now more hungry than we used to be.

The independent life that ≠Oma Djo and others describe to us from the past is in sharp contrast to the present situation at ǀKaeǀkae. More than one person tells us that because the Botswana government brought food aid during the recent drought and asked people not to hunt and gather anymore, many people have become demoralized. ≠Oma Djo says:

They . . . told us, the old people, not to go collect food. They told us to just sit and get government food, but now it no longer comes. We sat and sat waiting for it until we were weak. Then we tried to go out and gather food with our pitiful old feet and our pitiful shoes. It killed us! . . .

They don't want us to eat our own food, just to sit and eat government food. But where is it? The shoes they said they'd buy—where are they? The blankets they said they'd bring to cover us—where are they? They said money would come for us to buy cows—where is it? In other nǃores people have gotten money, but we just sit here. We need to eat so we'll be alive! Old people are dying today.

This is why I say ǀKaeǀkae is like Tjumǃkui [in Namibia]. What happened over there was that the [Afrikaner] government [prior to Namibian independence] gathered all the Juǀ'hoansi together and said, "We will feed you at Tjumǃkui." So the people forgot about bush food and ate only the mealie meal [corn meal] they were given. The government wanted them to leave their nǃoresi. Then [some of the Juǀ'hoansi] . . . said, "We refuse this. We're going to leave Tjumǃkui and go back to our nǃoresi, and hold fast to them.

Kxaru Nǃa'an, offering her insightful opinion with her typically sharp wit, summarizes the desperate side of the situation at ǀKaeǀkae: "They say strong people will get work and weak people will get food." She does not have to say that there is little work for the strong, even with schooling, and the government has proven an unreliable source of food, even for the weak.

The distrust of the government runs deep. N≠aisa Nǃa'an and her husband, ≠Oma Djo, recount an interaction with "government people": "These government people wanted to interview us about our lives," says ≠Oma Djo, "but we long ago spoke to them, saying 'Yo! You haven't brought food to the old people here.' But the government people didn't write [our words] down on paper and just left." "They didn't write our names and just went away," N≠aisa interjects for emphasis. "We're dead," she states. "We refused to speak to them about our lives."

The Juǀ'hoansi of ǀKaeǀkae, like the Bushman peoples of Botswana in general, have not been so fortunate as to return to their nǃoresi. When South West Africa became Namibia in 1990, political history favored the Nyae Nyae Juǀ'hoansi just across the border from ǀKaeǀkae. During the years leading up to that event, the Juǀ'hoan people's Nyae Nyae Farmers' Cooperative assisted a major back-to-the-land movement that eventually restored thirty-five communities to their more or less original territories. Ironically, the apartheid "homelands" policy of South West Africa had protected the Juǀ'hoansi's area from overgrazing and encroachment by cattle-owning ethnic groups.

In Botswana, however, the independence process had occurred some twenty-four years previously. At that time, Botswana made a lasting commitment to regard all ethnic groups as legally "equal" and gave no land or resource tenure protection to groups unable to establish these rights for themselves. In practice, this meant that groups with a strong central authority—for the most part pastoralists like the Tswana and Hereros—received license to expand as far as they were able, often into areas historically used by Juǀ'hoansi and other Bushmen. In recent

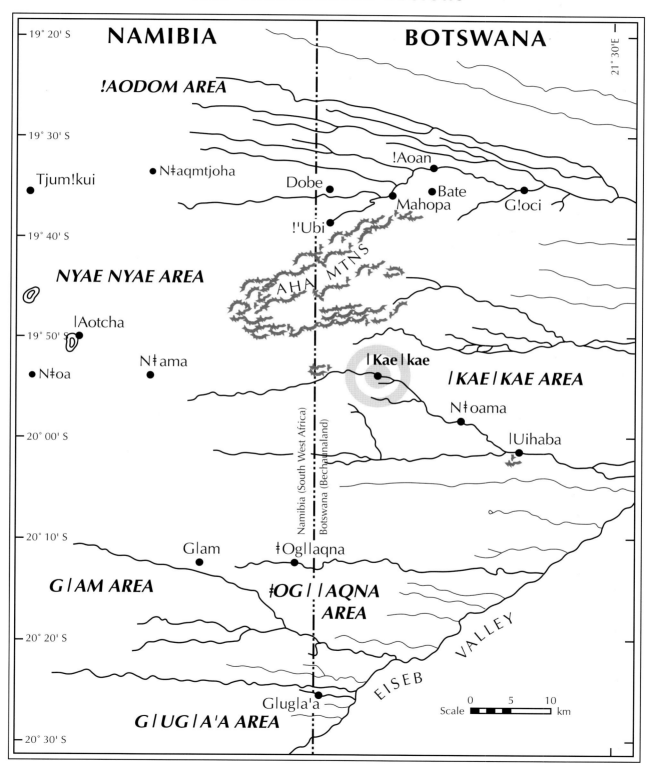

THE DOBE AREA
AND SURROUNDING REGIONS

NAMIBIA   BOTSWANA

19° 20' S

21° 30'E

!AODOM AREA

19° 30' S

!Aoan

Tjum!kui   • N‡aqmtjoha

Dobe   • Bate

Mahopa   G!oci

19° 40' S

!'Ubi

AHA MTNS

NYAE NYAE AREA

|Aotcha

19° 50' S

|Kae|kae

N‡ama |KAE|KAE AREA

• N‡oa

N‡oama

|Uihaba

Namibia (South West Africa)

Botswana (Bechuanaland)

20° 00' S

20° 10' S

G|am   ‡Og||aqna

G|AM AREA   ‡OG||AQNA AREA

EISEB VALLEY

20° 20' S

Scale   0   5   10   km

G|ug|a'a

G|UG|A'A AREA

20° 30' S

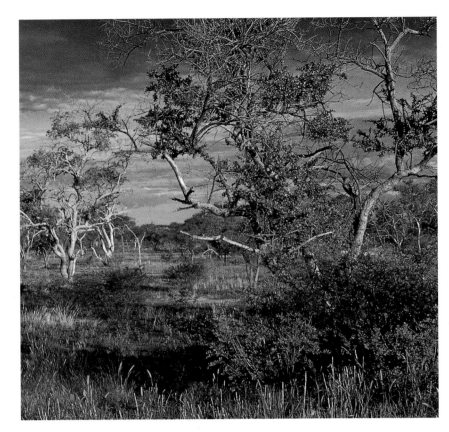

THE KALAHARI ENVIRONMENT IN THE LATE 1960S, LUSH AND GREEN FROM THE RAINY SEASON.

OPPOSITE: THE DOMINATION OF THE OLD ǀKAEǀKAE WATERHOLE BY HERERO AND TSWANA LIVESTOCK TURNS THE ONCE LUSH LANDSCAPE INTO A DUSTY FLATLAND AS EARLY AS 1968. THE DEFOLIATION AND DESERTIFICATION OF THE LAND IS EVEN MORE WIDESPREAD TODAY.

years their expansion has created a new level of outside pressure on once-isolated places like ǀKaeǀkae. This pressure has now alerted the Juǀ'hoansi to the need for positive action.

But such a realization took a long time to build. Because of ǀKaeǀkae's remoteness, the Tswana and Herero presence grew slowly over a number of decades. But, as in nearby Dobe and !Aoan, a relationship of servitude to cattle-owning people had had time by the 1980s to embed itself deeply in Juǀ'hoan self-conceptions at ǀKaeǀkae. All social reckonings had to be made in a context of relative powerlessness in the face of these peoples who were perceived as "masters." Juǀ'hoansi had pride in their own traditions of course, but they could not help but notice the wealth disparities that grew during the 1970s and 1980s. The gulf between themselves and the Tswana, the ruling ethnic group, and between themselves and the Hereros, the rich cattle owners of their area, gave many Juǀ'hoansi pause for

thought about the viability of their own traditions in a changed era. ǀKaece "China," a man with a lot of experience working for Hereros, offered this pointed and poignant assessment: "If you work for a Herero, he calls you *matjuange,* which means 'my son.' That's your death sentence!"

At the same time, Juǀ'hoansi like ≠Oma Djo tended to blame the outsiders for causing disruption in their communities and to take a resigned attitude toward new social problems. This seeming resignation may be understood in terms of their long tradition of extreme social tolerance for each other. Earlier, this tolerance worked; their society as a whole was nurturant and committed to mutual survival. In the new, demanding situation of economic confrontation with outsiders, their old social skills of sharing and facilitating communication did not serve them as well. Their social tolerance permitted outsiders to take advantage of them. ≠Oma Djo described the insidious arrival of cattle to the land:

We were just on our land, drinking our water from the ground. Then some Herero comes along with a few cattle, asking for water to keep those cattle alive. We cannot refuse them, for there are so few cattle. But then next season, there are several calves and they too need water. Again, we cannot refuse, even though there are now more cattle. Finally, we see what is to be—the cattle have multiplied into many and all of them need water. And now we cannot decide that enough is enough. The cattle have taken over our place and sucked the land dry of its water.

Ju/'hoansi began falling behind the newcomers to their area in virtually every arena of "modern" life: they were being held back in local representation, in land rights, in access to agricultural training and subsidies, in schooling, in public health, and in employment opportunities.

Developments over the years since Dick Katz first vis-

ited |Kae|kae in 1968 had taken several forms. There had been changes in subsistence options and patterns for local people; in the amount and pervasiveness of government presence; in the number of drilled boreholes for water,[3] the number of cattle, and other challenges to the environment; in patterns of visits to the area by outsiders; and in national and international political affairs that had a bearing on the Ju/'hoan people. All these changes took place very rapidly, and their effects were hard to integrate. Historically, Ju/'hoan society had not needed a mechanism to slow down or redirect such change, and appropriate mechanisms could not come about overnight.

HISTORY OF EARLY CONTACTS

The earlier history of Ju/'hoan and other Bushman peoples has been a long one of increasing dispossession of their land and resources. That the intrusions that occurred roughly before the 1960s were more gradual than those after the 1960s does not diminish their cumulative negative effect. To better understand the impact of the changes in the decades since the 1960s, we will examine this earlier history, emphasizing contacts between Jul'hoansi and various outsiders. In so doing, the process of change as a continuous, ongoing phenomenon with important historical roots becomes clear.

Much of ǀKaeǀkae's earlier history has been affected by what happened just over the "border" with South West Africa (now Namibia). In fact, the whole area on both sides of the border may be regarded as a regional unit both geographically and socially. The international boundary, though not actually fenced until the mid-1960s, cut the Jul'hoan population arbitrarily into two rough halves.

The first recorded contacts between outsiders and Jul'hoan people came during the 1850s. Early Jul'hoan trade occurred with both Black pastoralists (Hereros and Tswana) and White travelers and colonists (the British, Germans, and Afrikaners); the trade included salt, meat, hides, feathers, and crafts. The Bushmen were hunters, guides, and messengers for visitors to their area. In the 1860s Herero pastoralists expanded northward into Nyae Nyae when firearms became available; and in the 1870s, Tswana first came from the east to the area of Dobe and Gǀugǀa and presumably to ǀKaeǀkae itself.

In the decade of the 1880s both German colonialism in South West Africa and the British Protectorate of Bechuanaland (corresponding to the Botswana of today) were established. From 1885 to 1895 the Ghanzi Farm Block 125 miles (200 km) south of ǀKaeǀkae was settled by Afrikaner farmers, dispossessing Naron, Gǀwi, and other Bushman peoples. Some became squatters on White farms.

A Nama and Herero uprising against the Germans in South West Africa occurred from 1904 to 1907; it led to greater dispossession of Bushmen over a wide area. Herero refugees from the uprising escaped through the Jul'hoan area, some settling later in Dobe and ǀKaeǀkae. Today, descendants of these refugees have become the pastoral patrons of some of the Jul'hoansi, employing them to care for their cattle in an arrangement that resembles medieval serfdom.

Even before the arrival of the Herero refugees and as early as 1900, wealthy Tswana had involved some Jul'hoansi in *mafisa* cattle keeping. *Mafisa*, a Tswana word, entails a relationship in which one cares for the

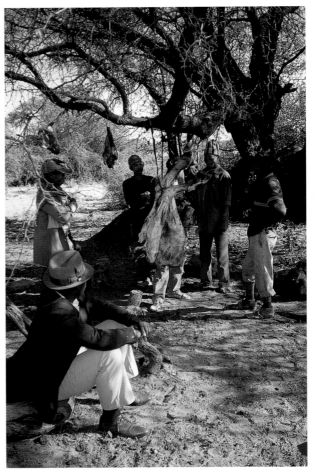

stock of another in return for milk to drink and a calf of one's own at the end of each year. A patron-client relationship with strong paternalistic overtones is implied in mafisa. By 1973 about 20 percent of Jul'hoan families in Botswana had some involvement in mafisa.

The Hereros, on the other hand, tended not to use the mafisa system. Regarding themselves as consummate hands-on experts with cattle, they often employed Jul'hoansi only to do milking and rarely paid in stock at the end of the year. "Wages" from the Hereros were usually confined to milk, food, and some cast-off clothing. Furthermore, since among Herero people milking is considered women's work, employing Jul'hoan men to perform this labor was seen by Hereros as somewhat demeaning.

Partly because their hunting and gathering territories were compromised, but partly also because it seemed to offer some advantages over lives perceived as arduous, Bushman peoples had seen some appeal in taking up labor and residence with Herero and Tswana cattle owners.[4] But, as we heard in detail from many ǀKaeǀkae people, Jul'hoansi had become bitter about this work by the 1980s, complaining that cattle promised in payment for herding work for Tswana were regularly not being paid, and that relationships with Herero families were filled with frustrations and broken promises as well. Many a complaint session centered around whether working for the Hereros or the Tswana was the lesser of two evils. Tending other people's cattle had become one of many disappointing economic options explored by the Jul'hoansi in their effort to compensate for a shrinking land-base and dwindling wild food resources.

The early twentieth century brought many challenges to Bushman peoples livelihood. In 1908 diamonds were discovered in South West Africa, leading to greater European immigration and further Bushman dispossession. After 1910, drought-related hunger led to stock theft by Bushmen, which resulted in hundreds of anti-Bushman patrols by the German administration. In 1915 Germany surrendered South West Africa to South Africa, and settlement there by South Africans led to more dispossession.

Then, Tswana from the Lake Ngami region were given permission in 1917 to graze their animals and use water in the Jul'hoan area located in the Nyae Nyae area (in South West Africa). They traveled through the ǀKaeǀkae and Dobe areas to get there. As they were told that they could not hunt, the Tswana pastoralists began to employ local Jul'hoan hunters to get them meat. Tswana cattle herds were sent out to the ǀKaeǀkae area, managed by Herero herd boys. This powerful cultural and economic combination had a telling impact on the environment there. Some local Jul'hoansi resisted this incursion upon their wild foods, which cattle trampled and grazed. Police were sent from both Grootfontein in South West Africa (254 miles or 410 kilometers away) and Maun in Bechuanaland (153 miles or 247 km away) to "quell" the resistance.[5]

During the 1920s, the South African administrative presence also affected the lives of Bushmen in South West Africa through stock theft and vagrancy proclamations, the creation of apartheid native reserves, residence and land allocation controls, and the curtailment of their economic activities. A 1927 act actually made it criminal to carry a Bushman bow and arrow. Another act that same year limited to five the number of "native" families that could live on an Afrikaner farm, reducing the problem of squatting but increasing the problem of homelessness for Bushman peoples whose land had been appropriated.

By 1934 Hereros had occupied naturally occurring water pans at ǀKaeǀkae, !'Ubi, !Aoan, and Mahopa. This put great local pressure on the water resources of the Jul'hoansi, who felt they had little alternative but to work for the occupying Hereros. In 1935, however, because of ethnic tensions the Hereros were evicted by Bechuanaland police and sent east. Then, in 1936, slavery was officially abolished in the protectorate.[6] A 1920s report by Isaac Schapera had influenced the British Parliament and the League of Nations to inquire into "the slavery question" in Bechuanaland. There was international criticism, for example, over the beating deaths of some Bushmen and their desperate labor conditions.

The response of the protectorate government was to make largely insignificant efforts at controlling "nomadism" by establishing a few Bushman settlements, though not in the northwestern part of the country (then known as Ngamiland) where the Bushmen had been living. In general, there was no effective creation of employment for Jul'hoansi, no real intervention on human rights issues, and no real positive effect on their overall socioeconomic status. Discrimination and injustice persisted.

In 1948 Isak Utugile, a Tswana, was appointed headman of the Dobe area.[7] This was the first moment of a detectable central protectorate government presence there. Almost simultaneously, "native affairs" in South West Africa was put directly under the South African Parliament in 1949. Both events testify to the centralizing colonialist spirit of the times in southern Africa, and they had similar effects on local Jul'hoansi on both sides of the border: further dispossession and further loss of autonomy. The Jul'hoansi's hold on their land and independent way of life was palpably slipping.

The first visit of the Marshall family from America to the Nyae Nyae region and the Dobe and ǀKaeǀkae area—lands situated on both sides of the border—took place in 1950. Lorna and Laurence Marshall and their children, John and Elizabeth, had a profound effect, slowing down the rate at which Jul'hoansi were losing their land—at least on the South West African side. Partly as a result of their fine anthropological and film work, the Schoeman Commission recommended in the early 1950s that a Bushman homeland be established there. The Jul'hoan toehold on this land remains today, though Jul'hoansi there are still fighting for clear legal tenure.

Until 1953, the Jul'hoan area of Nyae Nyae was occupied only by them, and they formed the then-largest population of hunter-gatherers in southern Africa. In 1954 there was a major influx of Hereros to the region from Makakung, some 100 miles (160 km) across the border in Bechuanaland. Through the rest of the 1950s there was resistance to Herero settlement, some of which was aided by the South African police, as protectionist policies toward the Bushmen had by that time been well established in South West Africa.

The years of 1959 and 1960 saw the beginning of the administration of the Bushmen by the homeland of South West Africa rather than by remote South Africa; a Bushman Affairs Commissioner was appointed in an administrative center, Tjum!kui. Bushmen were encouraged to move to that center with promises of rations and employment. A rural slum was thus started at the same time that the South West African government issued a twenty-year ban on ethnographic investigations, perhaps because they found the implications of the previous ethnography threatening. In 1961 a Dutch Reformed Church mission and a trading store were established in Tjum!kui. Then in 1963 the Odendaal Commission in South West Africa recommended setting aside two areas for Bushmen, one of which was a fraction of the former Nyae Nyae area. Other peoples were given the large areas over which the Jul'hoansi once freely hunted and gathered.

CHANGE QUICKENS: EVENTS SINCE 1963

In 1964 there were no government food programs, no boreholes, no trading store, no school, no clinic, and no resident civil servants (apart from Tswana headman Isak Utugile and his assistants) in the Dobe area. Headman Isak's office was a *kgotla*, a traditional Tswana outdoor court and decision-making place. It consisted of a homemade chair in the middle of a compound with a low fence of thorn trees. Hunting and gathering provided the Dobe people with over 85 percent of their calories, compared with roughly 30 percent now. Though a government presence in the Dobe area began to be felt slightly as a result of the government-commissioned publication of the "Bushman survey" report by George Silberbauer in 1965, the direct influence of the government remained minimal.

Change at ǀKaeǀkae began accelerating in the late 1960s, and the direction of these changes became more and more destructive as key events took place. In 1967 the first trading store was opened at !Aoan, about 31 miles or 50 kilometers north of ǀKaeǀkae, and was occasionally thereafter stocked with basic goods; it also became a source for sugar and other ingredients for making

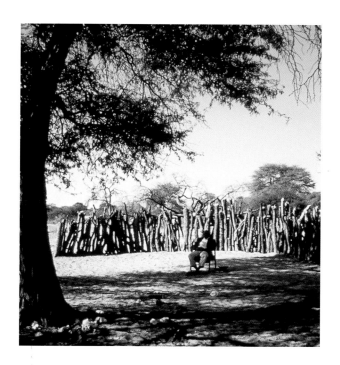

SITTING AS THE JUDGE IN THE KGOTLA, THE TSWANA-BASED COURT SYSTEM IMPORTED INTO ǀKAEǀKAE, THE HERERO HEADMAN IS SUPPOSED TO SETTLE DISPUTES AMONG THE HERERO, TSWANA, AND JUǀ'HOAN RESIDENTS.

tablished border posts "to watch for SWAPO"—the South West African People's Organization—which eventually liberated the country from South Africa in 1990. Many area Juǀ'hoansi were eventually recruited during the 1980s to track and fight in Angola with the South African Defense Forces. Tragically, these military jobs were an offer many couldn't refuse, but the Juǀ'hoansi lacked access to information to understand the implications of their participation on the side of the oppressor, South Africa.

At these South West African police camps along the border, the enforced sedentism of employment created a dependency among Juǀ'hoansi on trucked-in foods. A large group of people living at one place would quickly decimate the wild foods growing in the area. Along with mealie, or corn meal, sugar was part of monthly Juǀ'hoan police rations at the camps.

Sugar, especially brown sugar, was used to brew beer, something consumed only rarely in previous Juǀ'hoan experience. Though the paternalistic South West African officers were against drinking, there were parties when they were away. In some cases these border posts have become villages in their own right since the war, and they are experienced as areas of alcohol abuse even today.

Drinking was prevalent at Tjum!kui, the South West African administrative center established for overseeing Bushmen; a store selling alcohol was opened there under a government subsidy. Young men from ǀKaeǀkae would cross the border and travel some 75 miles (120 km) to Tjum!kui on foot in order to drink.

Drinking was also prevalent at !Aoan (on what had become, in 1966, the Botswana side of the border) whenever a truck arrived at the store there with sugar. Much beer brewing and drinking followed until the bags of sugar were used up. Many ǀKaeǀkae people also went to !Aoan, only 17.5 miles (28 km) from ǀKaeǀkae, in order to drink, but the supply at !Aoan was less reliable than at Tjum!kui.[8]

A recent land-use planning report by the Namibian government shows that even in the Nyae Nyae Farmers' Cooperative villages on the other side of the border from ǀKaeǀkae, there is still a large preponderance of wild

home-brewed beer. Two years earlier, a border fence was erected between the British Protectorate of Bechuanaland and South West Africa. It had a stile, put up by the South African police—and tolerated at that time by the British protectorate government—so that Juǀ'hoansi with relatives could visit on either side of the fence. Nonetheless, the border fence eventually began to obstruct the free exchange and visiting between ǀKaeǀkae people and their relatives in South West Africa. It also began to symbolize the tensions in the area generated by the upcoming independence of South West Africa from South Africa.

South West African government forces were at this time ever more closely containing the Juǀ'hoansi and other Bushmen. Game reserves were created in the north of their area in !Aodom and Caprivi and a "homeland" was declared for Bushmen under Act 46 of 1969.

In the early 1970s the South West African police es-

vegetable foods in the diet—despite the fact that these Nyae Nyae villages now have water points and small herds of cattle. This preponderance of wild foods is absent among ǀKaeǀkae people, highlighting the comparative severity of their nutritional situation. The causes for this deterioration are complex and interwoven: drought-relief foods, which created dependency for a while, have been withdrawn; bush foods are being trampled and eaten by pastoralists' cattle; people are often spending what little cash they can get on alcohol and tobacco rather than food; the government is asking people to settle in one place for purposes of administration, causing bush foods to be eaten out around them; the people's ability to buy and keep cattle is circumscribed; and water and land rights, which could allow cattle keeping, are denied them because of their relative political disempowerment.

Poor nutrition has had predictably negative effects on health. The rapid change from a diet high in vitamins, good-quality protein, and complex carbohydrates to one emphasizing sugar and other highly processed foods has meant lowered resistance to infections in general and the potential start of blood sugar problems of a kind now being experienced by many postforaging peoples of the world.[9] The combination of lowered resistance and increased contact with outside disease vectors has seriously compromised the health of the Juǀ'hoan population. In 1974 mobile clinics from Maun began to make regular visits to ǀKaeǀkae. Already at that time, about 10 percent of the Juǀ'hoan people had to be treated for tuberculosis. While the availabililty of services from a biomedically oriented clinic began providing some valuable resources, the biomedical model introduced new levels of oppression. Not only are there abuses of the model, for example an overuse of antibiotics, but the model, now a tool in Tswana hands, also conveys a racist judgment about the inadequacy of Juǀ'hoan life and knowledge that goes far beyond targeting their approach to healing.

The fact that the use of tobacco is virtually universal from adolescence on does not help the tuberculosis rate or the level of health in general. Tobacco first became regularly available to the Juǀ'hoansi through traders in the first two decades of the twentieth century. Long before the introduction of alcohol into the ǀKaeǀkae area, tobacco had been an important part of Juǀ'hoan social rituals, and one of the first requests of every traveler into the area is for tobacco.

The opening of a school in !Aoan in 1973 marked another turning point for the Juǀ'hoan people of ǀKaeǀkae. Some Juǀ'hoan families responded to the opening of the !Aoan school by registering their children and solving transport, feeding, school fee, and clothing problems with the practical help of the Kalahari Peoples' Fund (KPF).

KPF was formed in 1973 by members of the Harvard Kalahari Research Group as an advocacy group as well as a means of providing financial and consultation support to Juǀ'hoan and other marginalized Kalahari communities. It was most active in the areas of agricultural development and strategic support to educational initiatives. KPF helped establish a boarding school–like situation where Juǀ'hoan mothers were paid to take care of and cook for children from distant communities. Transporting food for this remote school meal program was also handled under funding from KPF. This became a Botswana national meal program in 1974.

But many Juǀ'hoan children, including some from ǀKaeǀkae, withdrew when their own language was forbidden on school grounds and when they experienced corporal punishment, which is contrary to Juǀ'hoan parenting practice. Absenteeism at !Aoan in the range of 40 to 60 percent continued into the 1990s. Interethnic conflict among the children appears to have been a factor in the high dropout and absentee rates. Distance from their home communities was also problematic for those whose families did not live at !Aoan.

In 1976, a second school was established at ǀKaeǀkae. The school was designed for the entire community—Hereros and Tswana as well as Juǀ'hoansi. Local labor was used extensively, and all the bricks were made on the spot. The ǀKaeǀkae people as a community selected the site for the school building. And in January 1977, the school opened for Standard 1 (equivalent to U.S. grade three),

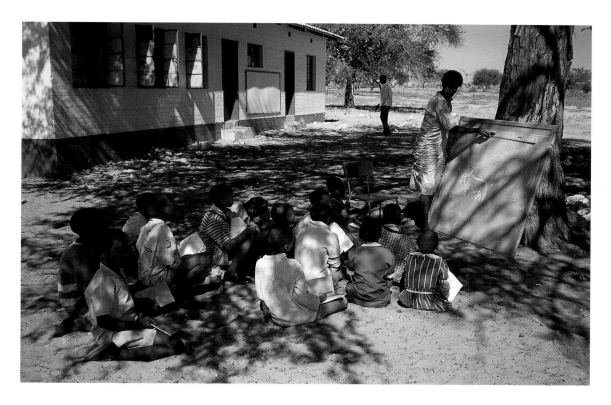

THE TSWANA TEACHER HOLDS HER CLASS OUTDOORS AT THE |KAE|KAE SCHOOL.

with all eligible first-time students in the community en-rolled—including children up to twelve years in age.

But by April 1979, only one room had been completed, although Standards 1 through 3 (U.S. grades three through five) were now being taught by a single teacher. Attendance was still quite good at that time, probably due in part to the fact that the school fostered sensitive interethnic relationships among the different groups of |Kae|kae children. Attendance was also encouraged by the school food program, which actually provided more than a single child could eat; each student could then share that ration with an extended family. The food was prepared daily by a local Jul'hoan woman. An association of parents and teachers was also begun that raised funds for the school and provided modest after-school activities and entertainment.

By 1984 all six standards (U.S. grades three through eight) were functioning at the school, the four-room school building was nearly complete, and there was a headmaster (the original teacher) plus two teachers. The building was completed in 1987, by which time another teacher had been added and several graduates were away at secondary school.

Racism continued to plague the Jul'hoan people. The Jul'hoansi's economic disadvantages in Botswana were finally addressed at the national level with the appointment in 1974 of a Bushman Development Officer within the Ministry of Local Government and Lands. The Bushman Development Program, headed by Liz Wily, became part of Botswana's National Development Plan. The program sought to redress the disadvantages experienced by marginalized Bushman communities, arguing that they needed more time than other groups to learn to exercise their options as Botswana citizens. The program was very active on behalf of Bushmen in the area of land use and allocation.

In 1975 the Tribal Grazing Land Policy was launched in Botswana, leading to land-use planning and zoning intended to aid all citizens equally. In actuality the policy was used to further dispossess Bushmen of traditional lands. When wealthy Tswana would want to expand cattle production, they would form borehole syndicates, which receive preferential treatment in the staking out of ranches in remote areas.[10] Ninety-nine-year leases, which can be bought and sold, make the possession of these leases practically equivalent to private tenure.

By the late 1980s this drilling was approaching the Dobe area. The Jul'hoansi had not then—and have not today—the financial resources to participate in a syndicate, and few cattlemen of other ethnic groups will open participation to them in any case. Compounding this situation are continuing logistical barriers, such as the Jul'hoansi's lack of access to information about where and when the land boards meet, as well as their lack of transportation to attend such meetings. As a result, Jul'hoansi cannot communicate their desires effectively to the local land boards. Being able to attend any of the government-sponsored meetings that are now shaping directions for their lives is always problematic. As !Xuma from Dobe says:

> When the government picks people up for meetings, they forget us. . . . Isn't a Jul'hoan a person whose father was the owner of his n!ore? Has he left his n!ore and gone to anyone else's? This is a matter of the heart.

When they contrast their situation with that of the recently nationally enfranchised Jul'hoansi of Nyae Nyae, the |Kae|kae and Dobe people often become deeply indignant. As Xumi N!an'an said:

> They always talk about "Batswana" ["people of Botswana"], but where are "BaSarwa" ["Bushmen"] supposed to be in that? . . . The land board is what they use to take our land away from us.

Tshao, another |Kae|kae man, added:

> The reason is that we're Jul'hoansi. The ones who are Black call themselves "the owners of garden-

ing," and they run the land board. Those of us who are Jul'hoansi are not represented. . . . They say that we're Batswana but they don't mean it. The only ones on the land board are Black people.

There has been increasingly bitter controversy at |Kae|kae about wells and planting lands supposedly registered in the mid-1970s with land boards on behalf of Jul'hoan people and thereby secured for them, wells and lands that have never materialized. The Jul'hoansi believe the registration papers were intercepted by wealthy Tswana and Hereros from the mostly nonliterate Jul'hoansi.

Kxaru N!a'an talks about this process of getting permission—"papers"—to dig wells, a process that now symbolizes the Jul'hoansi's ongoing frustration with their efforts at development.

> The government says we should get papers for wells in the bush. Those who divide n!oresi say people should separate and dig wells. But if they take too long, others will come and take the wells from them. So that's why we want to dig wells in the bush. But the Hereros are stopping us. We ask where we'll get a well so that we can live alone, just us Jul'hoansi. If there are many Hereros, they spoil the land.

Parallel issues existed on both sides of the border fence in 1976. In South West Africa there was a move to declare "Bushmanland"—the former homeland of the Jul'hoansi—as a nature conservation area in a patent bid to evict the people living there. And in Botswana, pressure to move was put on Jul'hoansi who were living in the grazing areas being considered for commercial ranches. The Tribal Grazing Land Policy consultation exercise conducted in Botswana increased information flow to rural areas such as |Kae|kae about the process of land allocation. But for many years, *knowing* what they needed to do to secure their tenure never enabled them in a *practical* sense to *secure* it.

In 1978 a drought symposium in the Botswana capital of Gaborone brought attention to rural peoples' problems; at that time recommendations were also made about land allocation. But a litigation consultant's statement that year about Bushman land rights was disavowed by the attorney general. The attorney general argued that Bushman land rights are assured both in Botswana's constitution and in various other state documents.[11] However, it was not clear in any of these documents that de jure (legally written) guarantees had been made in regard to Bushman tenure. Bushman people knew that their de facto (on the ground) land rights had been compromised all over the country.

Jul'hoan people voiced their anger among themselves at this treatment. Kommtsa from Mahopa spoke with fierce eloquence:

> We don't want a government that treats us like the woman who ate meat but only smeared her child's mouth with fat. When someone came to ask if the child had been fed she said, "Don't you see the fat around his mouth?" But in fact he was hungry.

All this while, Jul'hoan participation in the local Tswana-based court system, the kgotla, had been minimal because of the inequities between them and the Tswana and Hereros. All major decisions were in fact carried out by the kgotla councillors, none of whom was a Jul'hoan, though Jul'hoansi were the clear majority in the area. Even the Village Development Committees, which were set up in the late 1970s and included Jul'hoan members, were in actuality puppet organizations with no real voice or power accorded the Jul'hoansi.

The Tswana and Herero pastoralists are tribal peoples, speaking Bantu languages, with internal stratification in their societies. Jul'hoansi have found it difficult to escape a position at the bottom of these peoples' social strata. Jul'hoansi were not forcefully propelled into the cash economy, nor were they on any large scale enslaved by the pastoralists. But the real condition of their lives was one of virtual servitude as their options for self-reliance disappeared along with their land and resources.

Other outsiders who have had an influence on the Dobe area are missionaries, although compared with other parts of Africa, missionary influence in northwestern Botswana (Ngamiland) has been minimal. The Jul'hoansi take a frankly pragmatic approach to the social aspects of church attendance. In general those who participate do so as part of their patronage relationships with the Tswana and Hereros, who were Christianized long ago. Some syncretism is visible in the words and concepts used by the few Jul'hoansi with more extended contact with Christianity when they compare Christianity with their own religion. Certain healers, for example, recognize similarities between Jesus' healing work and their own.

The Jul'hoansi believe their God, called !Xu, is the same God spoken about in Christian teachings, as he is all-powerful and the source of nlom. !Xu puts healing power into the bodies of human healers. But they find these beliefs disparaged and patronized during their experience with missionaries. So beneath the surface, there is a great deal of anger among the Jul'hoansi at the cultural insult represented by White and Black missionaries and evangelists (mprofiti). Tshao N!a'an, in his typically cautious and gentle manner, voices a general feeling among healers: "My heart still hasn't desired [the Christian] church. I only know my own church: curing sick people."

Herero Christian church services are held on Sunday mornings and often last several hours; one such church exists in |Kae|kae. Church services are occasions for a great deal of visiting among Herero people, who dress for the occasion in their cleanest and most decorative German missionary attire—Western suits for men and the tight-bodiced, leg-o'-mutton–sleeved, and multi-tiered dresses for women. Most of the services are held outdoors, with people seated on the ground, perhaps under an arbor of cornstalks for shade. There is preaching in Herero by a local or itinerant preacher, and many hymns are sung in the Herero language to familiar German Lutheran hymn melodies. Like the famed cattle dance songs of the Hereros, each hymn trails off in a characteristic downswoop of falling notes and ends in a sort of hum or buzz.

Jul'hoansi who attend the services generally do not

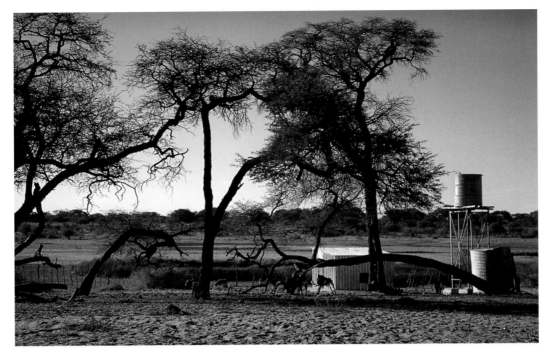

THE NEW WATER
SUPPLY FOR IKAEIKAE:
BOREHOLE WELL, WATER
STORAGE UNIT,
AND PUMP HOUSE.

sing, sitting with downcast eyes on the periphery of the crowd. Most Jul'hoansi attend these services in the context of their employment with the Hereros, and their Christian pretensions are just that—a pragmatic attempt to convince their employers that they are giving up their "heathen" ways.

THE CURRENT SITUATION: DILEMMAS AND CHALLENGES

In the final analysis, however, the Jul'hoan people's major source of dissatisfaction with their present situation remains their inability to establish their land rights. Land, they feel, would make a dignified and self-sufficient life possible. Without it they can aspire to nothing higher than political clienthood. IKaece NIlaq'o, a council member of the Nyae Nyae Farmers' Cooperative, articulates this fundamental belief:

> Land is something you don't divide. It's where
> your mother and father gave birth to you. All
> those little things your parents teach you to find
> and eat, things like *g//uia* and *g/o!'o,* all those

things nourish you while you grow up. When your parents die, you have children yourself and pass on what you know. What you know is your n!ore; you don't divide it.[12]

Years later, the situation in regard to Bushman land rights has progressed little beyond where it was when the attorney general rejected the litigation consultant's report in 1978. In practice, Bushmen without borehole funds have been awarded land as *groups* in the form of communal service centers and so-called Remote Area Dwellers settlements,[13] but they have a difficult time getting land as individuals. Moreover, the land that is awarded is not bigger in proportion to the number of individuals who apply as a group, so that extended family groupings are actually penalized for their degree of solidarity.

Without funds to establish water points, the Jul'hoansi have not been able to apply for grazing lands. The land they do get is usually in the form of residences and fields. Thus they are able to exercise their arable and domestic land rights, but are not able to secure larger blocks of land that would be suitable for either grazing or hunting and gathering. Hunting and gathering itself has not been defined in Botswana as a legitimate land use.

It would be hard to say that the Botswana attorney general has gone against Bushman land rights. Nevertheless, by the attorney general failing to take a stand, poor treatment of the Bushmen continues because such treatment is not challenged legally. There currently are no grounds on which Bushmen could state that they are being denied land rights.

Examining the complex and mounting evidence we have just sampled in this chapter, it is hard to overestimate the pressures that face the Jul'hoansi from all sides in this last decade of the twentieth century. Whichever way they turn there are problems for them, either because of competition by others for their resources or because of the challenges they face in a changing social and political environment.

In general, the Jul'hoansi face deprivation, dispossession, and demoralization, as is true for Indigenous peoples all over the world whose land and resource base is exploited and threatened. The situation has been destructive—and threatens to become even more so. But it is not hopeless. Jul'hoan strengths remain and provide positive forces to counteract the downward spiral. Glaq'o, ≠Oma Djo's son who has lived for years on the Namibian side of the border, offers these observations about the process and accomplishments of the Farmers' Cooperative:

> If we maybe sat and thought and listened, we'd say: "Let's not let Black people 'ride' us too much, because that's driving us backward. Let's work on trying to go forward. Let's try to gather our thoughts together to be one people."
>
> For instance, that we Jul'hoansi on this side [Namibia] today have boreholes is because we've gotten together to do something. People here now have water. Otherwise we'd be sitting among the trees with no water.

The healing dance stands dramatically among the Jul'hoan strengths, a very special and spiritual way of "getting together" to be "one people." Releasing boiling nlom for the healing of the people is felt to be quintessentially Jul'hoan. Nlom and the healing dance, the Jul'hoansi say, is "our thing"; neither can be taken from them. In the joyful gathering of community at the dance, in the daring spiritual journey all undertake, the Jul'hoansi have a buttress against adversity and a source of positive growth.

In summary, we can say that in the last twenty or so years, the Jul'hoansi have seen very rapid accelerations in the processes of change they were already experiencing as a result of outside pressures that began about 120 years ago, in the 1870s, with the arrival of colonial explorers and of pastoral peoples for seasonal grazing. This increased degree of change was unprecedented in Jul'hoan lives because of their prior relative isolation and the stable relationship with their environment that had evolved. Once they capably combined low levels of technology with high levels of information and expertise to live. Now technological advances such as machinery to dig wells, plows, and mechanical ground transport have had a major impact on their fragile ecosystem. Social and legal issues such as stratification, domination by neighboring groups, legal and political disenfranchisement, and an extremely repressive land tenure situation have made life gradually less and less secure. The Jul'hoansi of today indeed find themselves in a situation in which the government and other outside forces increasingly control their lives: "We used to direct ourselves . . . but now the government directs us."

"But at least we have our nlom," the Jul'hoansi go on to say. And it is to that nlom, the Jul'hoan spiritual energy and healing power, that we now return in the next chapter. Nlom and the Jul'hoan spirituality it epitomizes are, of course, not all that the Jul'hoansi have to meet these changes, but it is what we wish to focus upon in this book. Their life-enhancing values, community insights, and political skills are just a few of the many strengths they can draw upon. But perhaps nlom can serve as a stimulant in the entire mix of ingredients working toward healthy and sustainable social change.

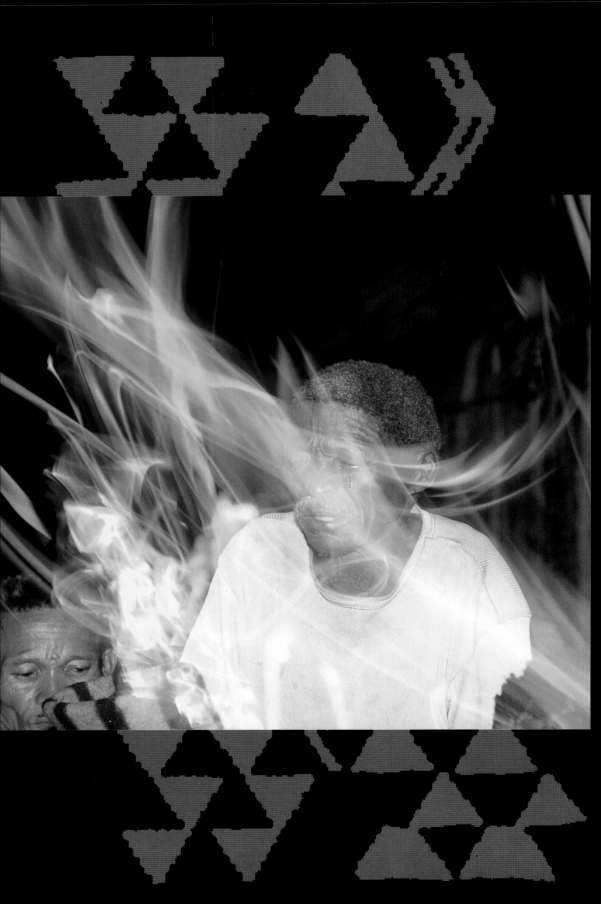

≠Oma Djo is a Jul'hoan Bushman in his eighties who is recognized in both Botswana and Namibia as a very powerful healer. His words show us that the healing power of nǀom is clearly alive and well among the Jul'hoan people, particularly for its older practitioners.

Nǀom is just the same as long ago, even though it keeps on changing. It's like this: if you have nǀom, you know things just by sitting and waiting. You see how things are and talk about them. Things like whether people talk to each other well or badly, and how the land is lying. You hear things like God [!Xu] saying, "Take good care of each other."

Sometimes you sit and say to yourself, "Uh-oh, this person is sick." !Xu will say, "This person will be mine [I'm about to kill him.]" And you say, "Don't say that: let him live." But !Xu refuses and takes him. Or sometimes if someone is sick, you can cure him so that he stays alive. The owners of nǀom can talk to !Xu about things, but ordinary people can't. Ordinary people can't really know if someone is going to die.

I'm old and going blind but when I'm doing nǀom, I can see everybody just fine. . . . I go all around at night and check on everyone, even at all the other villages, even when no one is sick. Sometimes two of us do that together. We just check to see if all the children are well. Once I went over to the well at N≠oama at night and there happened to be a young girl there who really needed a healer, and I made her well.

≠OMA DJO, IN A STATE OF !AIA, AS SEEN THROUGH THE HEALING DANCE FIRE, NOW STIRRED UP AND REVITALIZED WITH MORE WOOD.

3

"BUT WE STILL HAVE OUR NǀOM"

The dance is still here at ǀKaeǀkae. It's doing well and is still healing people. If you're a healer, all you have to do is sit around and news will come to you.

Recent political change has in some ways affected Jul'hoan communities in their use of nǀom. More healers now speak of wanting payment for their services, where once what they did was free to the community. Some young men seem satisfied to go to dances to enjoy dancing or to watch others dance without trying to seek nǀom themselves, whereas before such a search was nearly universal. And some of those who drink alcohol come to dances drunk, disrupting the beautiful rhythms and atmosphere with their loud voices and uncoordinated movements. More important, though, ideas about nǀom are being used in the immediately pressing task of self-definition, a necessary response to the encroaching interests of dominating groups like the Tswana and Herero.

For the Juǀʼhoansi, health is a whole picture of right and correct relationships. They make no distinction among their physical, emotional, and spiritual needs. The healing dance, where nǀom is used, is their main method for treating sicknesses of all kinds. The dance brings the community together for its most profound spiritual journey.

ANCIENT AND ENDURING VALUES

The benefits of nǀom are diverse. Many have to do with maintaining the spirit of sharing that the people see as all-important. Over and over, the healing dance reinforces the idea of the abundance of nǀom for all who remain actively in community with each other—as a spiritual energy, nǀom exemplifies a renewable and available resource. Its structure is the same as the society itself; it foregrounds egalitarian relationships at the same time as it supports the emotions and well-being of the individual.

The messages of egalitarian social support are carried back and forth among the Juǀʼhoansi in many ways as they help each other to create understanding and community. Many of their ways of speaking to each other, including the way they dance with one another, underscore the vital need to make sure each individual is included and no one stands out above others in a way that will bring harm. Conventions of daily politeness, circumscribed behaviors regarding hunting success, and respectful attitudes toward kin are just a few of the ways that Juǀʼhoansi ensure harmony.

Their jokes, songs, and folktales speak of achieving social peace as well. To the Juǀʼhoansi this is as important a goal as learning the ways of hunting and gathering. In fact, they regard their social technology as one of the most practical tools they have. From an early age, children learn

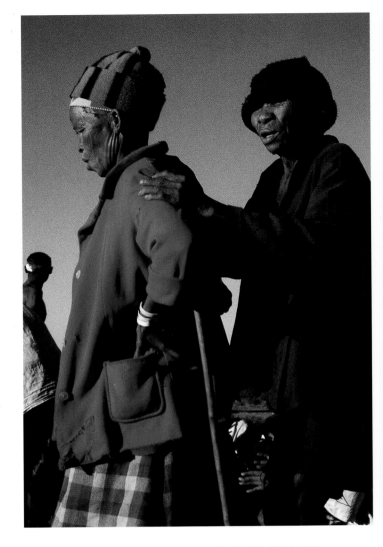

PEOPLE SUPPORT EACH OTHER AT THE DANCE. ǁXOAN (LEFT),

A STRONG PRESENCE IN THE HEALING WORK AT ǀKAEǀKAE,

LEADS AN OLD BLIND MAN AROUND THE DANCE CIRCLE.

OPPOSITE: FROM AN EARLY AGE, CHILDREN LEARN TO LIVE IN

ACCORD WITH OTHER PEOPLE. HERE YOUNG JUǀʼHOAN GIRLS SING

THE BEAUTIFUL HEALING SONGS FOR THEIR OWN PLEASURE.

THE SONGS CAN EXIST OUTSIDE OF THE HEALING DANCE.

to be in accord with each other and with their families as they learn about their environment. Small children sing of their delight in life in the mongongo nut groves:

E !xoana ka ≠'osi	We live in the groves
Te hatce ma ko dzui te?	And what little bird calls "dzui"?
Te e ku are te	And we're surprised,
Etsa mi di!uma	My little cousin and I,
G!ao ka g!!kaa te	On a gathering trip
Ee—uu, huu—ee.	for mongongo nuts.

Living with this sense of abundance is made possible by a great deal of detailed knowledge of the environment. Children learn this information from their parents through hands-on experience until they are able to provide serious subsistence themselves.

In John Marshall's film about her life, a Jul'hoan woman named N!ae reminisced about gathering and eating wild foods:

> When we were all living in the bush, I was a child, just a little child, only so big. We gathered so many different things. We picked /ore berries and struck down n≠ah.
>
> I loved to follow my mother. The two of us would be right beside each other. If my mother went gathering without me, I would cry because I was just a little girl.
>
> When we hit the n≠ah tree, the sweet berries fell. We'd all pick them up and pile them together to take home. I was such a big little woman then. Most things we dug. Our arms ached. We pried out the ≠ube root and dug g!xoa, the water root, from deep in the ground. In the forest we gathered g//kaa— mongongo nuts. There was so much dshin [morama beans] in the fall. . . . We had to taste things. Some of them were bitter. Some people ate plums. Some people didn't. In winter the berries dried but there was cucumber in the spring. And the beans you call "wild coffee," and different insects. And when the year grew warm, the trees oozed sap. . . .

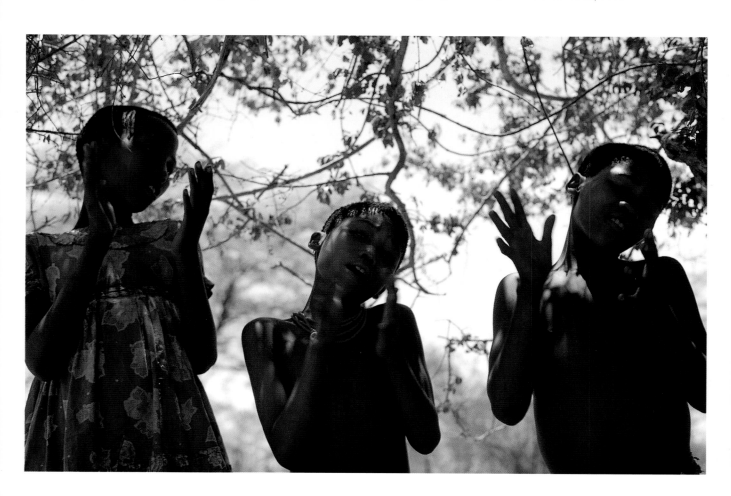

That was the food we ate. Those were the things that made us good and full and gave us many different tastes. My mother would open the baobab fruit and ask if we wanted some. Even if you hadn't worked, if hunger grabbed you, you could eat. And when we used up all the food and the year turned hard and hot, we traveled to another place. Those things we did long ago, before we knew about money.[1]

In their hunting-gathering–based life, Jul'hoansi learned from doing. They also learned from listening to reminiscences of older people and from folktales. They learned from each other about animal behavior, the location of bush foods, and good social attitudes. If we look at their stories, we see they are not didactic in the sense of purposefully instilling a lesson. Nevertheless, they are brimming with environmental details in a world of revealing human relationships. This was a most effective way for Jul'hoan children to learn.

All of the environmental information the children learned and used as adults was extremely *local*. Jul'hoan people, and hunter-gatherers in general, feel uneasy if they are far from their home areas. Their ecological adaptation is a finely honed instrument, utilizing a great fund of specialized knowledge about a given area.

Children grew up knowing how their society's rules about land and resources protected their livelihood. As Tsamkxao ≠Oma put it:

When my mother and father bore me and I was on this land, I looked at the land and they told me, "This is your father's father's n!ore." My mother said, "This is *my* father's father's father's n!ore, and I hold rights in it, and so through me do you."

So it is with my people. All of us are related, and we greet each other, and we understand each other. We live together.

We sit together and are related and greet each other and understand each other. We agree together about who is going to live together in this

n!ore and who is going to live together in that n!ore.

We are not a people who buy land. We ourselves do not buy land. Instead we are *born* on land. My father taught me about his father, who taught him about the foods of our land. Your father's father teaches you. People have taught each other and taught each other and taught each other. People have died but the teaching has gone on.[2]

Like most Indigenous peoples of the world, the Jul'hoansi did not buy and sell land. For them it was a spiritual entity, one they must treat with respect so it would nurture them. Animals, being living beings, would not respect arbitrary human boundaries. So the n!oresi had to be penetrable to allow the hunters to pursue game wherever it went. Yet the n!oresi had to be defined to some extent so that human stewards could watch the health of the land, gauging the use of water and food resources relative to the needs of their groups and visitors over time.

"Those who live on the land and know it well are its best protectors," said l'Angn!ao. Bushman peoples have had a reputation for being good conservators of their land and in fact see themselves this way. They rarely kill more animals than can be fully used. But it may be that they have been able to live lightly on the land—not having a heavy impact on its vegetation or on its surface through erosion—precisely because of their low population densities. With higher populations, they and other hunter-gatherers can adversely affect their environment, chiefly by burning.

Jul'hoan beliefs and teachings draw explicit parallels between the necessity of respecting natural providence and the necessity of sharing with others. Children are taught that the bounty of the bush is God-given and not to be squandered thoughtlessly. They are also taught that their most important resource is the goodwill of their neighbors; there is an imperative to share.

This imperative is taught to children from infancy. Mothers make sure that small children learn that part of whatever is put into one of their hands must immediately

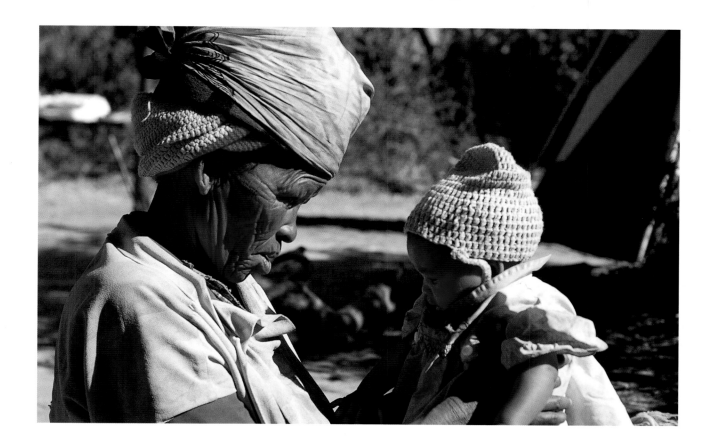

THE OLDEST GENERATION IS ALWAYS INVOLVED WITH THE YOUNGEST

GENERATION. HERE ǀXOAN EXCHANGES LOOKS WITH HER GRANDCHILD.

go out the other hand to someone else. Equalizing and leveling are two main themes in Juǀ'hoan society, constantly reinforced in songs, stories, rituals, and the conversations and behaviors of daily life. Lorna Marshall wrote in her article "Sharing, Talking, and Giving" of this constant flow of equalizing and relatedness.[3] She discussed how talking smooths social relationships; how good manners emphasize minimizing oneself and never flaunting one's abilities or experiences; how meat-sharing and arrow-sharing underscore the need of each member of the group to rely on every other member; and how gift-giving creates and cements trust.

All of these messages are told in the healing dance as well, regardless of recent changes. What happens in the present must be understood in terms of this subtext of

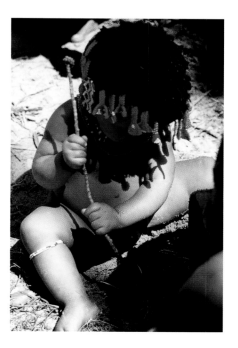

VALUES AND KNOWLEDGE ARE LEARNED AND PRACTICED

THROUGH PLAY EARLY IN A JUǀ'HOAN CHILD'S LIFE.

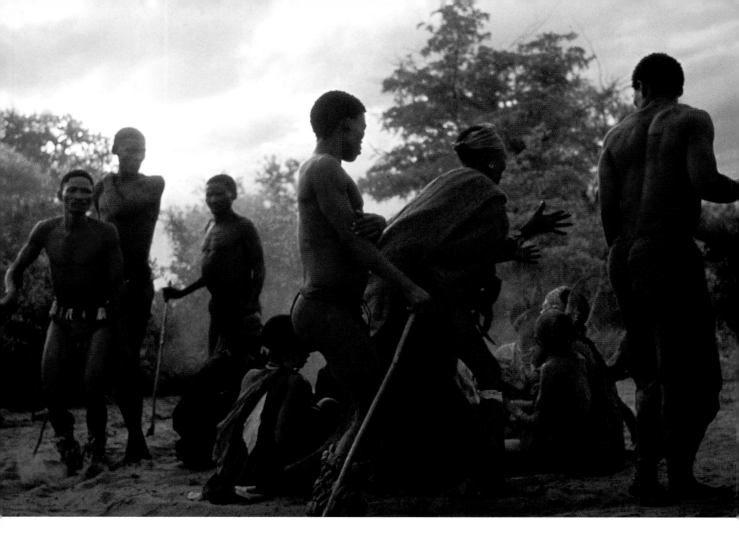

ancient values. The Jul'hoansi are constantly weighing contemporary changes against judgments they would have made using these traditional values. Nǀom grows by being shared freely and is diminished by competition or hoarding. In this synergistic quality, nǀom echoes the very essence of traditional Jul'hoan sociability.

FINDING THE DANCE'S HISTORY

Affirming its importance in promoting harmony and spiritual balance, the Jul'hoansi say the dance has a long history in their traditions. It is easy to see from the healing dance visible in ancient rock painting and the elaboration of ideas about healing that this beautiful, unifying form of art and spirituality has provided perennial strength.

THE HEALING DANCE PICTURED ABOVE IN 1968 MIRRORS THE ROCK PAINTING FOUND IN THE DRAKENSBERG MOUNTAINS SHOWN OPPOSITE. THIS PAINTING IS BELIEVED TO BE SEVERAL THOUSAND YEARS OLD.

One can see similarities between the healing dances today and how they were depicted in the rock art of previous centuries. Look, for example, at the photograph above, which shows a recent dance in the ǀKaeǀkae region, juxtaposed with the paintings on page 53—which may be several thousand years old—from the Drakensberg Mountains of South Africa, where Bushman people lived until they were decimated by the colonial encounters of

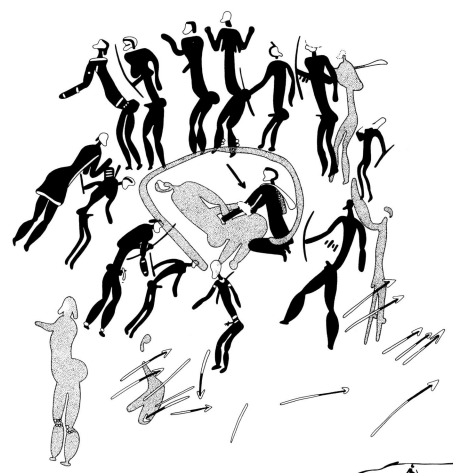

the late nineteenth century. Many familiar features of the contemporary giraffe dance, the primary community healing dance in the ǀKaeǀkae region, are faithfully depicted in these paintings, including the characteristic bent-over posture of the forward dancing motion and the seated women clapping and singing in a circle around the fire. The painting at the bottom of this page shows men leaning on carved sticks they often use at the dance to add balance and style to their dancing. These features of the depictions are naturalistic and have what seem to be narrative referents.

Less-tangible characteristics of the dance are also portrayed in the rock paintings, the large number of which make us aware that much more is occurring in these paintings than the mere depiction of an observable

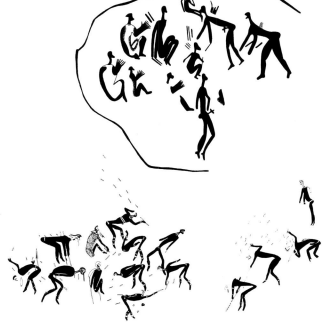

dance scene. South African scholars David Lewis-Williams and Thomas Dowson have used tracings and analyzed the symbols in the rock art images to establish that much of the ancient art was preoccupied with spiritual transformation.[4]

The southern Bushman people of the Drakensberg of South Africa and Lesotho sometimes varied the form of the healing dance as do contemporary Jul'hoansi. At times, one or more healers danced in the center while the women stood around them. Missionaries described such a dance around 1836:

> The movement consists of irregular jumps; it is as if one saw a herd of calves leaping, to use a native comparison. They gambol together till all are fatigued and covered with perspiration. The thousand cries that they raise, and the exertions that they make, are so violent that it is not unusual to see someone sink to the ground exhausted and covered with blood, which pours from the nostrils; it is on this account that this dance is called *mokoma,* or the dance of blood.[5]

Some features of mokoma appear in readily distinguishable form in the rock art. At times, blood is depicted flowing from the nose or healers may be shown raising a hand to their noses (see figure at left). The bending forward posture may be attributed to the painful contraction of the stomach muscles that many healers describe. Some healers are portrayed stretching back their arms, which is a posture assumed when asking the gods to put more nǀom into their bodies.

The naturalistic features depicted in the art are commonly accompanied by elements that go beyond a purely naturalistic description. For example, healers are depicted with antelope heads or with long lines coming out of their heads (see figure below). Sometimes the healers also have antelope hoofs and hairy fringes around their bodies; often, they are depicted in fanciful relationships with antelopes, especially elands, and with huge carnivores, as on page 55, reminiscent of contemporary healers' travels as lions.

Reflecting on the meaning of these metanaturalistic elements, Lewis-Williams and Dowson extract a set of

BELOW: FIGURES EXHIBITING CHARACTERISTIC BENT-OVER HEALING DANCE POSTURES.

OPPOSITE: PAINTED SCENES OF HEALERS WITH PHANTASMAGORIC HEADDRESSES AND AS COMBINATIONS OF MEN AND ELAND ANTELOPES, DEPICTING THE TRANSFORMATION OF JUǀ'HOAN HEALERS IN THEIR ALTERED STATES OF CONSCIOUSNESS.

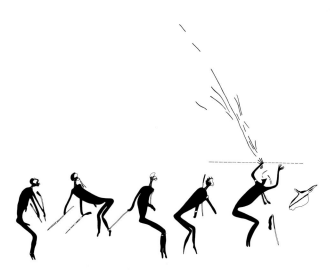

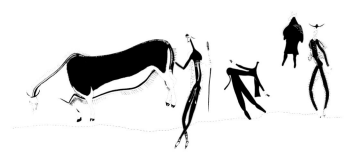

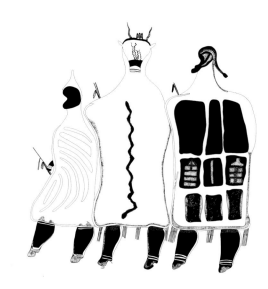

Though the roots of the dance are ancient, the dance expresses a vital and dynamic healing tradition. Change is essential to keeping that tradition alive. One way of understanding these processes of change is through the life of an individual healer. Here again, ≠Oma Djo can teach us a great deal. He reminds us that "n|om is just the same as long ago, even though it keeps on changing." His lifetime of intense association with n|om illuminates the fluctuations and evolutions that can occur in the use and understanding of n|om while emphasizing its enduring spiritual core.

We are talking with ≠Oma Djo early one morning as the sun is burning off night's chill. He is smiling, displaying his good mood for all to see, and speaks with a feeling of satisfaction.

> In the morning, you may see me arriving nicely with a happy heart. You'll know that in my night travels [to check on the people] I have found everyone well. But if my heart feels bad, you know someone is sick.
>
> Today I feel fine—everyone got up well this morning, and talked well together.

Yes, today ≠Oma Djo feels fine; he performs his healing work with dedication and skill. But life has not always been "fine" for ≠Oma Djo. There was a time when he gave up healing because he thought he might be harming people, and there was a time when others criticized him for seeking payment for his healing, which goes against Jul'hoan tradition.

≠Oma Djo is in his eighties. He has lived many of the changes experienced by his people. ≠Oma Djo's personal journey is a journey through his people's spirituality and social change. When ≠Oma Djo was growing up, the land was fertile; it fed the people. As a young hunter able to provide food for his family, he "gave birth" to his children. As the land has been changed, Jul'hoan subsistence has become more difficult. "The land is our life, but it is now dead. . . . it doesn't feed us anymore," is how ≠Oma Djo puts it. "It is our way to take care of ourselves. We can

values and ideologies that were important for these ancient Bushmen. Central to this set of values is a focus on enhanced consciousness. The work of Lewis-Williams and Dowson is corroborated by other data, including ethnographic description and folklore. If not its defining characteristic, the process of enhancing consciousness therefore seems both central to the healing dance and a dominant link between ancient and contemporary forms of the dance.

Other features in the rock art—painted "lines of force" linking humans and animals or healers and those being healed—point to an emphasis on meaningful transformation as experienced in the healing dance and recall the many ways in which the dance comments on social values of harmony, equality, and spiritual connectedness.

no longer do that." The Juǀ'hoan tradition of healing has changed, too, as it faces new challenges and creates new opportunities. The healing dance must transform to remain vital in the changed landscape of ǀKaeǀkae.

≠Oma Djo's path on the healing journey reflects these challenges and opportunities. His relationship with nǀom, while expressing times of confusion and doubt, has persisted, blossoming today into strong visions of the future.

≠Oma Djo has never been shy about describing the power of his nǀom. The process of becoming a healer among the Juǀ'hoansi has certain typical features. For example, nǀom can come to the people from God, though older healers typically pass nǀom on to those seeking it. The first "drinking" of nǀom does not occur until the mid-twenties, especially for the men. Exceptions to this usual process of learning are associated with powerful nǀom.

Though ≠Oma Djo's father had nǀom, he did not pass it on to his son. This is ≠Oma Djo's story about the special way he received nǀom:

When I was about fourteen or fifteen, I was asleep. God grabbed me by the legs and sent me out into the bush at night. Out there, he gave me a small tortoise and told me: "Leave this tortoise here. Then in the morning get your father to degut it and put nǀom into it, and that will be your nǀom." And then God took me farther and I was crying in the dark. My father came looking for me and found me crying and carried me back to the fireside.

In the morning I said: "Father, come and see this tortoise. Fix it for me and put nǀom in it and give it to me because this is what God has given me. Fix it and give it to me so I may keep it, so that when you are dying, I can use it and I'll save you." But my father refused. He just killed the tortoise, roasted it, and ate it.

Then the skin of my father's throat parted, and we could see his windpipe exposed. God said to me, "For what your father has done, I'm going to

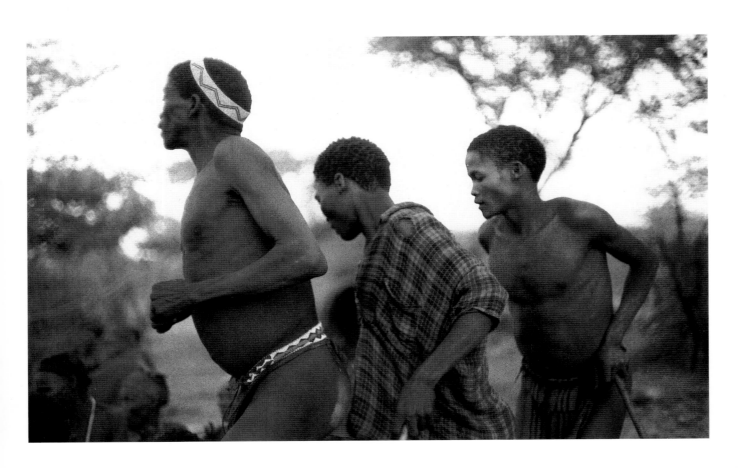

kill him. The thing I gave to you that he ate is killing him." And I refused and I said, "My father won't die." I took another tortoise with nǀom in it and dropped burning coals into the shell. And then I put the shell to my father's lips and he drank the smoke. The same day the skin above and skin below came together and closed and my father lived.

Then God said to me: "See what your father's arrogance has done to him. You tell him to stop that and not to do it again or else I will really kill him next time."

And that's how I got the nǀom that I have. That's where I started it, and today I carry the people in different camps. If someone is sick, I go to them.[6]

≠Oma Djo's early vision and gift of nǀom were both unusual and startling. So were some of the immediate effects. "I danced only after this experience," he says, "and !aia came only after this experience—but *right* after!" He adds that twice after the vision, God took him out to the bush alone and he went into !aia. The first !aia for Juǀ'hoansi is a time of especially strong fear. But ≠Oma Djo's two solo and God-induced experiences of !aia were different: "How could I be afraid during these experiences of !aia? God killed every thought. He wiped me clean. Then he took my soul away whirling. My thoughts whirled." It is this very whirling that so frightens the typical learner, even sometimes the older healers.

When he was in his late fifties, ≠Oma Djo was a controversial healer. Stressing the personal and individual power of his nǀom, he also refused to pass nǀom on to others, claiming that he thereby would only lose some of his own power. These attitudes were very much against the traditional and widely accepted Juǀ'hoan emphasis on

the communal roots and power of nǀom and the sharing of nǀom with whoever sought it. And most difficult for others to accept was ≠Oma Djo's expressed desire to be paid for his healing efforts. As elements of a cash economy began appearing in ǀKaeǀkae, his individualistic approach to nǀom seemed intended to establish his "professional" status. By emphasizing the power of his *own* nǀom, he sought to convince others that his services were worthy of pay.

Even as he professed a desire to be paid for his services, ≠Oma Djo continued to heal the people in the traditional Juǀ'hoan way—freely, as part of the general exchange that characterized the Juǀ'hoan sharing of resources. But he healed in his own way, a way that often was difficult for the people. For example, his favorite time to enter !aia was at sunrise. After a long night of singing and dancing, when everyone was tired and ready to end the dance, ≠Oma Djo would call upon the women to once again raise their voices to the heavens and propel him toward !aia. This they did, not wanting to refuse a healer's request to help the people; but there were grumblings and reservations that were expressed more openly in the days after the dance.

Despite the way in which ≠Oma Djo dramatized the power of his nǀom, he was widely recognized in the community as a healer of power. Yet even ≠Oma Djo went through a period of profound doubt and confusion.

≠Oma Djo had two wives. Both got sick, and even though he worked hard in his efforts to heal them, both died. In the Juǀ'hoan way if someone close to you "dies in your arms" and if you are unable to heal them, you and the community begin to question the power of your nǀom. ≠Oma Djo wrestled with this situation, trying to understand his losses, trying to understand his role as a healer.

My wives were withholding their spirits from me [as I tried to heal them]. I saw nothing from them. I said to myself: "God is today cheating me of these people. It must be that they will die."

I questioned myself, saying, "if my nǀom is like this, that my wives have defeated me and died"

IN THE DAWN LIGHT AT THE END OF AN ALL NIGHT HEALING DANCE IN 1968, !XAM AND ǀKAECE, TWO YOUNG MEN SEEKING TO DRINK NǀOM, DANCE BEHIND ≠OMA DJO, A STRONG AND EXPERIENCED HEALER.

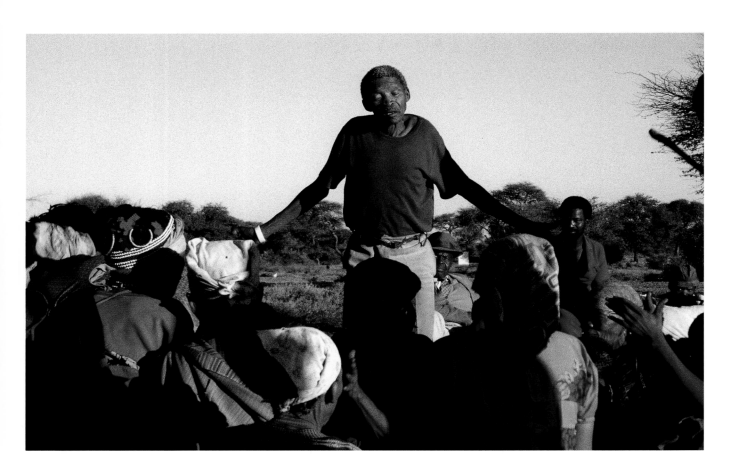

GOING INTO !AIA, ≠OMA DJO PLEADS WITH THE
SINGERS TO CONTINUE HELPING HIM WITH THEIR
STRONG SINGING.

. . . I thought my nlom was bad so I refused it, I left it. Then I just lived for years without doing nlom. When people were dancing, I just slept. I didn't go. And my heart felt bad. Nobody came to me. I just stayed alone.

Then when we were starting the well at lUihaba, people brought nlom to me again and asked me to heal. The [spirits] told me I shouldn't keep thinking always about my wives, that my heart should be happy and I should heal people again. They said, "You yourself will die one day; now leave off thinking about those people. Let's dance and heal people. You should enjoy yourself with people."

I was surprised when this happened. "Has that which has left me now returned?" I asked. So I agreed with it. I didn't fear it [this second time], I just agreed with it. I had left off just because I was unhappy that my wives had died. But at that time I was already a g!aeha [an experienced healer] so when nlom came again at lUihaba I just went on and healed and didn't fear.

From this trial of loneliness and doubt, ≠Oma Djo has emerged as a newly potent and highly respected healer. The freshness of his new healing work is captured by his own description of how he came back to nlom. "Only recently have I begun afresh, when I felt nlom coming back to me in my sleep. I said to myself: 'Maybe I can at least heal myself.' And since then I felt it and do it."

Today, the healer who was controversial is unquestionably loved and respected. His healing power, always considerable, is now seen as one of the most powerful at lKaelkae, a standard by which healing efforts are measured. ≠Oma Djo has become the healers' healer, the man other healers turn to for help in particularly difficult cases, the man who is a repository of the most sacred traditions of healing.

By reinventing traditional healing in his own life, ≠Oma Djo is nourishing traditional Jul'hoan healing for his people. Though he still *talks* about refusing to help others because they don't pay him, his uncomplicated enthusiasm for healing and his dedication to helping others defines his actual work.

> When people are sitting around talking about someone who's sick, your heart makes a sound like /'hi!, and there's a tapping in your fingers. You can't resist jumping up and going right to the sick person. It's like the nlom itself takes you there.
> I just see how the sick person is and heal him.
> . . . I don't just do a little nlom. I do it right until the person is fine again before I leave the dance.

If someone is sick, now ≠Oma Djo comes without requesting payment, and it is said by others, "He will do it right." And what happened to his favorite time of !aia? "When we dance all night, the sun comes up, and then I stop." The women singing at the dance appreciate this, adding their respect for ≠Oma Djo as the community's healer.

≠Oma Djo is no saint or even an ideal Jul'hoan. Not only does he retain his many human faults and frailties, but the Jul'hoansi, who do not allow anyone to have such an exalted status, make him the butt of as many jokes and teasing maneuvers as anyone else.

But ≠Oma Djo does offer a profoundly important possibility. "At first," he says, "[when I was younger] I 'sat lightly,' my words weren't strong. Now I say little, but my words are stronger." Others do listen to ≠Oma Djo; his words, particularly about healing, advise others. And like all Jul'hoansi, he is now deeply involved in the social changes swirling about him: the loss of land, the domination by Tswana and Herero cattle owners, and the disempowering presence of the government at ǀKaeǀkae. He too speaks out against this loss of land, of culture, of self.

His eloquence about healing remains in his talk about the land and its destruction. Will ≠Oma Djo's newly gained respect as a healer enable and encourage him to speak for the people about their land and their dwindling capacities for survival?

≠Oma Djo is nearly blind. "Both my eyes are bad, but I see a bit out of the right one. I think I'm going blind. But when I'm doing nlom, I can see what's troubling others, I can see everybody just fine!" Can ≠Oma Djo's ability to "see," made possible by nlom, be translated into a generic ability by the people to see their own "troubles" in order to act? Where will this spiritual seeing lead? Who will follow in ≠Oma Djo's footsteps?

THE EDUCATION OF HEALERS

The ancient heritage of the Jul'hoan healing dance—flexible but enduring—serves as the basis for the education of healers. The apprenticeship of young seekers to older healers in the learning of nlom has been, at least until recently, as durable as any in the Jul'hoan tradition.

Though boiling nlom is painful, the Jul'hoansi still seek to become healers. Dabe, a young man in training during the 1960s, expressed the motivation that prevails:

> We Jul'hoansi seek nlom even though it's painful because we can help people. If someone is very sick and almost dead, with nlom we can bring them back to life. That's why we seek nlom.[7]

During the 1960s, more than half of the men and women who sought nlom, in fact, were discouraged by its pain and their fear of it. Nevertheless, seeking nlom is a powerful cultural theme that animates Jul'hoan people of all ages. Long before they try seriously to become healers, Jul'hoan children play at !aia healing. A group of five- and six-year-old children may perform a small healing dance, imitating the actual dance with its steps and healing postures and falling down as if in !aia. A parent or another close relative, always a Jul'hoan healer, is usually one's healing teacher. Teachers are viewed as ordinary people rather than intimates of the gods when not in !aia. They do not demand obedience from their students or a

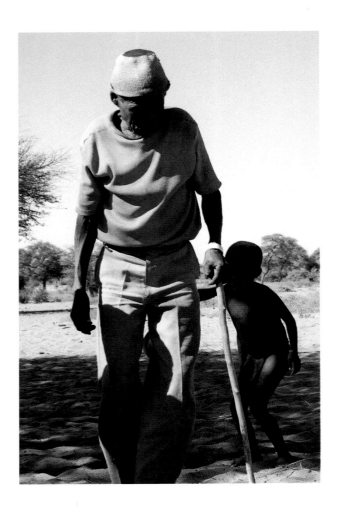

THE TEACHING BEGINS EARLY AS A YOUNG BOY FOLLOWS

IN ≠OMA DJO'S FOOTSTEPS AROUND THE DANCE CIRCLE.

long apprenticeship; in fact, the teaching relationship is often quite informal, with vague and permeable boundaries. Teaching is primarily by example.

The key to becoming a healer seems to be the willingness to accept boiling nǀom. "I want to be like [imitate] my father!" is the passionate cry of grown men who have become healers. Sometimes they call this phrase out while in !aia, stating their transition toward becoming an active healer. The passion and desire to heal are very im-

portant; still, these qualities cannot be coerced. When they appear spontaneously in a young person, they are celebrated by the whole community.

To heal depends upon developing a desire to "drink nǀom," not on learning specific techniques. The healer's education stresses not the structure of the dancing but the importance of dancing so one's "heart is open to the boiling nǀom"; it stresses not the composition of the healing songs, but singing so that one's "voice reaches up to the heavens." Nǀom is not "put into" someone who will not accept it; the student must seek to receive it, pain and all.

The active desire required by seekers of nǀom prompt some critical questions we ask ourselves when we return to the Juǀ'hoansi: Will we still find younger people as passionate about developing nǀom as they had been in the late 1960s? What alternatives might the people be using or thinking of using? What impact, for example, will the newly available clinic medicine have had upon the Juǀ'hoan approach to health and healing?

In the late 1960s, young people's doubts expressed about nǀom dealt with their fear of nǀom and therefore their ability to "drink nǀom"; this condition persisted into 1989. But the power of nǀom and its relevance and importance to their lives was never questioned. During our 1989 visit, however, young people are clearly in a period of intense transition. They see the value of their traditions but they also see their traditions being ignored by the wider Botswana society. And they see most intensely how their people are being denied access to resources. Our impression, however, is that many young people still seek nǀom with passion, though it is a passion at times riddled with doubts about their economic future and thence some doubts about the relevance of nǀom.

There is also a sense of unease among older people about the new generation of potential healers. In particular, healers like ≠Oma Djo and Tshao Matze express concern that many young people's aspirations no longer turn toward healing. They wonder what will happen to their communities if no one learns from them how to heal. ≠Oma Djo puts it this way:

They want to [learn] but they're bad and don't dance; [they] just sit around. Some of them are good young men but they just don't know how to do [nǃom]. They dance but don't put their hearts into it. It's as if they were just singing for themselves and when others sing for them they just talk and don't dance properly.

Tshao Matze adds:

The kids of today, if you say you'll teach them well, and you teach them, and teach them, and teach them, they think you're just fooling around. They don't remember that [without the dance] people will die.

Some of the frustration and disappointment ≠Oma Djo and Tshao Matze feel about the young points to actual changes in the last twenty years. An indifference and lack of seriousness toward nǃom is apparent in some of the young people. And if seekers of nǃom "don't put their hearts into it, we know nǃom will not come to them." Still, some of their frustration expresses the classic pattern of looking to the past as the time of the "true" or authentic tradition and seeing the present generation as diluting or losing that tradition. In 1968, for example, healers, including the older ones, spoke glowingly of deceased healers—"the healers of long ago"—as the real and the most powerful healers.

As to the clinic and its medicines, we find that in 1989 people have begun to identify certain illnesses as needing the treatment offered by the clinic. Tuberculosis, for example, is considered by many to be an illness for which the clinic has powerful medicine. Many discuss the nature of the clinic's medicines and what kind of nǃom they might have. And many use the clinic, especially for treatment for tuberculosis and pre- and postnatal care. But no one is ready to dismiss the power of the healing dance and Jul'hoan nǃom. Though the clinic is seen to have a kind of nǃom, its applications are perceived as quite limited, allowing the Jul'hoan traditional dance to continue on as the primary healing resource for the community, the place of first resort when sickness or problems emerge.

NǃOM AND ITS CHANGING CONTEXTS OF MEANING

We ask ourselves a number of other related questions, many having to do with social and spiritual effects of the great changes that had come to ǀKaeǀkae in the past two decades. We want to find out whether the land and resource dispossession of the Jul'hoansi, which has had an impact on their system of sharing among themselves, might have affected the ways in which they have traditionally shared nǃom. Do neighboring villages, for example, still come together for mutual benefit in healing dances, or have "hoarding" and competition developed in regard to nǃom as it had to some extent in regard to economic resources?

Our impression is that the healing dances in 1989 are more local, occurring more often only within the context of a particular camp and with fewer visitors from other camps. In 1968 it appeared there were more occasions during which several camps or villages joined together to put on a dance. From conversations we heard about the dance, people seem to have become less interested in spending the long night of the dance in the company of others from outside their camp. Perhaps the dance functions less as a greater community gathering. Yet there is not a *new* sense of hoarding or competition in regard to nǃom. The lessened desire to spend time with others may be a reflection of the increased general tensions running through ǀKaeǀkae.

We also want to know whether the spiritual intensity of nǃom has changed in some way. Are more or fewer healers experiencing the most powerful manifestations of nǃom, including traveling out of the body as lions to heal others or sitting at home and healing themselves? In 1989 the powerful manifestations of nǃom seem more frequent. In 1968, only a few—and then only the oldest and most seasoned—spoke of experiencing these more intense levels of healing. In 1989, most of the mature healers do so, and not just the oldest ones.

Perhaps the new ambiguity and doubt about seeking nǃom seen among young people has been balanced by increased intensity of nǃom in the veteran healers. As a result, it is possible that the traditional emphasis in !aia on "seeing properly" and seeing with "steady eyes" might provide a generic process of healing *all* that the Jul'hoansi see wrong in their environment.

The way the dance has evolved over many centuries seems to have forged a powerful tool of social and spiritual technology. We believe it is a way in which the voices of Jul'hoan people, as a group and as individuals, have been reliably heard for a considerable period of time. The dance encodes in its very demands on young learners all the lessons needed to be good Jul'hoan individuals, such as that selfless commitment can coexist with personal delight and joy.

As we seek to understand the relationship of the Jul'hoan healing tradition to the social changes that whirl about them, we must constantly return to the education of young Jul'hoansi to become healers: How many are learning to be healers and what are they being taught in these complex times?

We must look to the older, more experienced healers to understand the relationship between healing and social change. As ≠Oma Djo says, "If you have nlom, you know things. . . . You see how things are." The experienced healers also have the authority of age among the Jul'hoansi, as well as being teachers of those seeking nlom. But the seekers of nlom can give us further insight into the future of the healing dance, nlom, and the Jul'hoansi.

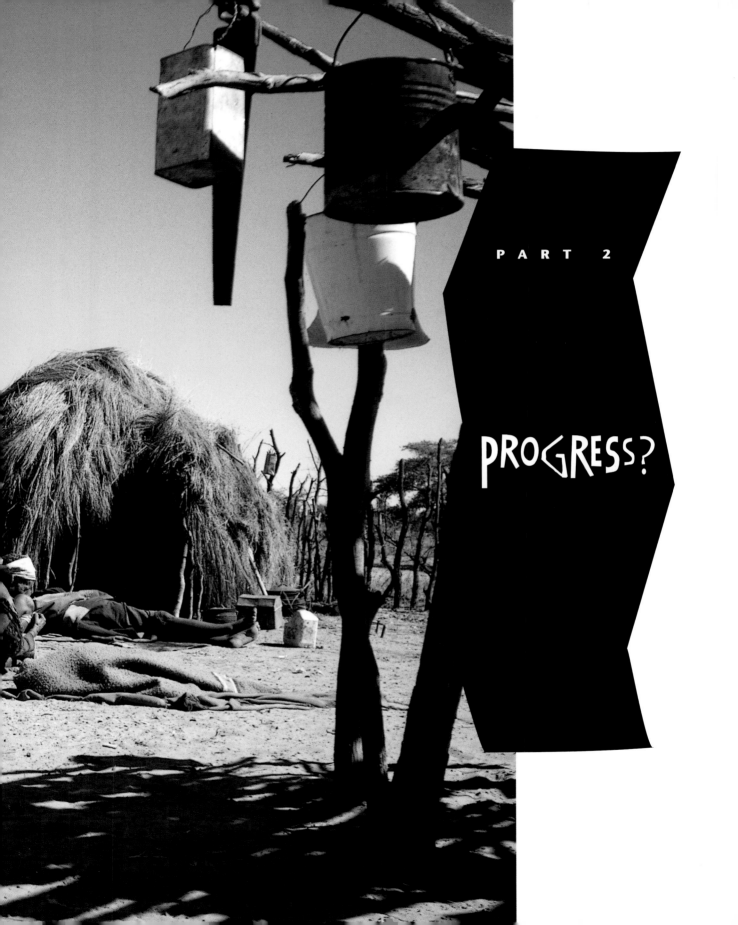

PART 2

PROGRESS?

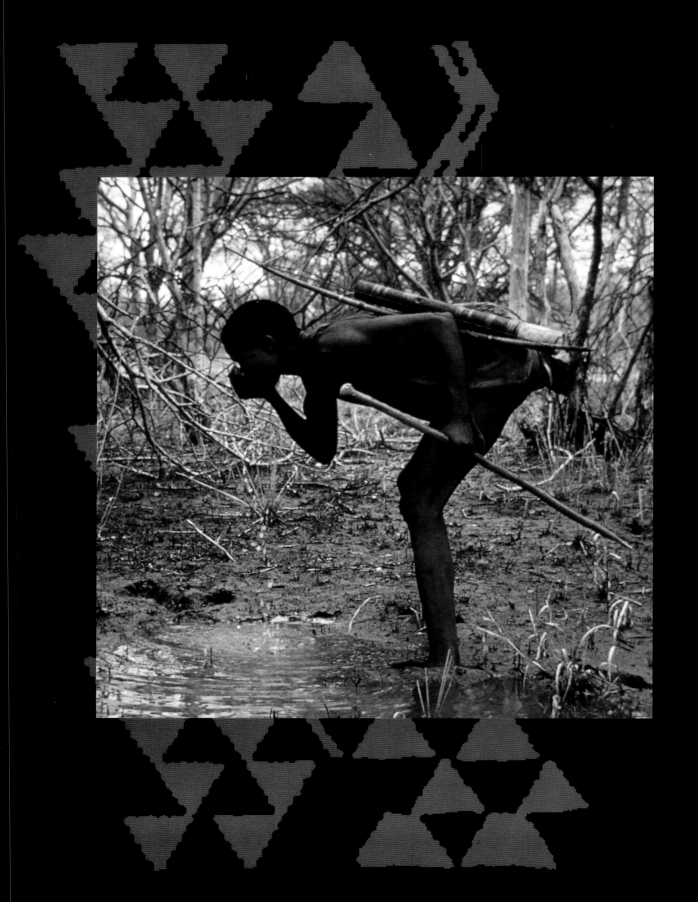

At the most basic level of Jul'hoan existence sits the land—their home, what the Jul'hoansi call their n!ore. The n!ore is where you exist—physically, emotionally, spiritually. As Tsamkxao ≠Oma puts it:

> A big thing is that my food is here and my father taught me about it. I know where I can drink water here. My father said to me, "These are your foods and the foods of your children's children." If you stay in your n!ore you have strength. You have water and food and a place.[1]

The n!ore feeds you with bush foods, social supports, and spiritual sustenance. "Our n!ore is who we are," says ≠Oma Djo.

The traditional Jul'hoan way of hunting and gathering is characterized by the government as "subsistence" living, implying a "lower" standard of living in terms of Western ideals of economic prosperity. Moreover, hunting and gathering is considered an unreliable source of food and an economically and politically counterproductive activity because it takes Jul'hoan people away from all the government institutions meant to "help" them. How could the schools "educate" or the clinics "cure" if the people are out foraging in the bush, providing for themselves? And so the government promises food as an inducement for people to stay put, to stay close to these government services—but these promises are made and kept in a discontinuous fashion.[2]

A more basic reason that government and cattle owners want to keep Jul'hoansi close to settlements has to do with control. If Jul'hoansi spread out over the land hunting and gathering, it is harder to make a case for allocat-

4
HUNGRY PEOPLE ARE EASY TO COERCE

ing that land to incoming cattle people. The Jul'hoansi also become a cheap labor force, hungry squatters around the settlements of others. Jul'hoan people become "settled," "sedentized," and "civilized."

But large government food shipments, initiated during a drought of the second half of the 1980s, have been reduced in the late 1980s to smaller deliveries to a few high-risk sectors of the population like tuberculosis patients and the elderly. Lists in hand, the government driver goes only to the camps of those now earmarked for food. The food consists primarily of cornmeal, refined sugar, salt, tea, and a few other food items, which

HIS BOW AND ARROWS SLUNG OVER HIS SHOULDER, AND CARRYING HIS DIGGING STICK, !KAECE PAUSES FOR A DRINK OF WATER WHILE HUNTING IN THE EARLY 1960S.

does not add up to a balanced diet. Any positive effects have been countered by the damaging dependency created, and the unrealistic expectations fostered.

When the government food is delivered and distributed, the contrast with traditional Jul'hoan food distribution patterns is stark. The amount of food brought in a government shipment would be equivalent to a good-sized animal, like a kudu. Traditionally, when a fresh kill is brought in, all the people gather about the butchered animal visiting, joking, and offering (usually unsolicited) advice and complaints as individuals wait for their share. Now, only the select few for whom the government shipment is intended gather around the delivery truck, surrounded by some of their relatives. Once the pile of food is unloaded, it is taken directly to the home of the recipient, usually by the younger relatives who are there. At best, all others just watch—and at a distance.

Traditional food distribution is a ceremony of inclusion, which ensures that all are fed as fairly as possible. Government food is dumped unceremoniously on the ground by a driver and then carted away by the recipients, who try to avoid contact with the nonrecipients, perhaps fearing their jealousy or requests for food. Though there is a secondary distribution once the food reaches the camp, as each recipient takes care of relatives, there are also bad feelings, as the food has not been gathered by the people but given to them by the government. The act of that giving is itself often begrudging and tainted with negative judgments. Drivers can be heard to complain about whether people really deserve this "free" food, and there are often arguments, with the people complaining to the driver that someone or other was wrongly left off the list or that the amount or kinds of food delivered are inadequate.

The delivery of government food is not a happy exchange. Participating in a ceremony of exclusion, the recipients cannot even feel grateful, for they are now being pitted against their neighbors who have gotten nothing. The food program takes on the all-too-familiar look of a handout. Only the traditional Jul'hoan commitment to sharing rescues some measure of dignity and

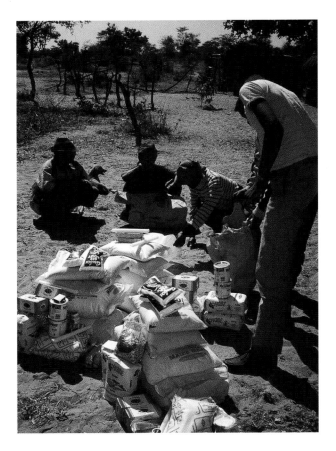

A GOVERNMENT FOOD SHIPMENT FOR A JUI'HOAN CAMP

SITS ON THE KALAHARI SANDS.

integrity to the arrival as recipients pass out the food to relatives. Compared with the skill, independence, and community negotiations surrounding the traditional hunting, gathering, and distribution of food, the government food program seems dehumanizing. But each shipment represents food, and since their bush-food resources have dwindled, the people cannot refuse. They are coerced into the unpleasant exchange.

While the actual food that comes from the government feeds people, it also feeds problems. Tea, sugar, and salt are somewhat addictive and of questionable nutritional value, especially when used in the large quantities the Jul'hoansi do whenever possible.[3] In addition to any physiological addiction to these Western food items, the more insidious addiction is to what is perceived as "superior" food, better than any bush food obtainable.

Since the government food items cannot be obtained from the bush, the Jul'hoansi are seduced into a cash economy as they seek to replace depleted supplies. Trucks, outfitted as traveling stores and stocked with these low-quality items, as well as eagerly sought-after high-fat and sugar-based snacks like bags of chips and bottles of soda, come periodically to ǀKaelkae. But the Jul'hoansi have little or no cash at hand to fill their new "needs."

Tshao Matze explained this chronic oppression:

> In this land, we who are Jul'hoansi are dying. . . . We just have to look at our land, ǀKaelkae, and see it being taken from us right before our eyes. . . .
>
> The Botswana government says they are our government, but why are they killing us?
>
> If we plant melons, we don't get to eat them. If we plant corn, we don't eat them. The Herero and Tswana cattle go in and eat them. They've taken our land.
>
> The government says we should buy food with money instead of gathering food. But where is this money supposed to come from? There's a little work sometimes, but the Hereros and Tswana people get it. This is discrimination. This is what we see and hear.

Most important, the promised food is not always delivered. ≠Oma Djo bears witness to the disastrous consequences:

> The government told us, the old people, not to go collect food in the bush. They told us to just sit and get government food, but now it no longer comes. We sat and sat, waiting for it until we were weak. Then we tried to go out and gather food with our pitiful old feet and our pitiful shoes. It killed us!

The death that results is not just from hunger but also from the loss of opportunities to teach the young people about hunting and gathering as the old people are "encouraged" to go less and less to the bush. "They don't want us to eat our own food, just to sit and eat government food. But where is it?" asks ≠Oma Djo.

Though the government sees settlement as a sign of progress, in fact it represents an "assimilation" of Jul'hoan people into a social structure that has reserved a place for them at the very bottom of the ladder. The people who once had provided for themselves are becoming beggars in their own land.

While living in the bush, Jul'hoansi survived with a minimum of clothing and shelter, but they never felt or looked "poor." Instead, they were adapting effectively. Now living in settlements, their minimum of clothing is almost exclusively Western and in threadbare condition. Housing is often decrepit. Instead of the grass-thatched houses of the bush, whose construction materials were readily available, Jul'hoansi seek to imitate the permanent mud-walled Tswana dwellings. But since the Jul'hoansi don't always have resources such as cow dung to bind the mud for walls and are thus unable to complete these dwellings properly, their "new" homes often remain in a half-built or deteriorated condition. The Jul'hoansi are looking increasingly like urban poor. The terrible irony is that what appears threadbare to a Western eye can remain a highly valued possession to a Jul'hoan simply because it is of Western origin.

Food and the threat of hunger it masks becomes the ultimate weapon over people, allowing for the manipulation of their lives. Hungry people are easy to coerce. The struggle over food is a symbol for the many struggles Jul'hoan people are facing; taking away a people's land and the food it provides is an essential step in the process of colonization.

Agricultural and pastoral peoples the world over regard foraging with disdain. In the Botswana case, the supposedly irresponsible "nomadism" of the Jul'hoansi and other Bushmen—necessary for their successful foraging—has been used as a weapon of criticism against their culture. In actuality, settling so-called nomads has caused untold hardship and privation and has disrupted

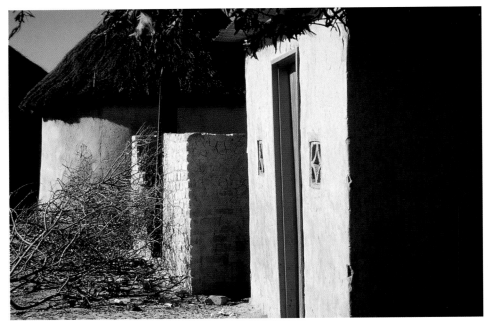

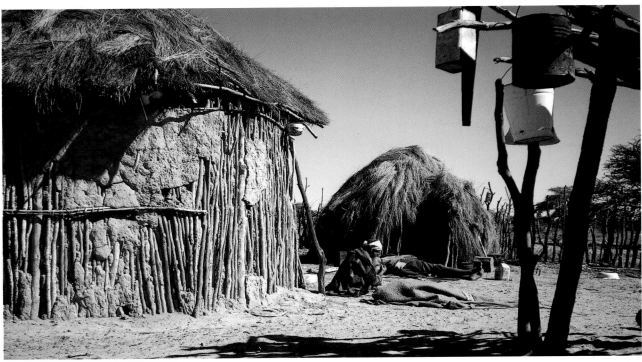

sustainable land- and resource-use patterns in many places.[4]

It is hard to dance on an empty stomach. But sometimes it is all the Jul'hoansi have these days. Dances themselves were not used traditionally to ask the gods directly for food in times of scarcity. Instead, dances could arise when people were feeling anxious, as when interpersonal problems flared due to privation and hunger.

Today, people say they sometimes dance because there

is no food and "there is nothing else to do." But they also dance when their stomachs are full and they are at ease with each other. Therefore, dancing when they are hungry is not simply a comforting spirituality. It may actually be a response to an extreme situation, one with a point of no return. Within limits, dancing and healing generate extra energy to tide people over during tough times. But if there is not a reasonable economic alternative available to take up the slack caused by the loss of foraging territories, knowledge, and incentive, then the healing dance and Jul'hoan spirituality as it exists today will be hard pressed to continue.

The Jul'hoansi are resisting loss by demanding their land and resource rights and thinking more critically about food handouts. In many areas of Jul'hoan life, there is a quiet resistance from people struggling to regain their power, a resistance that may eventually become truly powerful. Kommtsa is unyielding in his comments:

> We don't want a government that treats us like the woman who ate meat but only smeared her child's mouth with fat. When someone came to ask if the child had been fed she said, "Don't you see the fat around his mouth?" But in fact he was hungry.

Many Jul'hoansi now own animal stock, and some have put in gardens. As a result, they cannot leave their settled villages because of the substantial daily labor requirements of upkeep and because of their general desire to protect their valuable capital investments. They are caught and even sometimes compromised by the economic adjustments they've needed to make to settled life. But they express an understanding of the trade-offs and still think the new settled life offers benefits.

There are other Jul'hoansi who feel bush food is the only "real" food. They turn to the bush for sustenance some or all of the time, and see this activity as their way

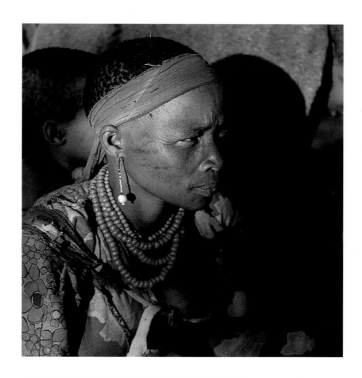

HAVING SUNG ALL NIGHT WITH HER BABY ON HER BACK, !XOAN, A MEMBER OF !AI!AE N!A'AN'S GROUP, BASKS IN THE WARMTH OF THE RISING SUN AFTER THE DANCE HAS ENDED.

to remain Jul'hoan. Many of these "back-to-the-bush" people are the strongest supporters of the healing dance.

As an arena where Jul'hoansi feel proud of their strengths and traditions and realize one thing that makes them quintessentially Jul'hoan, the healing dance can counteract the denigrating effects of eating from the government's hand. If the dance helps build up their strength as Jul'hoansi, it could also help them turn the food they get, from whatever source, into their own food, food they deserve and earn. Then hunger will not be their constant enemy and point of greatest vulnerability.

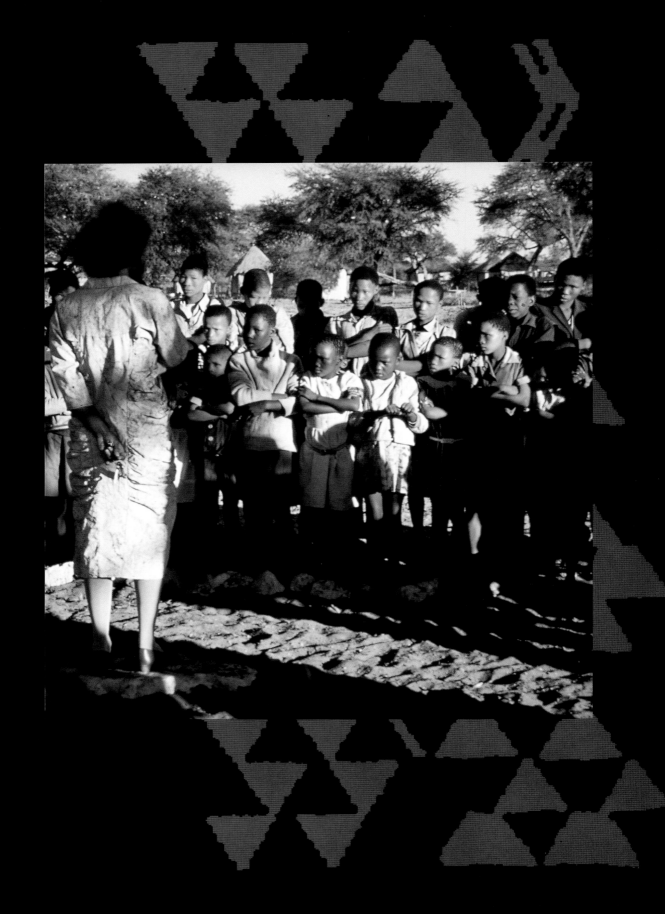

‖Kae‖kae now has a school. The government is proud: "We have given them education," say the bureaucrats, assuming the self-evident importance of education. This assumption is not shared by the Jul'hoansi, for whom the idea of school is new and has yet to prove its value. In fact, the school remains in conflict with their traditional approach to education and may even undermine essential elements of their traditional approach to healing. Perhaps only when Jul'hoansi themselves become teachers in the school will their healing dance be supported— though by then it could be too late.

The espoused aim of the government for the ‖Kae‖kae school is to bring Jul'hoan people into the mainstream of Botswana life. One primary aspect of that goal is the possibility of wage-based employment. As the present headmaster states:

> The aim of the school was basically to meet the educational needs of the BaSarwa [Jul'hoan] people. The village of ‖Kae‖kae is one of the remotest villages in Botswana, far from big towns where development takes place.

The headmaster expresses the government view on development, tying it into an urban-oriented capitalistic model. Participating in such models of development is a recipe for disaster for most Jul'hoansi. They will be consigned to the lowest position in the social structure, since they do not have access to the necessary capital resources.

The value of education as a way to build self-esteem and identity, skill and intelligence—a path toward empowerment—is not emphasized by the government. Yet this path is critical for a people like the Jul'hoansi,

THE TSWANA DEPUTY HEADMISTRESS ADDRESSES THE

UNIFORMED STUDENTS OF THE ‖KAE‖KAE SCHOOL AT

THE MORNING ASSEMBLY.

5

"THE SCHOOL OWNS OUR DANCE"

whose feelings of unpreparedness and inadequacy in the face of recent socioeconomic changes provide added fuel to the present situation of disempowerment. The sense of empowerment is especially important to those few Jul'hoansi who are not only attending school but succeeding in it and going on to the higher levels. ‖Ukxa, for example, received his Junior Certificate in 1987, a high school diploma roughly equivalent to completion of the eleventh grade in the United States. He told us:

> When I first started school, I thought it wouldn't help me. Then when the school days went by, I

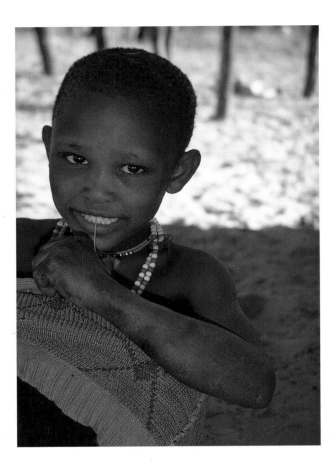

A YOUNG JU/'HOAN GIRL. CAN THE EMPOWERING
POTENTIAL OF EDUCATION BE FULFILLED WITH HER AND
OTHER JU/'HOAN CHILDREN?

realized that schooling can help a person grow a
bit and can improve somebody's life.

This evaluation of schooling is echoed by the four other
IKaeIkae area Ju/'hoansi who have by 1989 achieved
advanced status in their education by completing their
Junior Certificate: Kxao Jonah IOIOo (also known as
Royal), Tci!xo NIIaq'u, IAi!ae IAice (also known as
Benjamin), and Tshao Xumi (also known as Geoffrey).

IUkxa and the others definitely connect this empowering effect of education with its promise to qualify them
for employment opportunities. And for them, employ-

ment is an opportunity to serve their people better and
improve the life of their communities. Teaching back in
their home communities is their aim. Empowerment is a
merging of individual and community needs.

Certainly a cadre of Ju/'hoansi with advanced schooling functioning as teachers in local schools could be a
powerful and positive influence on the direction of social
change now sweeping the IKaeIkae area. But severe problems exist, threatening to frustrate such a scenario. First,
there is the deep conflict between schooling and traditional Ju/'hoan teaching, including the failure of the
schools to recognize the value of Indigenous knowledge.
And second, there is the undelivered promise of schooling—thus far, jobs are only sporadically available to
advanced Ju/'hoan students.

CONFLICTS BETWEEN SCHOOLING AND TRADITIONAL JU/'HOAN EDUCATION

There is a school at IKaeIkae, but is it an opening to education or an obstacle for the Ju/'hoansi? The school is run
by Tswana teachers with a Tswana-based curriculum,
teaching in a pedagogically constricted fashion. No curriculum is value-free, and, without being acknowledged,
the curriculum reinforces in Ju/'hoan children a sense
of inferiority as it generally ignores the strengths of
Ju/'hoan culture. Though the Ju/'hoansi are recognized as
one of Botswana's distinct tribes, the schoolbooks'
description focuses on their hunting-gathering skills,
presenting them as quaint habits of an exotic people
whose skills are unrelated to the needs of the contemporary world. The Ju/'hoan healing dance, the heart of the
culture, is not discussed at all. Fundamental cultural values such as sharing and egalitarianism are ignored.

The IKaeIkae teachers describe how they supplement
the official curriculum to make the school more relevant
to Ju/'hoan children. But their supplementary teaching
does little to add to a positive image. For example, while
recognizing the existence of the healing dance, the teachers restrict its purported functions and value. As the current headmaster states:

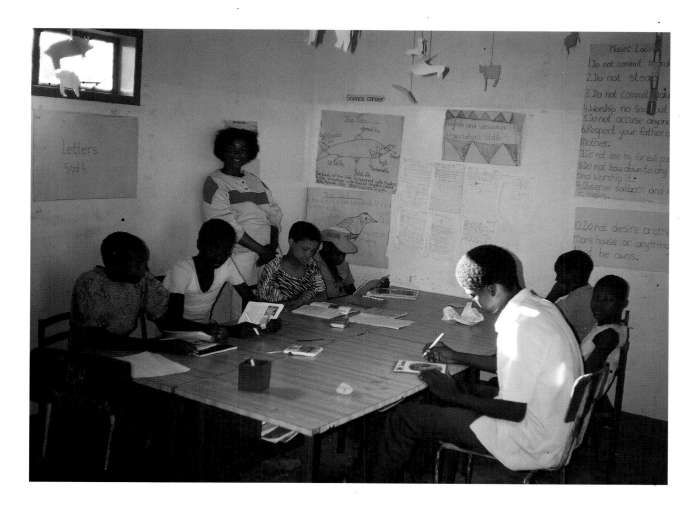

The [Jul'hoan] healing dances are good to a certain extent. But sometimes they are dangerous; especially when a healer is in !aia, he can fall on the fire and get injured . . . and he can run wild and therefore be dangerous to himself and others. The healing dances are good to the extent that some people really are cured of their ailments; they are good for anyone who wishes to attend them either for illness or for any other purpose. But I would advise someone to visit the clinic first before one goes to the healing dance, since modern medicine works faster than traditional medicine.

And though the headmaster says that he "does not mind getting treatment from the healing dance," he adds that he has "never been healed by these dances," and while teachers occasionally go to dances, he says he does not

IN THE UNFAMILIAR ENVIRONMENT OF FOUR SQUARE WALLS, DESKS, AND CHAIRS, THE TSWANA DEPUTY HEADMISTRESS TEACHES A CLASS OF OLDER !KAE!KAE STUDENTS.

"remember any of [his] teachers ever attending a dance."

Furthermore, all the teachers lament the negative effect of the dances on school attendance. They attribute absences on the day after a dance to the fact the children participated, stayed up too late, and were too tired to go to school. Teachers caution their students not to go to healing dances during the school week.

The school becomes equated with education; it has no place for traditional Jul'hoan patterns of learning that give Jul'hoan children the life skills they need.

Traditionally, Jul'hoan children are taught to become contributing community members, proud of who they are. It is a system of education that respects each child's rhythms of learning and tolerates individual growth, allowing children to learn through their own mistakes. The school's lockstep procedures, emphasis on universal standards, and rewards for successful outcomes—with mistakes consigned to the category of "errors"—all violate these traditional principles of education. Jul'hoan children are being judged according to culturally meaningless criteria such as learning that must conform to the content of some "universal" curriculum and forced and regular attendance that must conform to the rhythm of some external schedule. They are being judged and found wanting.

The cultural oppression experienced by Jul'hoan schoolchildren at the hands of their Tswana teachers must be seen as part of the larger context of their socioeconomic oppression. At the same time, any one particular teacher can make a difference, especially the headmaster. During the mid-1980s, a Tswana headmaster named Mr. Seelapilu helped establish an atmosphere at the ǀKaeǀkae school that was more congenial to Jul'hoan students and more respectful of their culture.[1] For example, Jul'hoan children were allowed to speak their language rather than being punished, as was typical at other schools implementing the government policy of assimilation. The ǀKaeǀkae kids responded positively, with an attendance rate reaching over 90 percent at one time.

THE UNDELIVERED PROMISE OF SCHOOLING

"People who have children can be taken care of by their children, if the children get jobs after school," Kodinyau,

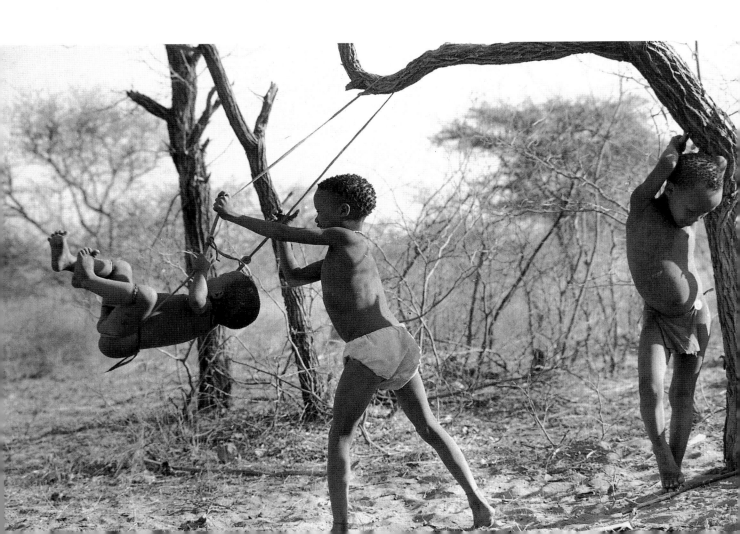

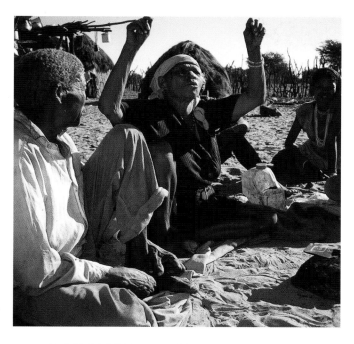

AS ≠OMA DJO LISTENS, N≠AISA N!A'AN, WHO HAS LIVED NEARLY SEVENTY YEARS, EXPRESSES HER VIEWS ON THE CHANGES SHE HAS WITNESSED.

OPPOSITE: TRADITIONAL JU!'HOAN EDUCATION RESPECTS EACH CHILD'S RHYTHM OF LEARNING AND INCORPORATES "PLAY" INTO EVERY ASPECT OF LEARNING.

a |Kae|kae elder, affirms. A man moving boldly into new patterns of economic adaptation such as owning goats and planting a small field in back of his home, Kodinyau expresses the economic justification for schooling. One hears that justification often. In fact, schooling as a way to employment is the only fully articulated rationale for the school that is shared by both the government and the people.

With few exceptions, the rationale remains theoretical. Jobs in the |Kae|kae area are generally limited, and throughout the region access to jobs is severely limited for Ju!'hoansi, regardless of educational achievement. As Tshao Matze observes, existing jobs usually go to Tswana and Hereros "while our Ju!'hoan people are passed over." Though "many kids from |Kae|kae have been to school,"

says Kxao Tjimburu, they don't get jobs. "The land of the Tswana has no help for us," he concludes.

Old N≠aisa N!a'an offers a firm judgment about the present value of schooling:

> This [|Kae|kae] school can't help kids with anything. Because when the school closed for holidays, the teachers took away the [kids'] school uniforms and put them back in the school.
>
> There were two boys who passed Standard 7 here at |Kae|kae and then went on to secondary school but they didn't get jobs. They are named |Ukxa and Tshao Xumi. They finished school in 1987 and didn't get any jobs until this year [1989]. And that is when they got their first job, working for you [as translators].

As she describes the way the uniforms are retained as school property, N≠aisa N!a'an is commenting on the larger issue of the discontinuity between school and community, questioning the commitment of the school to work with and serve that community.

Lack of employment opportunity is particularly painful for Ju!'hoansi who have worked hard at school to receive their Junior Certificate. |Ukxa puts it this way:

> I think most [Ju!'hoan] people in |Kae|kae see education as a useless thing. . . . If you know that education can do better for someone, then all the children may have to attend school, but today only a few do. [Because] when a student is about to finish school or when they are doing Standard 7, they have to leave school with no hope of a good job and have to go to the cattle post to work [for the Herero or Tswana cattle owners]. That means the people take education as a useless thing.

|Ukxa's own experience with schools underlies this judgment. A personable and talented young man, he has not been able either to find steady employment or to further his education. For example, he hopes to enroll as a Senior Certificate student, which calls for an additional year or two of high school in Maun. Recently he received

a message from the Ministry of Education to come to Maun to enroll, but when he arrived, no spaces were available. |Ukxa is beginning to doubt the value of schooling; if his disappointment continues, he too might label school useless.

In some cases, schooling does lead to employment. Such instances are restricted to very few graduates. Kxao |O|Oo worked in 1989 for a Jul'hoan craft collective, which bought items from the |Kae|kae region, such as beaded leather pouches and drums, then sold them to non-Jul'hoansi through a store in Maun, the closest town. Recently he has been hired as a teacher in Namibia. He sees schooling as imperative· to avoid what has become demeaning work at the cattle post.

> The Tswana and Herero people regard Bushman
> people as their slaves. They want us to take care·of
> their cattle and they pay us low wages. I really hate
> this. . . . I used to tell my uncles that I didn't want
> to stay with them because they were looking after
> Herero cattle. I don't want to waste my energy
> watering [other people's] cattle. . . . My uncles said
> there is nothing they can do. . . . If they are to sur-
> vive, they have to look after Herero cattle.

The |Kae|kae school, like many in isolated Indigenous communities, too easily functions as a weapon of cultur-al imperialism, more dominating because of the weight of the government resources behind it and its promise of a better life for its graduates. A concerned and sensitive staff can lessen such imperialism and open doors of opportunity for Jul'hoan children. Even when operating within a paradigm of cultural imperialism, a school can offer new opportunities, at least in employment, to a few graduates. Most important, literacy can be a powerful ingredient in a people's struggle for self-determination no matter how inhospitable the conditions of its origins.

ARE RESIDENTIAL SCHOOLS THE ANSWER?

According to school officials, the Jul'honsi are not inter-ested in the school. Teachers, for example, point to spo-radic and low attendance as evidence that the Jul'hoansi do not "understand what schools are all about," nor are they "serious about the purpose of schools." Employing a form of "blaming the victim," the teachers interpret the "attendance problem" as a sign that Jul'hoan parents are neglectful of their children.

But attendance reflects the Jul'hoan community's ambivalence about the school's value, not a lack of con-cern for their children's welfare. Attendance is also affect-ed by the Jul'hoansi's commitment to their culture and traditional means of subsistence. Children still are expected to help with foraging. Spending a day in the bush to secure food takes precedence over school. Everyone in the village—including children—partici-pates in the healing dances. Again, the health of the peo-ple takes precedence. Attending school may be impossi-ble after a late-night dance.

Attendance is certainly not a true measure of the Jul'hoan commitment to education or even to formal schooling. At issue is a conflict between the Jul'hoan land-based economy and the wage-based economy implied by formal schooling. That conflict must be resolved before schooling can become a positive factor in Jul'hoan life. As ≠Oma Djo expresses the conflict:

> Kids have to be fed. We can go live in the bush
> and get food. Those who have no children can go
> eat there. But the government people will accuse
> us of taking our children out of school and running
> off. How are we supposed to be in two places at
> once—out [in the bush] getting food and staying
> with our kids at |Kae|kae?
>
> Lately we haven't been eating anything. The
> government people were giving us mealie [corn]
> meal but now they've stopped. What will we do?
> They don't really know anything about our needs
> but just talk as if they do. So we have to just sit
> [and do nothing]. The [government people] them-
> selves are the ones who stopped the food. If they
> want our children to stay in school, they must pro-
> vide the parents with food.

PROGRESS?

The government has not reflected fully on why there is an "attendance problem." Overlooking the complex discontinuities between schooling and Jul'hoan culture, they instead have come up with a "solution." Residential schools are seen as a way to make formal schooling a real part of Jul'hoan life. "We must free those Jul'hoan children from the influence of their parents," the regional officer of education says. "Otherwise they don't attend school. Those parents really don't understand the value of education."[2]

Throughout the world, residential schools have become a part of government strategies to "educate" or "assimilate" Indigenous peoples and other groups who are outside the "mainstream." With residential schools, formal schooling will become an even more powerful influence on Jul'hoan communities. There is mounting and indisputable evidence about the devastating effects of residential schools that rip the children out of their cultural context. The loss of language, self-esteem, dignity, and cultural identity often leads to cycles of alcohol and drug abuse, family violence, and sexual abuse among adults.

Among Jul'hoansi there is an intuitive resistance to this solution. As Kodinyau asks, "How will we speak with our children when they come home from these schools?" He knows that in the future Jul'hoan traditions could become objects of scorn rather than respect and the healing dance seen as a quaint ritual or even an embarrassment.

Ti!'ae and her husband, ≠Oma !'Homg!ausi, wrestle with the complex issue of residential schools, trying to put a positive light on it. "It's better for kids to stay away from their mothers," suggests ≠Oma !'Homg!ausi. Ti!'ae agrees, adding that then "the kids will work better. [But] I don't know whether they will forget the language of the Jul'hoansi and the things of their parents," she immediately wonders. Kxao Tjimburu asks, "What if the kids come home and fight with their parents, who don't understand Tswana?" referring to the language of instruction in the schools. "Then they'll come home and teach their parents," Ti!'ae responds optimistically. "If they forget their language," adds ≠Oma !'Homg!ausi, "we

will teach them again." But when the possibility is raised that the kids will not want to return home after residential schooling, both Ti!'ae and her husband are clear. "That would be bad," they say.

CULTURAL PRIDE AND CULTURAL APPROPRIATION

In the early 1980s, the deputy headmistress began working with a ǀKaeǀkae school club whose activities included performing traditional dances. The headmaster, Mr. Seelapilu, encouraged her to enter the club's dance troupe in the traditional ethnic dance competitions. These are sponsored by the government to encourage cultural appreciation in the schools. The ǀKaeǀkae group was eventually named the ǀUihaba Dancers, after famous caves near the village. Within less than a decade, the ǀUihaba Dancers demonstrated both the school's promise to be a positive force for Jul'hoan identity and culture and its tragic failure to fulfill that promise.

"I can no longer support that ǀUihaba dance group," said Xumi Nǃa'an, "because the school now owns our dance." Xumi Nǃa'an is a respected elder who is dedicated to improving conditions for Jul'hoan people through schooling. His son, Tshao Xumi, is one of the few Jul'hoansi who have graduated from the ǀKaeǀkae school and one of five in the region who have attained Junior Certificate status. The son attests to the importance of his father's support. Other respected members of the Jul'hoan community are beginning to share Xumi Nǃa'an's concerns; in one more way the school is becoming an enemy.

In three short years, the situation with the ǀUihaba Dancers has changed dramatically. When the dance group was first formed and entered the government competitions, people of ǀKaeǀkae, especially the Jul'hoansi, were quite pleased. Wearing traditional Jul'hoan dance outfits, complete with leather garments, beadwork, and dance rattles, the troupe performed dances based on the traditional Jul'hoan healing dance. The songs were based on both Jul'hoan healing and initiation songs. However, there was no healing in the dance, nor any !aia or behav-

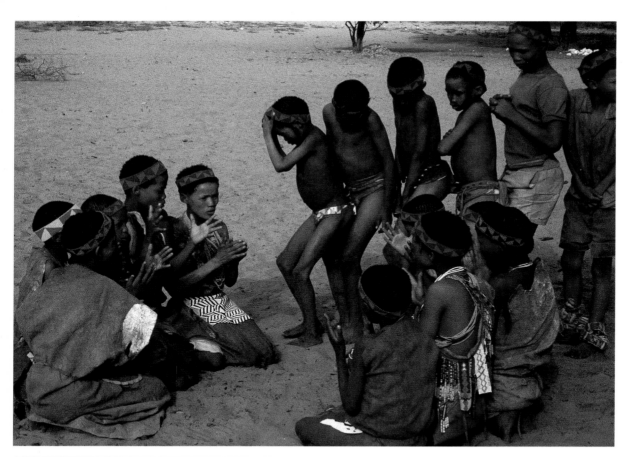

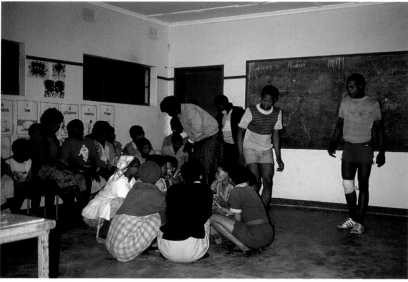

THE ǀUIHABA DANCE GROUP, WEARING TRADITIONAL JUǀ'HOAN DANCE OUTFITS, PRACTICES AT ǁKAEǁKAE. AS OF 1989, HERERO CHILDREN NO LONGER PARTICIPATE IN THE GROUP.

LEFT: UNDER THE SUPERVISION OF THE TSWANA DEPUTY HEADMISTRESS, WHO KNOWS VERY LITTLE OF THE JUǀ'HOAN DANCE TRADITION, THE ǀUIHABA DANCE GROUP PRACTICES IN A ǁKAEǁKAE SCHOOL CLASSROOM.

ioral imitations of the !aia experience. As Xumi said, "There is no nǀom in that ǀUihaba dance. It's meant only as a dance."

The troupe included Juǀ'hoan and Herero dancers. Juǀ'hoan healers and other elders played an important role in instructing the troupe. The ǀUihaba Dancers, who expressed the beauty and vitality of Juǀ'hoan traditions, gave particular pride to the Juǀ'hoansi at ǁKaeǁkae. The headmaster saw the group as a tangible success of his effort to promote racial tolerance at the school.

In 1986 the |Uihaba Dancers won at the district level, at the regional level, and then amazingly at the national level. They went all the way to the national finals and won first prize. Little |Kae|kae . . . the first prize. A truly singular achievement. The peoples' pride expanded, and their joy was overwhelming.

Events then began turning in a different direction. The Tswana teachers, who had always had ultimate control over the dance troupe, now began exerting more total control. Recalling her early involvement with the group, the deputy headmistress says that, "assisted" by several Ju/'hoansi, she "began by improving upon the traditional Ju/'hoan dance and thereby perfected it." By 1989 the Ju/'hoansi are no longer even "assistants." Their presence has become peripheral. |Xoan and her husband, Tshao N!a'an, who were the central figures in teaching the original dance troupe, are now no longer consulted. "That Tswana teacher does not know how to sing the songs," laments |Xoan. Furthermore, Herero schoolchildren are no longer in the group. The special pride the Ju/'hoansi felt in seeing children from this usually dominating group wear Ju/'hoan garments and perform a Ju/'hoan dance is dissipated. The school has also begun gathering up and storing the finest dance regalia for the yearly competitions. Some of the most beautiful ritual attire is no longer available for the actual village healing dances.

Most devastating to the Ju/'hoan people, especially those who had eagerly supported the |Uihaba Dancers, is that the prize money won by the group in the competitions never leaves the school grounds. "Shouldn't we people, we who dance that dance, shouldn't we be getting some of that money . . . we who need it so much?" Xumi N!a'an's angry question has a receptive audience among those gathered at his campfire. In fact, when several schoolchildren request some dance rattles for the next competition, Xumi N!a'an refuses.

Is the |Uihaba dance group helping to preserve Ju/'hoan traditions, as the government seems to think? From the evidence in 1989, we are doubtful. The troupe, in fact, may be diluting the healing dance. The dance adaptation, though it has similar movements, has no connection with healing. Without its heart—the n|om and the healing—the |Uihaba dance expresses only a shell, a form. When spiritual ceremonies are transformed into ordinary entertainment vehicles or, worse, tourist attractions, the ceremonies suffer. Audiences generally wish to have light, undemanding entertainment. Seeing

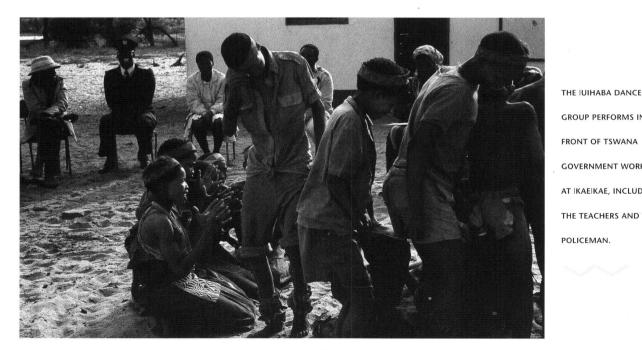

THE |UIHABA DANCE GROUP PERFORMS IN FRONT OF TSWANA GOVERNMENT WORKERS AT |KAE|KAE, INCLUDING THE TEACHERS AND THE POLICEMAN.

"THE SCHOOL OWNS OUR DANCE"

the |Uihaba dance troupe performing a light entertainment adaptation of the healing dance could bring the actual dance into some question. The dissipation of the pride Jul'hoansi felt in the early days of the troupe could make such questioning more likely.

On the other hand, there are many examples where the spiritual core of a ceremony turned into entertainment is consciously removed or deeply hidden because performers wish to keep their spiritual traditions from abuse. That may be happening with the |Kae|kae Jul'hoansi. Then the |Uihaba troupe could be effecting a renewed appreciation of the value of n|om.

As he considers the way the school has taken over instruction of the dance and now keeps dance regalia and prize money for itself, Xumi N!a'an's anger is clear: "The school owns our dance. It is no longer ours." At the same time as he expresses his resistance to this situation, adding "we will now dance for ourselves," he implies that the school does not own the heart of the dance—the n|om.

SCHOOLING AND HEALING

The relationship between schooling and healing can be examined on many different levels. The school itself must always be given primary importance. The |Kae|kae school remains a vehicle of cultural imperialism and the healing dance becomes one target.

None of the teachers openly criticize the dance. Several speak of its healing value for the Jul'hoansi, and one teacher talks about how she would go to the dance to be healed if she had an illness. But they don't attend many dances or seek treatment when they do. They believe the clinic provides more efficient and often more effective treatment, and always recommend it as the first line of defense against illness. The implicit judgment is that the dance is "primitive" and, in time, the clinic's "modern medicine" will prevail. Among Hereros and other Tswana living at |Kae|kae, there is respect for the dance, albeit a respect tinged with fear. These villagers may attend the dance when ill. Because they truly fear its power, they avoid criticizing the dance. Yet, given their perceived status and power in the village, the teachers'

skeptical attitudes carry great weight.

The |Kae|kae school, like so many government schools in rural, undeveloped parts of the world, is also an advocate for a Western approach to hygiene. Village life is portrayed as filled with dirt and germs that spread diseases. Though some hygienic lessons are obviously sound, some merely reflect a limited cultural notion of cleanliness. In the attempt to sweep the village "clean," the dance is not immune from criticism. Not only does the dance prevent people—especially the children—from getting enough sleep, but conditions of the dance, such as sleeping outside at night during the dance, are seen as unhealthy.

Another way of considering the relationship between schooling and healing is to look at the educated elite, those most advanced in their schooling. There are at present many areas of conflict between schooling and healing for these educated elite. One conflict is quite pragmatic: the time spent in school, especially advanced schooling away from home, makes it difficult to attend dances at times. Kxao |O|Oo describes the dilemma: "I did try going around to the dances, but I never felt the n|om rise up because I spent most of my time at school. I would come back too late [for some of the dances]."

Another area of conflict is more profound. Instances of confusion or doubt about the more advanced functions of n|om appear among the elite as they begin applying their school-learned knowledge of the universe. Kxao |O|Oo describes his impressions of healers' out-of-the-body travels:

> I had never heard of their traveling around during the night . . . and it is still hard for me to explain. I don't know how the healers pull out of their bodies or spirits. It's still hard to understand.

Kxao |O|Oo is not alone in his inability to explain these healing journeys, but he is more articulate than most and more analytical. Still, Kxao |O|Oo attributes his lack of understanding more to a shortage of time for learning than any inherent impossibility of such night travels. "It is hard to explain," he says, "though I know it happens." Kxao |O|Oo also desires to learn how to climb the threads to God's village, another function of boiling nǀom he finds hard to understand. Yet he appreciates that this is possible only to those who already have learned to drink nǀom.

> If I want to try to learn to climb the threads to God's village, first of all I have to learn to heal people. After that, the healers will teach me how to use that thread. I am willing, but it is hard. It will be very difficult because I spend most of the time at Maun [working for the craft cooperative] and don't have a chance to come back to my village and stay with the healers who can teach me.

Climbing the threads also attracts the interest of ǀUkxa. But he expresses even more doubt than Kxao ǀOǀOo about this function of nǀom and healing:

> Climbing the threads is something I knew nothing about until I heard it [in the research interviews we had with healers]. . . . I think this climbing is something like magic . . . [and] it is hard for me to believe. . . . I think it may happen, that it is true that the healers climb these threads. All of them say they do, so maybe it's true they do, but I'm not sure.

When ǀUkxa speaks about healers turning into lions during their healing work, his doubt is even more concrete.

> I have only heard about Kxao Tjimburu being able to change into a lion, and I don't believe that. I hear that Bushmen [healers] can turn themselves into lions, but I don't believe that human beings can turn into lions. I don't believe that.

The doubts and confusions expressed by both young men should not be overemphasized or overinterpreted. They merely point to another area of potential conflict between schooling and traditional healing.

Since neither has learned to drink nǀom and neither is seeking to or is an active participant in the dances, they are not privy to the arena in which such advanced func-

tions of nǀom are described and taught. In fact, research team members who translated our interviews with healers told us they learned many things about nǀom for the first time during the interviews. Kxao ǀOǀOo says:

> The ways of nǀom are new to me. My father didn't do nǀom. My grandfather didn't teach me these things. When I was a bit grown, he died. So today [as we are doing this interview with a healer] is the first time I'm hearing these things.

But those less-schooled young people who also would not know *how* these advanced nǀom functions occurred nonetheless would *believe* they *did* occur.

More important, both Kxao ǀOǀOo and ǀUkxa express belief in and respect for nǀom. As Kxao ǀOǀOo states:

> I think healers are very helpful because if you get sick and don't have a healer, who is going to heal you? . . . If the healers can teach the young men and girls [to heal], it will be helpful [for the people] because then they won't forget their culture.

ǀUkxa is more ambivalent, though others, even without schooling, phrase their belief in nǀom in terms of its efficacy.

> Oh, yes, I believe in nǀom. I believe in it sometimes, and sometimes I don't believe in it. Healers can heal a person and a person gets better, but sometimes the person will be just the same. So sometimes I believe in nǀom. Sometimes I don't.

Significantly, however, ǀUkxa and Kxao ǀOǀOo, like their less-schooled age-mates and other community members, turn to the healing dance for help with their own and their families' problems and illnesses. Their actions tell us that nǀom remains their most important and primary healing resource. Whether the doubt expressed in their words will eventually affect their actions is unclear. Whether they will find the time—and motivation—to pursue the healing work is also unclear, though both express a desire to learn more about healing.

In 1991, Kxao ǀOǀOo proposed a very compelling

N≠AISA, A STRONG SINGER AND DANCER AND THE WIFE OF THE HEALER KXAO TJIMBURU, IS ONE OF MANY ADULTS WITH MUCH KNOWLEDGE TO PASS ON TO THE NEXT GENERATION.

VILLAGE SCHOOLS ALLOW JUI'HOAN CHILDREN TO START SCHOOL IN THEIR OWN COMMUNITIES. HERE, YOUNG BOYS RELISH THE ENJOYMENT OF PLAYING A TRADITIONAL JUI'HOAN HAND GAME.

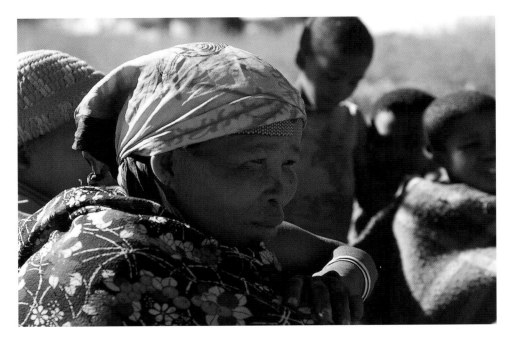

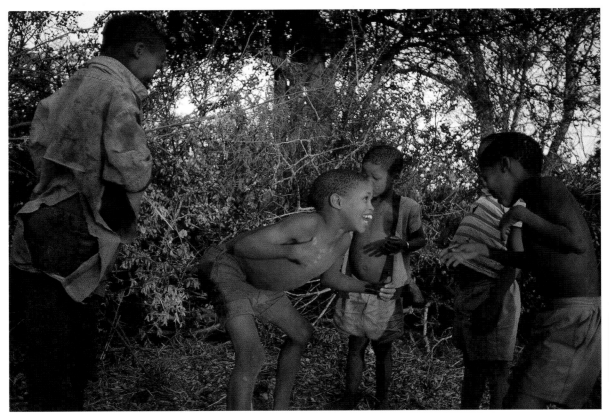

PROGRESS?

future when he was asked whether he, as a formally trained teacher, thought nǀom could still be of help to the Juǀ'hoansi. By then he had begun teaching school in Namibia under that government's affirmative action plan.

> There are old people still around who can teach the young people to do nǀom if they want it. It's like bush food: young people can still learn from their mothers how to gather it. Some children want to be with their mothers and fathers in order to learn. I want them to have a chance to do that as well as go to school. . . . I think children should do both things, learn the things of the old days *and* the new things.

Around the time of Kxao ǀOǀOo's remarks, alternative, community-based schooling called the Village Schools Project had started in Namibia; it remains a worthwhile experiment. In contrast to conventional schools—which are alien to Juǀ'hoan culture, language, and subsistence patterns—the new village schools allow Juǀ'hoan people to contribute to the creation of curriculum in their own language, and young children start school in their own or nearby communities where they can live with kin.

These new community-based village schools are designed to provide Juǀ'hoan children with a nurturant environment and social bridge to the Namibian school system. The first three years of school are in the Juǀ'hoan language, and the curriculum is based on their culture, emphasizing the self-initiated, organic changes it is undergoing. Children can then generalize the skills of literacy and critical thinking learned in their own language to English, the new language of independent Namibia. Furthermore, school schedules are tailored to support genuine economic needs and interests, including some foraging activity. Kxao ǀOǀOo's comments reflect his excitement with the philosophy of the Village Schools Project, which takes important steps toward resolving the conflict between schooling and traditional Juǀ'hoan education.

Botswana may one day follow the lead of other countries in promoting relevant, realistic, and spiritually nourishing educational approaches. For example, with governmental attitudes and policies demonstrated in the Namibian Village Schools Project and with persons like Kxao ǀOǀOo as teachers, a ǁKaeǁkae school could become a strong supporter of the healing dance. The numerous, and at times irresolvable, conflicts between schooling and healing could be acknowledged more sensitively and a relationship of respectful exchange established.

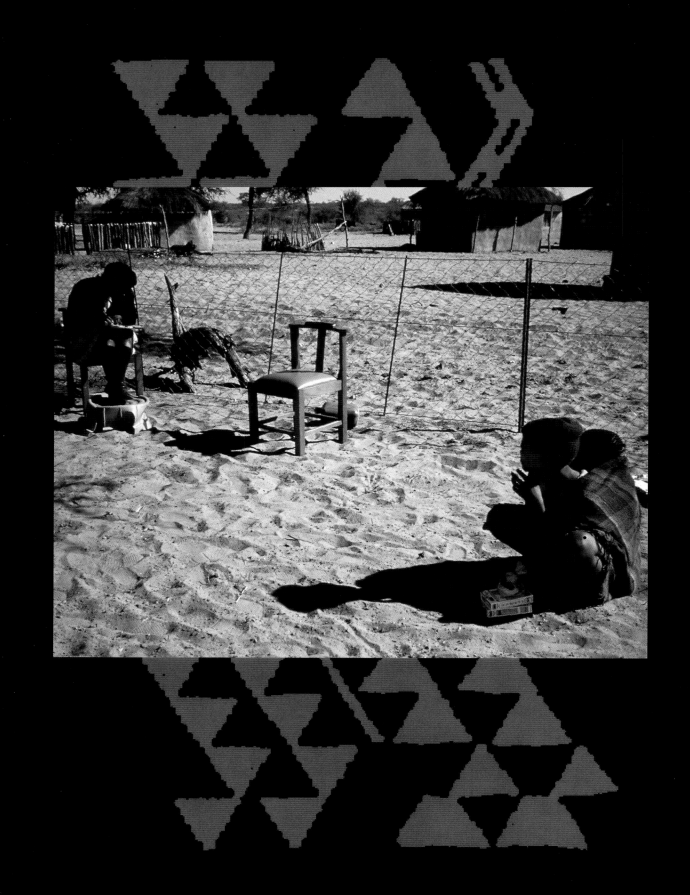

With its institutional yellow paint and fenced-in courtyard, the rectangular concrete building that houses the |Kae|kae clinic sits formal and aloof in the Kalahari sands. Part of the complex of government buildings that includes the school and residential quarters for teachers, the clinic is set apart from the village and the people. Inside the clinic is a small room with a bed for one patient to stay overnight, a dispensary with shelves loaded with medicines and pills, and a record room, where the Tswana nurse spends most of her work time entering patient data, turning individual Jul'hoansi into health statistics. Throughout the clinic there are chairs and tables—and as little as possible of the sand that forms the everyday living place of the people.

To use the clinic, prospective clients must walk through a gate. Often, they come to a window in the dispensary, whose height requires many Jul'hoansi to look up to the nurse inside in order to state their needs. Other times, they go directly to the nurse if she is sitting outside. In that case, clients sit in the sand at a distance from the nurse, who remains in her chair above them. In both approaches, the status and power difference between the nurse and the client seeking help is made clear.

The clinic has a preferred response to illness—pills and injections. Penicillin, for example, is commonly administered for a variety of ailments. On the door of the larger clinic at !Aoan, there is a sign that expresses government policy: "You don't always need injections or capsules." The sign is largely useless; not only do most Jul'hoansi not read, but most patients of the clinic are in fact given either an injection or a pill whenever they visit—and these powerfully symbolic exchanges function

REINFORCING HER STATUS, THE TSWANA NURSE SITS IN

A CHAIR WHILE ONE OF HER JUI'HOAN PATIENTS SITS

BELOW HER IN THE SAND.

6

DOES THE CLINIC HAVE N|OM?

as a wedge for the biomedical model into Jul'hoan life.

In contrast to the starkly bureaucratic clinic, the healing dance continues with its warmly human, intensely emotional atmosphere of community. Far from the clinic's square walls and chairs, the people come together in the sand to form a close-knit healing circle around the fire. Rather than rely on one supposed "expert" to dispense the limited materials of "modern medicine," the Jul'hoansi turn to boiling n|om, their spiritual healing power that covers all as it circulates from the healers throughout the dance.

How long can these contrasting cultures of help and

healing be maintained? The clinic and the Juǀ'hoan healers and their community will decide together. They will also determine what models of care will next emerge for the ǀKaeǀkae people.

The person who runs the ǀKaeǀkae clinic is officially called a "Family Welfare Educator," but in effect she is the local nurse. A Tswana woman who has been at the clinic since 1980, she is responsible for community hygiene and child care as well as the administration of medications. Among her most common tasks are treating diarrhea and dressing wounds. She also makes weekly school visits during which she looks for the symptoms of such conditions as skin problems, eye infections, and malnutrition.

The ǀKaeǀkae nurse presents a very complex ideological picture. Though she believes the healing dances can cure people, she is committed to a strict biomedical approach in her own work and neither refers people to the dances nor supports their going to the dances instead of the clinic. "We must get these people to come to the clinic first," she warns, "and quickly . . . otherwise they will keep getting sick." She sees the dance as a potential impediment, an obstacle to Juǀ'hoansi receiving the proper treatment at the proper time. "The [Juǀ'hoan] people are difficult to advise [about health matters] and slow to understand and accept health education. . . . It appears that health principles conflict with their traditional principles." She also sees the Juǀ'hoan way of living as being "dirty," an example of their failure to adapt to "modern" conditions. As a Tswana speaking about the Juǀ'hoansi, the nurse's warnings have strong undercurrents of racism. "How could they really believe in that dance?" she asks.

Yet the nurse herself believes Juǀ'hoan healers can cure.

Sometimes a critically ill patient, when taken to a healer, improved. Tshao Nǃa'an was once bitten by a snake and because we didn't have treatment for snakebites in our clinic, he was treated by one of the healers. Tshao Nǃa'an was able to recover the next day and he never received any clinical treatment.

But she emphasizes that this healing occurred without a healing dance. It is almost as if she sought to make the healing more akin to, or at least acceptable to, the biomedical model of intervention.

Interestingly, the nurse was herself once healed by a Juǀ'hoan healer:

I've never been healed by the healing dance. But once when I was pregnant, I experienced pains in my tummy. I was at our cattle post. A [Juǀ'hoan] healer was called to treat me. The healer massaged me and laid his hands on me. Later he claimed that there was a rough membrane covering my fetus and it was putting pressure on the fetus. That was the reason he gave why I felt the pain. He never prescribed anything for me. He only smeared me with the sweat from his armpits. But I was able to recover. I never felt pain again.

I was puzzled because when I asked whether the healer had gotten rid of that membrane, the healer said yes. But I never saw it being taken out of me. Yet all the same I was healed.

In describing her own healing, the nurse again emphasizes that there was no healing dance and pictures the healer's work, as much as possible, within the framework of a Western doctor treating a client. Most important, she stresses that Western medical help was unavailable on an isolated cattle post.

As the local ǀKaeǀkae nurse struggles to understand the Juǀ'hoan approach to healing, she naturally tries to accommodate it to the biomedical model of care that she is committed to. In trying to understand the experience of ǃaia, she turns to her own fear-tinged experiences in the church: "I compare the ǃaia to the trance that takes place during a church service. I think it's something like a spiritual possession." This comparison with spirit possession may help explain the Tswana nurse's deep distrust of Juǀ'hoan spirituality. In contrast to the process of boiling nǀom in which God, energy, power, and spirit all come from within human bodies, Tswana spirit possession involves being inhabited by an alien spirit. Seeking to understand boiling nǀom in

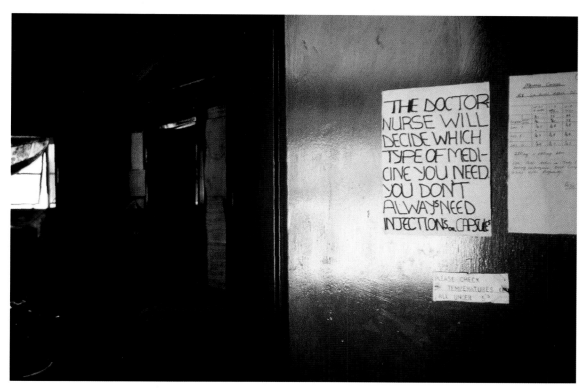

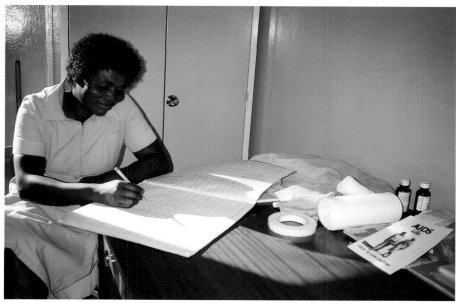

A SIGN ON THE !AOAN DISTRICT CLINIC EMPHASIZES WHO IS REALLY IN CONTROL OF HEALING DECISIONS, AS WELL AS THE TWO TREATMENTS OF CHOICE.

THE TSWANA WOMAN WHO IN EFFECT RUNS THE ǃKAEǃKAE CLINIC, AS WELL AS SERVING AS A LOCAL NURSE, SPENDS A LOT TIME WORKING ON HER CLINIC RECORDS.

her own terms, the nurse seems to regard it as an *alien* altered state, not to be trusted.

Though the ǃKaeǃkae nurse is open to many aspects of Juǀ'hoan healing, her behavior in administering health care either ignores or even denies these beliefs. The bio-

medical approach reigns supreme.

In comparison, the regional nurse, a Tswana man stationed in !Aoan, has a more accepting view of Juǀ'hoan healing, but his experience of the dance is extremely limited. Trained in the capital city of Gabarone, he is theo-

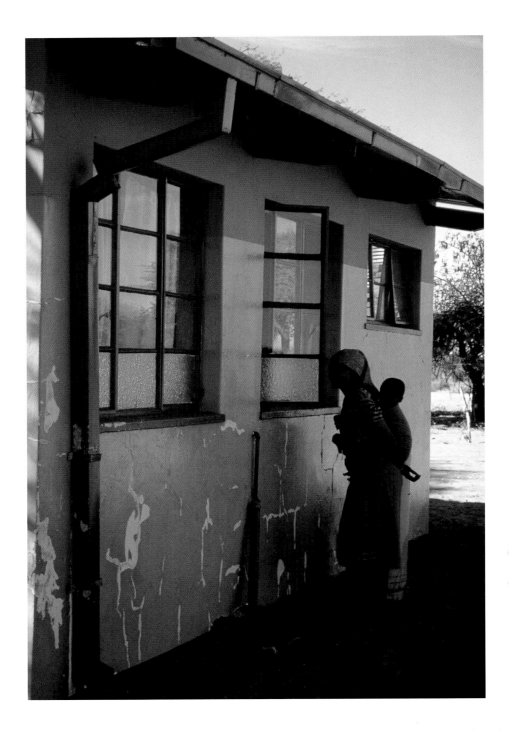

retically open to the dance but unable in practical terms to institute policies of collaboration or support. Though he supervises and is administratively responsible for the ǃKaeǃkae clinic, the local nurse runs it according to her own values and attitudes.

With a new mandate that everyone have regular medical checkups, the influence of the clinic on the community has increased. The view of the dance articulated by the local nurse is also supported by other local government institutions. The school's hygiene curriculum and

PROGRESS?

the teachers themselves reinforce the nurse's own ambivalence toward Jul'hoan healing. Pills and injections symbolize not only a manner to approach health and illness but also her way of living. The government seeks to assimilate the Jul'hoansi into the Botswana mainstream by largely denying the distinctive values of their culture.

The Jul'hoansi, on the other hand, assume a pragmatic, tolerant, and eclectic approach to health care. They are more accepting of the clinic, utilizing what is available according to their own notions of effectiveness. This approach to health care is common among traditional peoples when given the option of Western medical services and represents their effort to maximize the quality of their own care. The Jul'hoansi recognize that there is nlom in the clinic as well as their dance. As they articulate the nature of the clinic's nlom, they are beginning to define the specific value and role of the clinic in their lives.

"There are different kinds of nlom," ≠Oma Djo said. "There is the nlom in our healing dance, but there is also nlom in the clinic." ≠Oma Djo is generous in his assessment of the clinic at |Kaelkae, and he delineates the nature of the clinic's nlom, stressing its effectiveness for certain illnesses such as tuberculosis, while suggesting some of its limitations.

≠Oma Djo is building on traditional Jul'hoan values of humility about their own ways and acceptance of the ways of others, even those quite different from their own. When first exposed to Western medicines at the clinic in !Aoan, in 1968, Kxao ≠Oah said:

> [European medicine] is like ours. . . . If I were sick, and if the European healer were close by, I would go to him and drink his medicine. But if the European were far away and one of our own healers was close by, I'd go to our own and get healed.[1]

Kxao ≠Oah was a very strong, experienced healer, fully active in the traditional healing dance. Nlom had pervaded his entire life, and it was always his first option in times of illness. The broad, sparkling smile that crossed his face as he spoke of European doctors emphasized not only his desire not to offend practitioners of another way of healing, but also his easy acceptance of the pills and antibiotics. Kauh, a younger healer, expressed a profound humility toward his own Jul'hoan nlom:

> Maybe our nlom and European medicine are similar, because sometimes people who get European medicine die, and sometimes they live. That is the same with ours.[2]

Many Jul'hoansi will visit the |Kaelkae clinic, especially when they experience what have come to be identified by the people as "clinic sicknesses," which include tuberculosis, headaches, and infections. Meanwhile, the dance is the first treatment sought for nonclinic sicknesses and often for clinic sicknesses as well. Kxaru N!a'an, one of the |Kaelkae elders and a strong drum dancer, said that she goes to the clinic when she has headaches or chest pains, but then added, "When I'm really sick, I go to our own healers for them to heal me." Like most sensible people who are sick, the Jul'hoansi seek what they perceive to be the best of treatments. They will gladly use both their own healing dance and the clinic for a particular illness. The Jul'hoan values of humility and acceptance of others' ways facilitate this collaborative approach.

Does the clinic have nlom? The Jul'hoansi have already answered yes, because they realize the clinic has shown the power to cure certain illnesses. But having nlom in the clinic does not negate or detract from the nlom in their dance. Does the Jul'hoan dance have nlom? The clinic nurse seems to acknowledge the power of healers to heal. But she has not acknowledged the existence or reality of nlom and continually downplays the spiritual, community context of the dance. If others follow the lead of the Jul'hoansi, there is some chance the two systems of health care can survive together and even collaborate to provide the people with superior health care.

But a primary threat to a working relationship between the two health systems comes from the government bureaucracy. If the government remains fully committed only to the biomedical model, the Jul'hoan approach will be threatened.

But there are hopeful signs. As part of the worldwide recognition of the value and contribution of Indigenous healing practices, the Botswana medical school is considering the development of curriculum material about Jul'hoan and other Indigenous healing. The openness of the regional nurse to Jul'hoan healing is indicative of this shift. Government practitioners who shared his openness, especially if Jul'hoan nurses were introduced into the system, could turn these promising signs into a reality of collaboration. To accomplish this, the local nurse would have to be convinced that supporting Jul'hoan healing need not contradict or undercut her own biomedical practice.

The government has also sponsored regional seminars devoted to the topic of Indigenous healing. But thus far these seminars have not fulfilled their potential. The local |Kae|kae nurse has attended but has not discussed Jul'hoan healing there because she feels "people in the region already know about it." Most important, though Jul'hoan healers have been invited, they have yet to attend. The government usually notifies them about the seminars too late for them to arrange transportation. Such seminars could become points of open exchange and a foundation for effective collaborative healing efforts.

|Kae|kae Jul'hoansi sense the institutional power behind the clinic and wish to learn lessons from its apparent institutional longevity. Tshao Matze spoke about the young people:

The kids of today, if you say you'll teach them
along well, and you teach them, and teach them,
and teach them, they think you're just fooling
around. They don't remember that people will die.
The people at the clinic make sure to teach more
and more people, so that even if a doctor dies,
another one knows how to do medicine.

But the Jul'hoansi of today—they aren't like
those of us in the past who learned. If they were
people who'd put their hearts into it, OK, that'd be
fine. But they don't.

As Tshao Matze compares the education of young healers with what he understands about the clinic's Western medical education, he reveals anxiety over whether the traditional strengths of Jul'hoan society will continue.

In other parts of the world, Indigenous peoples have taken the opportunity to choose in their own way from their own and a Western, biomedically oriented healthcare system and to choose their own preferred sequence of treatment. Dick has seen such situations in the Fiji Islands, for example.[3] He has seen three principles at work in successful collaborations. First, there is a mutual respect between practitioners in the two systems. The Jul'hoansi have already offered their respect. Second, neither system can operate in an imperialistic fashion, claiming the ability to heal every illness. Again, the Jul'hoansi have never assumed such an attitude. Jul'hoan healers continually emphasize that they are not able to treat all illnesses, and most important, that any success or lack of success they have is ultimately due not to their own power but to the wishes of the spirits and the great God. Third, practitioners in each system must know how to make referrals to the other system. Here again it seems the Jul'hoansi healers are taking the lead, as they willingly go to the clinic and suggest that others do the same.

Whereas the Jul'hoansi are clearing the path for collaboration, the clinic and in particular the local nurse show little interest in traditional healing. She remains convinced that better hygiene and the "pills and injections" approach will eventually cure everything if only given time. And she has yet to refer any of her clients to the dance.

Can the clinic develop the necessary respect for the dance and initiate the exchanges that would provide the people with more and better treatment options? Put another way, can the clinic give up the power it has accumulated and share healing tasks with the people? Given that the growing world recognition of the value of Indigenous community healing is echoed by the regional nurse and some of the medical school administrators, there is hope.

But with this hope, caution must remain. It is

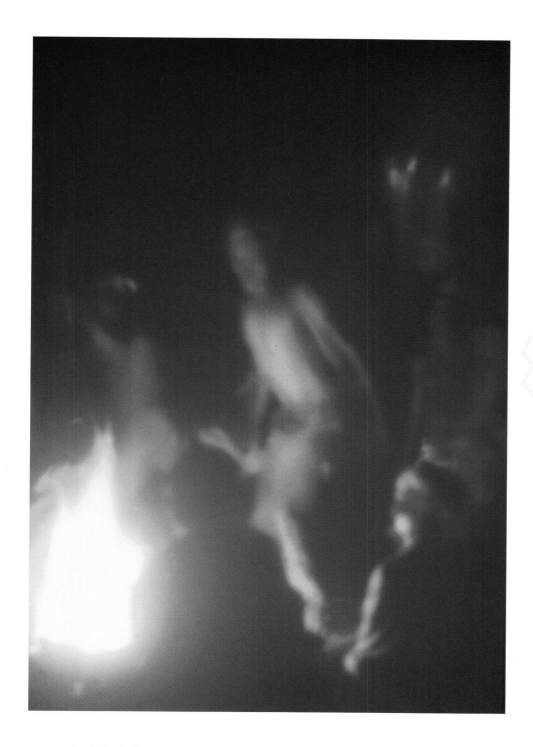

JUI'HOAN DANCERS AND SINGERS, UNITED BY THE GLOW OF THE FIRE, FORGE BONDS OF COMMUNITY AND ALSO CELEBRATE INDIVIDUAL CREATIVITY THROUGH THEIR PARTICIPATION IN THE HEALING DANCE.

extremely difficult for a government bureaucracy committed to "modernizing" the nation to support fully an Indigenous approach whose heart is spiritual healing. Seen by many bureaucrats as the "enemy" of progress, n|om and the healing dance are hard to accept, especially with their profound egalitarian, communal, and spiritual implications.[4]

Most of all, the aim for |Kae|kae health care should be

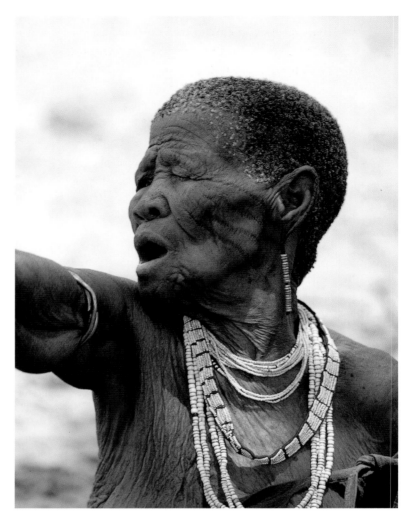

consistent with the Jul'hoan value of living with, even celebrating, differences whether they be in personalities, opinions, or ways of living. Research suggests that the most effective combination of care allows each different approach to healing to maintain its own integrity rather than constructing one unified system that merges or integrates approaches.[5] "Integrating" approaches seems to lead to the traditional, Indigenous system being subsumed under the Western system and eventually being stripped of its unique contributions, particularly its spiritual healing power. On the other hand, with the collaboration model, persons could participate in the healing dance even when they were being treated at the clinic, with the full support and encouragement of its staff.

But for such collaboration to occur, racist attitudes toward the value, indeed the reality, of Jul'hoan nlom and by extension Jul'hoan culture must be confronted and removed. Tshao Matze analyzes the situation succinctly:

> Black people have their nlom, and White people
> have theirs, and we Jul'hoansi have our own. But
> Black people are prejudiced and say Jul'hoansi are
> nothing-things, and don't know anything. How is it
> that you people [who come to work with us] from
> America know we have knowledge, but those from
> here do not know it?

IXoan N!a'an, a very old, charismatic woman who

healed frequently and most powerfully in the G!oci area during the 1960s, offered the grounding for healing systems—and people and their cultures—to work together.

> People were created by . . . [God] with different things to use, different skins, and different nǀom. The Blacks have their nǀom in divination and sorcery, the Europeans have their nǀom in pills and steel needles, and the Juǀ'hoansi have their nǀom in the . . . [healing dance]. Different nǀom, very different ways of living. But when you cut any one of them their blood flows the same color.[6]

As a well-schooled young person in 1989, Kxao ǀOǀOo offers a more pragmatic version of ǀXoan N!a'an's vision:

> I think the healers and the clinic should work together. Because sometimes with some of the sicknesses we need to go to the healers, and sometimes with some of the sicknesses, like malaria, we need to go to the clinic.

With a sense of mutual respect and humility and the aim to serve the people most fully, collaboration between different approaches to health and healing would be in the true Juǀ'hoan spirit.

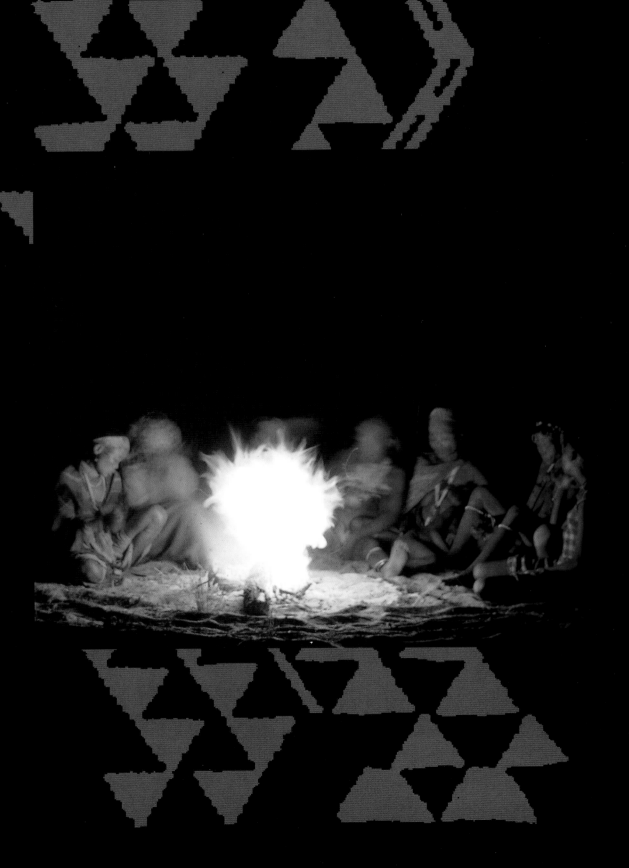

Mixed in the evening in large pots, the kaq'amakoq berries and other ingredients are propelled by the sugar and yeast to do their work throughout the night. By early morning the *!xari,* or homebrew, is ready. The drinking will soon begin.

Alcohol travels quickly into a people's heart.[1] It was only in the mid-1970s that it became widely available at |Kae|kae, yet its trail of destruction among Jul'hoansi people is evident. During periods when beer-brewing ingredients are available, it is easy to observe almost daily one manifestation of drinking: half a dozen or so Jul'hoansi walking home unsteadily in a ragged line from one of the Herero homesteads in the vanishing daylight, signaling the end of the !xari supply at the homestead. "If there is any money among the Jul'hoansi, people drink every day," comments |Kaece "China."

!Xari is made regularly only by the Tswana and Herero peoples. They are the only ones who can afford the non-local ingredients, including the sugar and yeast. They brew it not only for their own consumption, but also for sale to the Jul'hoansi, thus turning this !xari into a weapon of sociopolitical oppression. The scenario of alcohol devastating a disempowered group as it profits another group with greater economic and political power has tragically been played and replayed through-out the world.

!Xari has begun eating away at the Jul'hoan will, as well as their ability to live together in the close quarters of their traditional camps. Alcohol consumption among the Jul'hoansi introduces a new level of violence into the community. ≠Oma Djo gets right to the point:

ILLUMINATED BY THE HEALING DANCE

FIRE, THE WOMEN SINGERS

BOND TOGETHER DURING THE DARK

KALAHARI NIGHT.

7

"THE PEOPLE ARE DRINKING THE MEAT"

Today people are insulting each other and fighting [because of their drinking]. !Xari makes us fight, that's what it does. Our home has become a bad place [because of this !xari].

Xumi N!a'an adds his views:

!Xari brings you madness, anger, and death. Sometimes people look at each other and just start to fight. They might even kill each other. That's why I don't like it.

As one of the most vocal critics of drinking, Xumi N!a'an struggles to remain sober; he says he refuses !xari because of the "kind of work it does." When people ask him to come drink, he tells us he doesn't go because "beer is a bad thing":

> Sometimes people tell you there is only a little bit of !xari left, and [you should come, but people still] get angry and fight. I don't like that !xari—it's bad stuff.

As the Jul'hoan community tears at its own fabric, those in power—those who are making the homebrew—profit. Only those who already have *sufficient* money from selling cattle or drawing government salaries, for instance, make money from this enterprise. The cycle of dependence and economic exploitation becomes complete.

Traditionally, meat from the hunt was distributed freely and widely so that no one remained hungry in the camp. Some hunters like ≠Oma !'Homg!ausi and Tshao Matze still value that sharing ethic, though their distribution is more focused upon and limited to their own camps. But now other hunters often will sell most of the meat from a kill, and only the Hereros and Tswana can afford to buy it. Aside from the hunter and his immediate family, few Jul'hoansi now eat meat from such a kill. The money from selling that meat initiates a new wave of sadness and pain, as the hunter usually spends his income to buy homebrew for himself and his family. "The people are drinking the meat," observes ≠Oma Djo.

Sometimes there is a pot of !xari available in one of the Jul'hoan camps. Then the traditional Jul'hoan sharing ethic receives another blow, an especially perverse one. The brew, made by either Hereros or Tswana, is then turned over to a Jul'hoan to be sold to other Jul'hoansi. The pot of !xari sits outside one of the Julhoan homes, and the people gather around to talk, to visit, and to drink. But instead of this resource of !xari being shared, it is sold—and even close relatives of the one entrusted with the supply are expected to buy their drinks. The Jul'hoan in charge of the supply must "account" for the distribution of the homebrew and is cautioned against "free" drinks. Selected Jul'hoansi find themselves becoming entrepreneurs who unwillingly thrive off the misery of their own people, though even then they earn only a minimal compensation.

We cannot comment upon the precise extent of the drinking that goes on at |Kae|kae, among either the Jul'hoansi or the Tswana or the Hereros. Since so many Jul'hoansi do drink, and there is already an idea that drinking is "not a good thing," Jul'hoan people prefer not to talk much about alcohol use, wishing to avoid too public a criticism of others. There is, for example, a real hesitancy to identify any one person as "drinking too much."

Because we respected the people's own sense of privacy about drinking behavior, we did not intrude any systematic observational activities to document issues such as the number of drinkers and the frequency of drinking. But we noticed no apparent differences between women and men, or between healers as a group and others in regard to the frequency of alcohol consumption during the ordinary day. At the dances, however, healers rarely were drunk and, if they were, it was a cause for concern. But clearly alcohol has become a poison running through the Jul'hoan community, threatening to contaminate if not erode the healing power of the dance in the process. Kommtsa N!a'an is unyielding in his comments:

> If you drink a lot of beer you'll lose your n/om. Because beer goes into each part of your body, including your bones, so that after a while you just stop [doing n/om]. Beer makes your legs weak. All you see is the sand because you're lying on it all the time.

"The young people don't put their hearts into the dance [anymore]. . . . [It is now] !xari only," lamented ≠Oma !'Homg!ausi. "Heart," of course, is the essential ingredient in learning to "drink n|om." |Xoan, regarded as an especially strong singer over the five decades of her life, speaks with a quiet sadness: "It was much better for the singing when there was no !xari. Now the dance is weaker. !Xari has ruined the dance."

The young people see the same effects of !xari even with their briefer perspective. "In my growing-up years,"

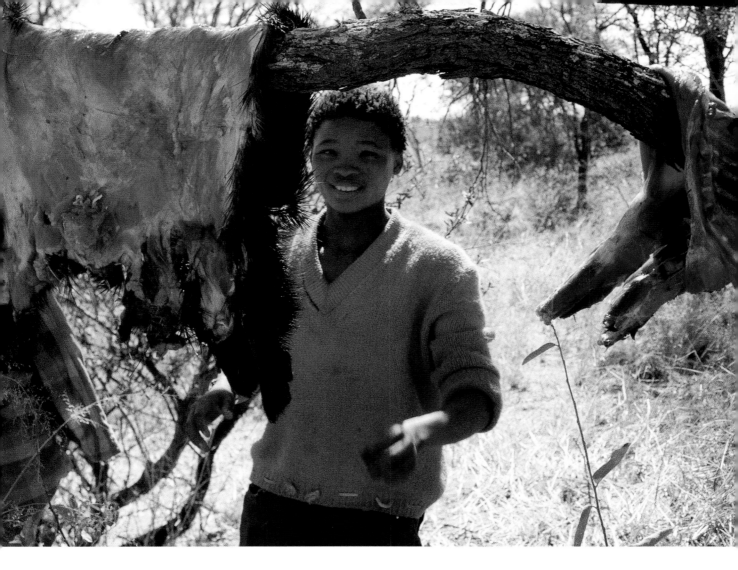

states Kxao ǀOǀOo, "the dances were powerful, but today they are weaker because of the !xari." A person whose education gives him a special view into possibilities for the future, Kxao ǀOǀOo remains pessimistic about the effects of drinking at ǀKaeǀkae:

> I think that if the people continue their drinking, in the years to come there will be no development, . . . and it seems as if the drinking won't stop. The drinking will continue and continue. [When I try to tell others to stop] they say, "No, we are just going on for a little while and then we will quit." But they don't.

In 1968, when there was no drinking at ǀKaeǀkae

TSHAO XUMI, ONE OF OUR JUǀ'HOAN TRANSLATORS AND A MEMBER OF THE RESEARCH TEAM, HANGS UP THE SKIN AND MEAT OF A PORCUPINE HE HAS JUST KILLED, PRIOR TO SHARING IT WITH OTHERS.

among the Juǀ'hoansi, people nevertheless knew about alcohol and its effects on the mind. Being drunk was universally considered a "bad thing." As Khallʼan, a strong healer from !Aoan said, a person who is drunk does not "know people. You start off talking nicely but then you can't finish." Healers in particular distinguished between nǀom and alcohol, making clear that the effects were quite different. "Nǀom is one thing, alcohol is something

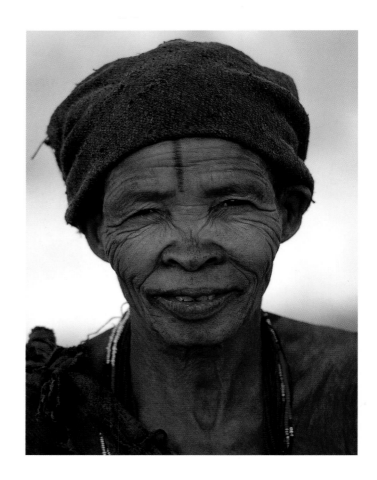

else," ǂOma Djo emphasized, "and they are two different things that don't belong together." He went on to state that though one could ǃaia from alcohol, it was not the same as nǀom ǃaia. Alcohol ǃaia had no connection with healing; at its best, it could provide relaxation or release. At its worst, it led to violence.

But though people in 1989 still retain a clear sense that nǀom and alcohol are "two different things" that do not mix, they have already witnessed many occasions during which alcohol has intruded upon and undercut nǀom and its healing functions. The "two things" *are* mixing—with tragic results.

During a large dance that occurs after a feast we put on to mark our imminent departure from the Kalahari, one of the younger but experienced healers arrives drunk. Struggling to maintain his balance, he moves awkwardly among the dancers, his bizarre and jagged movements a pitiful imitation of Julʼhoan dancing. Sometimes slumping onto other dancers, sometimes stumbling into their paths, his presence clearly interferes with the other dancers. Gradually, several of them try gently to encourage him to leave the dance and sit on the periphery. They put their arms around his shoulders and try to dance him away and talk with him, asking him to rest so the others can dance properly. He continually resists. Finally, efforts to get him to leave become more firm, and he is taken by the arm and partly led and partly dragged away.

As dramatic as the drunken behavior itself is the unwillingness of others to confront the drunk person and force him to leave. The Julʼhoan tolerance for differences and respect for individual independence, which prevent too quick or harsh a response, also allow disruptive behavior to carry on for nearly an hour. Equally dramatic is the power the dance structure retains, which ensures its continuity until he is finally gone.

On another occasion, during an evening drum dance held in one of the Julʼhoan camps, an experienced and powerful healer arrives drunk, begins playing the drum, and then begins to ǃaia. His unsteady movements do not prevent him from doing some healing work. Nobody tries to stop him, perhaps because he is an elder and his nǀom is so respected, and perhaps because his drinking does not on the surface interfere with his drumming and healing actions. Xumi Nǃaʼan offers another explanation of the drunken healer's behavior:

He drank enough !xari to be tipsy, but had just begun to taste it. Thus, he was still able to heal. But if he had drunk a lot, he wouldn't have been able to bring the nǀom he has. [What he was doing] would look like !aia, but it would all belong to !xari. He wouldn't "see" anything [in that !aia and therefore couldn't heal]. Then he would just leave off.

According to Xumi N!a'an, the healer who had been drinking did not pass over some line that would have made alcohol a definite detraction from nǀom. ≠Oma Djo seems to support Xumi N!a'an's position. "If I want to do my work well," he claims, "beer will never defeat me." But ≠Oma Djo emphasizes he is talking about a "little bit" of beer, and in fact we have never seen him even a little drunk at any dances and no one has ever reported him being in that condition at one. If judgments like Xumi N!a'an's are increasingly made, and therefore some mixing of nǀom and alcohol is allowed, the entire relationship of !xari to the healing dance will change. As there is no Juǀ'hoan tradition or experience in a strict and disciplined use of alcohol for healing purposes, the change would not bode well.

Many questions remain for us after witnessing dances such as those described above. Would participants at the large dance ever have allowed the dance to be fully disrupted? Throughout the young healer's drunken behavior, the dance continued; the singing and dancing seemed strong enough to ward off the disturbing effects of the drunken healer. And did the fact that we were hosting the dance make it a less-Juǀ'hoan occasion and therefore more susceptible to the intrusion of alcohol? In contrast, we never saw drunken behavior around any of the smaller healing dances performed inside one of the Juǀ'hoan camps. Perhaps these dances, always focused on one or more sick persons, had become a protected arena, which all understood were not to be violated with alcohol. But would there be a "first time" there, too?

Alcohol consumption has had a particular effect on some of the young Juǀ'hoansi's desire to learn to become healers. Their minds and hearts seem elsewhere, no longer focused on the dance.

At first, the Hereros were selling homebrew. We Juǀ'hoansi stayed together just fine, and the only thing we had was dancing. People danced and sang together. Every day. When the Hereros didn't bring sugar, everything was fine.

But now that the Hereros are traders, homebrew is here at ǀKaeǀkae. When I go home to my village, everyone is just in terrible shape. They sit and talk, talk, talk . . . they drink and go crazy. They drink until their speech sounds foul.

This is how one of the experienced healers, who struggles to remain sober, describes the situation in his camp, which has an unusually large number of adolescents and young adults.

When will alcohol be perceived by the Juǀ'hoansi as a community problem that needs to be resolved?[2] And, most important, when will alcoholism be viewed by outsiders not as another excuse to blame the victim but as a symptom of oppression? Such awarenesses mark the recovery of communities throughout the world from the devastating grip of alcohol abuse and seem particularly essential to the Juǀ'hoan people, especially if they are to avoid the more profound and pervasive forms of that abuse.

The traditional Juǀ'hoan tolerance for individual differences describe an outer limit on behaviors such as physical violence, which threaten the cohesiveness and survival of the community. As many of the elders are already suggesting, alcohol abuse must now be considered unacceptable. "We cannot let those who are drinking stop our dance," warns Xumi N!a'an, an elder whose dedication to the dance is legendary. "!Xari is killing us," warns Kxao Tjimburu, one of the most energetic of the ǀKaeǀkae healers, who likewise is committed to remaining sober.

Xumi N!a'an is particularly upset that some of the younger Juǀ'hoansi, following in the path of their parents, are also drinking. He sees the especially devastating consequences of such occurrences. Xumi N!a'an stresses that it is a "very bad thing" for children to watch their parents drinking.

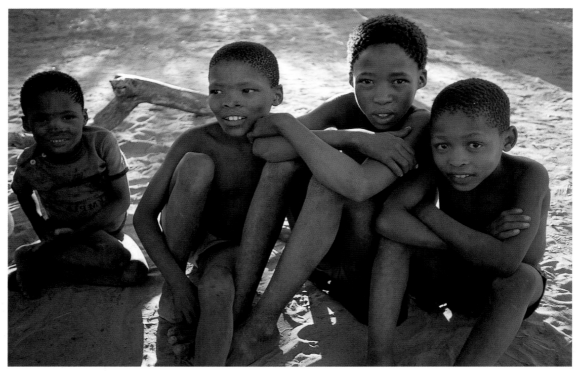

[In our way] when you "eat" something and a child just watches, and you don't give it some, that is bad. If you eat and don't give some to the child, that is death. . . . But if I see someone who gives !xari to children, I'll really fight them. I don't drink, and I don't want a small child of mine to drink.

If Kxao Tjimburu finds himself in a place where !xari is being served, he avoids drinking. "I refuse to 'eat' it," he states, "because it is not the type of food I want. I refuse it and sit awhile and, if I see they're doing bad things, I'll go away." ≠Oma Djo describes his response to drinking, typical of traditional Jul'hoan methods of avoiding conflict and criticism: "If I see people drinking, I never talk with them; I just pass by."

Across the world, particularly among communities of Indigenous peoples, there is a struggle to overcome the tragic consequences of alcoholism. There is often a pattern to that community struggle, a cycle that runs almost inevitably through a period of denial to the recognition that people and the community have hit "rock bottom,"

where nothing worse can be imagined. Often starting with one or two individuals, there is then a turning point, a refusal to continue on the path to further destruction and a courageous stand against the forces of oppression that nourish the community's ties to alcohol. With dedication, honesty, and humility, these few individuals fan the spark in others. With much pain and patience and often strengthened by a revitalized traditional spirituality, the weight in the community eventually begins to shift toward sobriety. A sober community becomes a possibility.[3]

No one can say where |Kae|kae will go in its dealings with alcohol. But even at these beginning stages of alcohol use at |Kae|kae, there are resisters to alcohol abuse. And some of the most powerful voices of concern are found among the healers. While emphasizing the link between alcohol and violence, they restate what the people have always known: alcohol and n|om are "two different things, which do not mix." By drawing attention to the potential destruction of the healing dance, their voice allows the people to see in a dramatic way how alcohol kills.

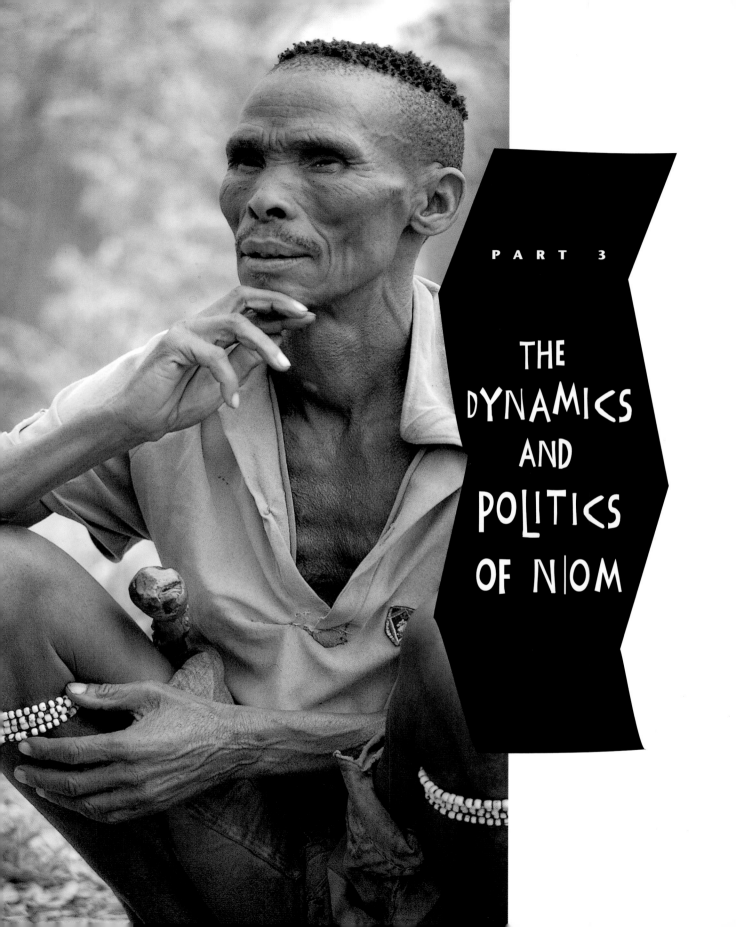

PART 3

THE DYNAMICS AND POLITICS OF N|OM

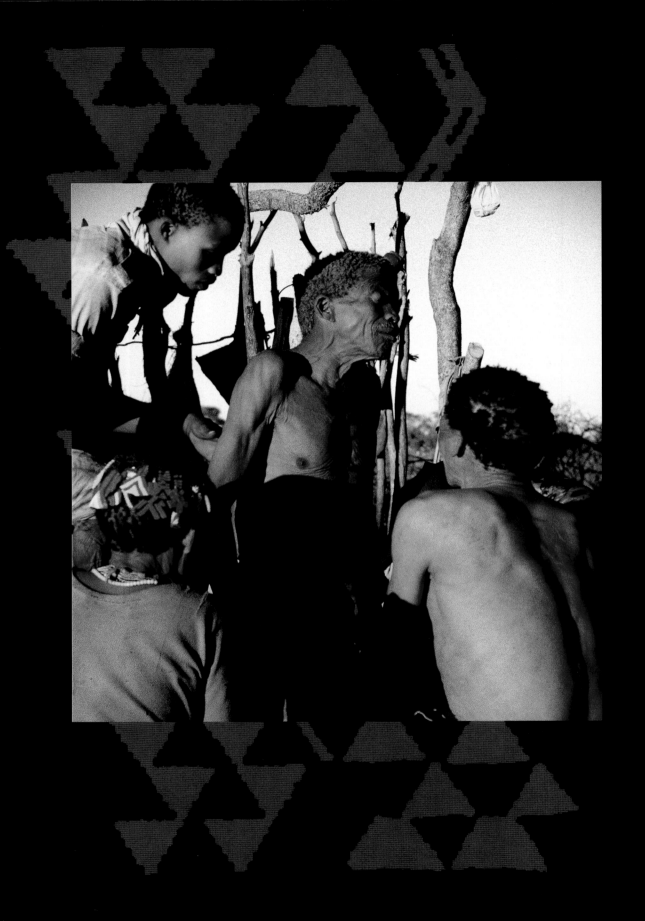

The healing dance persists into these times of threatened cultural disintegration. But it has changed in a dynamic relationship with the other trends. There is less focus on a cross-camp healing ceremony in which separate camps come together and more focus on individual camps putting on their own dances. Also, the dances in general seem shorter; during our stay in 1989 no dance lasts much beyond midnight, whereas in 1968, dances often went on into the early morning and at times until dawn or even further. It's as if the people are not as willing to spend the long nights together on their healing journey, as if a sense of connectedness has lessened. Also, there is more concentration on curing specific illnesses and less of the older emphasis on generic healing, of being together at the dance to recreate community, with the cure of particular illnesses being only one part of that experience.

Despite this apparent weakening of communal bonds, the commitment among individual healers to spiritual journeying seems to have become more intense, suggesting a deepening of the dance's power. The experience of !aia, the healers' state of transcendence that results from the nIom boiling inside them, remains rich and varied. In fact, we find that !aia reaches profound levels of challenge and liberation in even more healers today than it did twenty years ago. Spiritual journeys that used to be spoken of by only a few of the older, more experienced healers are now described by most of the older healers and some of the younger experienced healers as well. Now many healers turn into lions in order to travel

8

CLIMBING THE THREADS TO GOD'S VILLAGE

rapidly and with power, visiting faraway places to heal the sick. They go to God's village, risking their lives to rescue the sick person's soul.

Can this apparent increased individual commitment to the spiritual journey, to risking one's life in order to heal others, fuel the dance fire and bring people together through the dance? For though individuals speak of these journeys, they are in essence made and enabled by the community, which sends the healers forth on their perilous travels as their representatives to engage the gods in the pursuit of healing.

These transformations of consciousness in the dance

PEOPLE GATHER AROUND ≠OMA DJO, NOW DEEPLY IN

!AIA, TO HELP HIM AS HE STRUGGLES TO REGULATE HIS

BOILING NIOM.

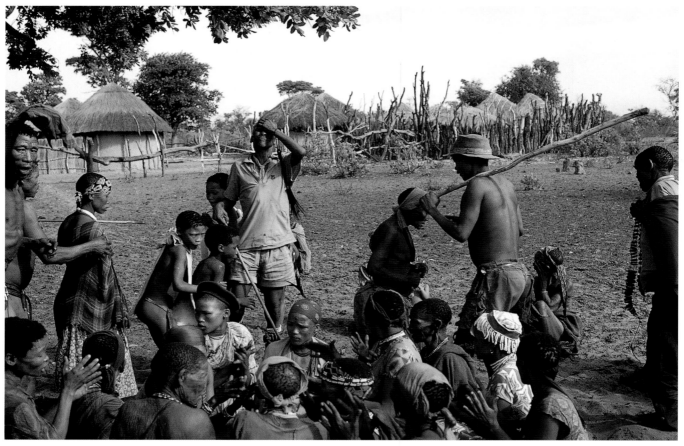

DANCING INTO !AIA, BLIND KXAO ≠OAH PUTS HIS HAND

TO HIS HEAD AS HE FEELS THE N|OM BOILING EVER MORE FIERCELY INSIDE.

clearly radiate life among Jul'hoansi today. But we want to ask if these same transformations already or can eventually also feed political evolution. Are suggestions for the direction of social change encoded in the spiritual experience of the healers? Can contacting the profound mysteries of their culture offer support for meeting the everyday confusions and frustrations that surround the people? Does the terrain of that spirit world offer guidance for the treacherous political landscape now confronting the Jul'hoansi?

All these questions are prompted by our knowledge of the challenges the Jul'hoansi face today and by our observations of the profound healing that always seems to have been available through n|om. Though such questions are ones that the Jul'hoansi themselves might not pose at all or in the same form, their "answers" are far from simple. In the rest of this chapter, we try to trace the threads of their answers, emerging, we hope, with a way of understanding our questions from a Jul'hoan point of view.

THE RAW POWER OF N|OM

The Jul'hoansi often reply to our questions with a story. They resist generalizing and stay with the concrete, enabling us to see, time and time again, the unmistakable raw power of n|om and !aia. N|om heals the people. ≠Oma !'Homg!ausi, a strong and dedicated healer, recounts how n|om, and the spirit world n|om comes from, saved his life:

One morning, I was walking around hunting. I heard a leopard talking, going "huh, huh, huh." I walked along and soon saw an ostrich. I lay down my bow and stalked the ostrich. The leopard was lying under a tree. So I got my bow and went after him [for his skin]. I chased him and he hid himself and lay down. I couldn't see him. I looked for him and he jumped at me. We fought. I had wanted to kill him for his skin. We grabbed each other and fought. He tried to bite me on my side. I got my arm in between so he tried to climb up me. Then I stabbed him with my knife, but I hit one of his bones. He sprang at me again. I threw him down. The knife tip was bent against the bone of the leopard. So I tried to choke him. I put my hands in his mouth. He bit me and I pulled my hands out. He bit right through my hand. I grabbed his mouth and then stabbed him in the side. He ran off and I chased him. And finally he died.

So I left him and started to travel home. I was all alone. Blood was pouring off me. My chest was open so that you could see my heart. Part of my lung was sticking out. Nlom was with me that first night. It is the reason I didn't die.

The next day I took care of myself. I scraped the blood out [of my wounds], because I wanted it to come out, not to stay inside my chest. If you just leave it inside, it kills you. I slept on the way, and another day dawned. There were waterholes, and I drank lots of water and died. When dawn broke I got up and finally arrived at my home.

Ten days later I was covered with sores and my hand was in terrible shape. Hunger and thirst killed me and I didn't know what I was doing. One old woman said I was too crippled and she'd have to leave me in the village.

It was then that my mother's father, who died ten years earlier, came to me and said: "What are you doing?" I had died and he told me to get up. He said, "I've already died and you aren't going to die also. Get up." And I got up.

≠Oma !'Homg!ausi means ≠Oma "Leopard Claws," a name he has earned. The scarred crevices and puncture wounds that appear on his chest, arm, and hand scream out the pain of his battle; his muscular physique, normal movements, and vigorous approach to activities document the miracle of his recovery. It is with that same vigor that ≠Oma !'Homg!ausi approaches discussions of politics and social change. He had been appointed to serve on the |Kae|kae village council, a body of Tswana, Herero, and Jul'hoan representatives formed for village government, but he resigned in disgust, feeling that his voice—and through him the voice of the Jul'hoansi—was not heard.

TENSIONS WITHIN THE COMMUNITY

When tensions and conflict emerge within the community, the Jul'hoansi often turn to the dance as a way of reducing or even resolving that difficulty. The Jul'hoan dance has a way of including human diversity, of allowing people with different points of view to coexist. It brings the diverse individuals of a camp into vital contact with each other in such a way that the uniqueness of each is felt as a contribution to group life rather than as a threat to it.

If there is bad feeling between two women, others will contrive to put them next to each other in the singing circle; participating in that form of sisterhood paves the way for a more enduring sisterhood to reestablish itself. The circular frame of the dance unites all the people into a single dynamic form.

At one dance, the circle of the singing women around the fire has not formed. Instead, the women sit so they form two curved lines, neither more than a quarter circle. These two lines wrap around opposite sides of the fire, and the gaps between the lines speak silently of a glaring rift. Each line contains predominantly women from one of two |Kae|kae camps involved in an ongoing dispute about a prospective divorce. The dance has no power; the singing is desultory.

Arguments begin between the two lines of women, shouts about each other's "stinginess" or "bad manners." The shouting escalates, dominating the dance for a moment. Then two older women, facing each other at opposite ends of the two lines, bring the angry exchange to a climax. Suddenly, as each feels some redress has been won, they agree to resolve their differences and move on with the dance. Each of the women grandly rises from her spot at the end of her line and moves around the fire toward the other. They sit down again, now next to each other. The other women follow their lead, merging to form one tight singing circle. The mood of the dance immediately lightens and laughter breaks out. The songs take on a new vitality, and very soon the dance ignites. Strong n!om is activitated within hours. A dispute that had poisoned the atmosphere of the village had threatened to poison the dance as well. Instead the dispute is overwhelmed by the circle of healing the dance stimulates.

Sometimes an unspoken tension in the community is expressed by the healers in !aia, and in this way the threat to the harmonious relations so valued by the Ju/'hoansi is dispelled. The chant that follows, sung in a drawn-out and intermittent fashion by one of the healers while in !aia, displays this tension-reduction activity in action.[1] The sick person being healed is described by the healer as being sick as a result of tension in the group. Some of the words of the chant have distinct reference to a specific social situation, namely a disagreement about cattle, being aired and alleviated through the dance.

> . . . Are you looking at each other?
>
> How is it that you are full adults, yet you refuse to give each other an agreement? What makes you tremble at seeing each other? What do you see when you look at each other?
>
> You people here who are arguing and glaring. You people who are arguing and glaring. You people who are arguing and glaring.
>
> What makes you do that is your argument about cattle. You are battling it out and you are killing each other.
>
> His blanket, help him put it over his shoulders; can't you see, he is trembling? Help him cover himself.
>
> He is exhausted; his arms are dry; his legs are dry. Help him take his blanket and cover him. . . .
>
> He lies there dying; while you sit above him wrangling and fighting and arguing and glaring, arguing and glaring, arguing and glaring. . . .

Ancient as the dance is, it can embody new realizations such as misunderstandings about recently introduced cattle. Dance is the one activity in Ju/'hoan life in which virtually all members of the group participate. Its greatest strength may lie in its inclusiveness, its ability to make a whole of whatever group is present, even as it expands for a newcomer. While a dance is in progress, it essentially fills the social universe, taking precedence over all other activities. The delight in being part of a shared activity and the feeling of community that is brought about by joining together to banish trouble from the group are important elements in the meaning of the dance circle.

People today speak of this social healing function of the dance, emphasizing how n!om eventually makes "everything right." They describe not only the reduction of tensions within the Ju/'hoan community, but the possible move toward harmony between the Ju/'hoansi and other groups. They point out that despite their long persecution at the hands of the Tswana and Hereros, they are hopeful of eventual peace with them. They say that in 1989 United Nations officials came to neighboring South West Africa to help supervise the independence elections, and these officials said to the ethnic groups there that "we should all be friends."

SPIRITUAL JOURNEYS

Healers mediate healing power and information about how things are in the spirit world and how people in this world can best relate to these spirits. Therefore, great attention is given to healers' accounts of what they have experienced, and no one's account of a genuinely altered state is treated casually.

Nearly twenty years ago, Kxao ≠Oah, a strong healer who was totally blind, told the memorable story of his spiritual journey to God's village and of the threads of the sky. Others listened intently. All regarded it as an important piece of the truth.

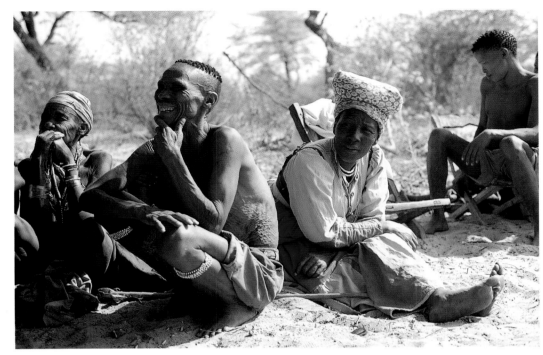

KXAO ≠OAH, THE
RESPECTED BLIND HEALER,
AND HIS WIFE N!AQE TU
(LEFT) RELAX IN THE SAND
WITH A HERERO WOMAN IN
THE WARM AFTERGLOW OF
A HEALING DANCE, WHEN
TENSIONS ARE ERASED.

Just yesterday, giraffe came and took me again. God came and took me and said, "Why is it that people are singing, yet you're not dancing?" When he spoke, he took me with him and we left this place. We traveled until we came to a wide body of water. It was a river. He took me to the river. The two halves of the river lay to either side of us, one to the left and one to the right.

God made the waters climb, and I laid my body in the direction they were flowing. My feet were behind, and my head was in front. That's how I lay. Then I entered the stream and began to move forward. I entered it and my body began to do like this. [Kxao ≠Oah waved his hands dreamily to show how his body traveled forward, undulating in the water.] I traveled like this. My sides were pressed by pieces of metal. Metal things fastened my sides. And in this way I traveled forward. That's how I was stretched out in the water. And the spirits were singing.

The spirits were having a dance. I began to dance it too, hopping around like this. I joined the dance and I danced with them, but God said to

me, "Don't come here and start to dance like that; now you just lie down and watch. This is how you should dance," he said, as he showed me how to dance. So the two of us danced that way. We danced and danced. We went to my protector and God said to him, "Here is your son." To me God said, "This man, your protector, will carry you and put nlom into you."[2] The man took hold of my feet. He made me sit up straight. But I was under water! I was gasping for breath. I called out, "Don't kill me! Why are you killing me?" My protector answered, "If you cry out like that, I'm going to make you drink. Today I'm certainly going to make you drink water. . . ."

The two of us struggled until we were tired. We danced and argued and I fought the water for a long, long time. We did it until the cocks began to crow. [Kxao ≠Oah softly sang a medicine song.]

That's how my protector sang. He told me that was how I should sing. So I sang that song and sang it and sang it until I had sung in the daybreak. Then my protector spoke to me, saying that I would be able to heal. He said that I would stand

up and !aia. He told me that I would !aia. And the
!aia he was talking about, I was already doing it.
Then he said he would give me something to drink.
. . . He made me drink it and said that I would
dance the dance I had learned. And so I have just
stuck with that dance and grown up with it.

Then my protector told me that I would enter
the earth. That I would travel far through the earth
and then emerge at another place. When we
emerged, we began to climb the thread—it was
the thread of the sky!

Now up there in the sky, the people up there,
the spirits, the dead people up there, they sang for
me so I can dance.[3]

Though a degree of cultural patterning is present in
many healers' accounts of travels into the spirit world,
the Jul'hoansi treat these experiences as unique messages
from the beyond. Because these journeys are accessible in
no other way than through !aia, narratives of these experiences are regarded as valuable documents.

Elements of the !aia experience suggest parallels
between spiritual journeys and political actions. The use
of "hot," powerful nlom for "cool," peaceful, harmonious social purposes is emphasized over and over in
Jul'hoan folktales about spiritual transformation. The
daring involved in spiritual journeying echoes the
courage necessary to challenge death in the dangerous
areas of everyday life, such as hunting, pregnancy and
childbirth, confronting capricious weather, and avoiding large carnivores.

Climbing the "threads of the sky" to God's village
offers an especially dramatic example of possible parallels between spiritual journeying and political action.
"We climb these invisible threads to God's village to rescue the souls of the sick ones, and bring them back to
our village," says ≠Oma Djo. Climbing these threads
requires profound courage as well as a knowledge of
spiritual technology. Healing the sick is thought to be a
perilous effort, linked by many metaphors of transformation to other areas of danger in daily life and social
interactions.

≠Oma !'Homg!ausi describes the dangerous nature
of that journey because these threads are very thin and
can break, but he displays his confidence in making the
journey:

Once, when I was still new to nlom, I was climbing
the threads but they broke . . . and I fell to the
ground. I was scared and didn't know what to do.
My father came over to help me. "Climb again,"
he said. And I did. Yes, this climbing, this is what
we healers do.

Kxao Tjimburu, who says the threads are no thicker
than a microphone cord, talks further about their fragili-
ty and the dangers of their breaking:

If the thread breaks out there in the bush, it just
dumps you there. If you see a healer who doesn't
come back [from his travels up the threads] then
you know it's the threads that have broken. You
have to wait until dark again. The [healer's] body at
home will just sleep. It's that the healer has not
returned.

He adds some practical words, but they do not necessarily instill a sense of security:

When you're traveling an old [thread] you can see
if it's going to spoil. But if it's a new one, you just
travel with it . . . [yet] somewhere the threads are
tight and somewhere they are loose, so they can
easily break.

And as ≠Oma !'Homg!ausi cautions: "The thread
always breaks, even far from the village, and then you
have nothing to bring you home."

≠Oma Djo puts the function and gift of these threads
into the perspective of one who knows about the work-
ings of nlom. Responding to the question of how such a
thin thread can carry healers, he says:

Isn't the thread a thing of nlom, so it just has its
own strength? You learn to work with it. You learn
to do it, to lie on top of it. You come to know it
well. You watch and watch where it's going until

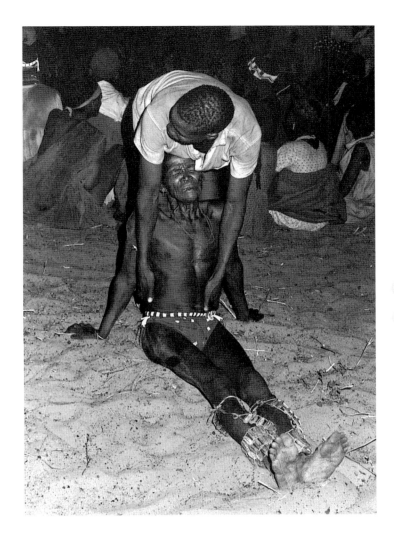

THOUGH AN EXPERIENCED HEALER,
KINACHAU IS OVERCOME BY HIS
TOO RAPIDLY BOILING NIOM;
HIS NEPHEW KXAO HOLDS AND
RUBS HIM, TRYING TO CALM DOWN
THE NIOM SO THAT KINACHAU CAN
"SEE PROPERLY."

you can see straight where it's going. . . . The one who helps you climb is !Xu [God].

Again and again we are prompted to ask if experience in these perilous but necessary journeys—these vehicles of transformation—prepares the people for difficult tasks in other realms of their lives. The "answer," as we continue to explore, has the nature of an unfolding.

"TO SEE PROPERLY"[4]

There are other transcendent experiences healers have, such as "seeing properly," that are further vehicles of transformation. During !aia, healers can "see properly," allowing them to view the insides of people so they can see the sickness and cure it. Kinachau, a respected and experienced healer, describes this process:

> You dance, dance, dance. Then nlom lifts you up in your belly and lifts you in your back, and you start to shiver. Nlom makes you tremble; it's hot. Your eyes are open but you don't look around; you hold your eyes still and look straight ahead. But when you get into !aia, you're looking around because you see everything, you see what's troubling every-body.[5]

IUi, an old, experienced healer, speaks of Glaq'o, who is still comparatively "young in !aia":

> What tells me Glaq'o isn't fully learned is the way he behaves. You see him staggering and running

around. His eyes are rolling all over the place. If your eyes are rolling around you can't stare at sickness. You have to be absolutely steady to see sickness, steady-eyes, no shivering and shaking, absolutely steady . . . with a steady gaze. . . . You need direct looking. Your thoughts don't whirl, the fire doesn't float above you, when you are seeing properly.[6]

G!aq'o acknowledges that he is not a g!aeha, that he is not a "completely learned" healer: "A g!aeha is a person who really helps people. He is someone whose eye-insides are steady. He can see properly. I heal people, but I can't see them properly."[7] In seeing properly, healers see where and what the sickness is, intensifying their treatment of sickness with their "absolutely steady" stare.

Proper seeing can become even more general. A healer can begin to see into and beyond many material manifestations. "Invisible" elements of the dance become "visible." ǀUi talks about this aspect of !aia: "You see the nǀom rising in other healers. You see the singing and the nǀom, and you pick it up. As a healer in !aia, you see everybody."[8] Others describe how they can see at a distance or can see what the gods want to tell the Juǀ'hoansi.

For proper seeing, the literal, physical act of seeing may or may not be involved. The eyes may be open, but they may also be closed. The experience remains one of enhanced perceiving and knowing.

What are the political implications of seeing inside others or seeing the "invisible" nature of things? How might the cutting edge of the "absolutely steady" stare, the "direct looking," be turned to other issues? And what are the different messages that can come out of seeing what the gods wish for the people? Is "seeing properly" a generic process, allowing for insight into various realms of everyday life? Could it extend to the present Juǀ'hoan sociopolitical situation, supporting a critical analysis, for instance, of power structures?

≠Oma Djo alludes to this possibility as he describes the things he sees inside sick people: "When God brings sickness he ties you up with sinews so your body is bound up with sinews; and other times your body is bound up with metal wires that come from Europeans." We asked ourselves if those metal wires are symbolic of a political sickness, a binding and disempowerment caused by political and economic exploitation? Again, we reflect on this question, talking with each other. Most important, we continue to listen to the Juǀ'hoansi tell their stories, hoping our questions willl enable us to hear more clearly what they might be saying.

THE STRUGGLE AND PAIN OF HEALING

In describing nǀom and !aia, there is always an emphasis on struggle, pain, and suffering. And because nǀom is painful and mysterious, it is greatly feared by the Juǀ'hoansi. Along with feelings of release and liberation, the experience of !aia brings profound pain and fear, especially as the nǀom begins to boil.

The nǀom burns as it boils fiercely inside the healer. "It is hot, this nǀom, just like fire," says Tshao Matze, "it burns our insides. That is why sometimes . . . we run from it."

Physical and psychological effects of the boiling nǀom merge. Healers typically sweat profusely, move about stiff-legged, or perhaps stagger on wobbly legs. Kinachau says:

Your footing gets bad, your legs become rubbery. You feel light, your feet don't touch the ground properly. It seems that you don't have any weight on the ground holding you steady. You have to work to keep your balance. You lose control over your body because you feel as if there are no bones in your body.[9]

The body trembles, especially the legs, and healers usually have a blank, glazed stare, sometimes grimacing with stomach pain. They often report their perception is "congested" and their thoughts "whirl."

The healing itself is also accompanied by intense pain. As healers put nǀom into the person being healed, draw the sickness out into their own bodies, and violently shake that sickness out from their own bodies, they show their suffering by crying, wailing, moaning, and shriek-

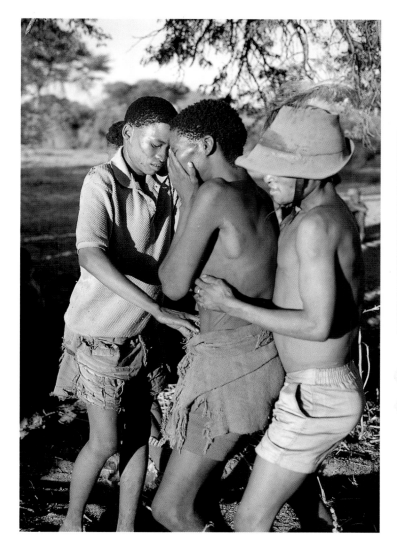

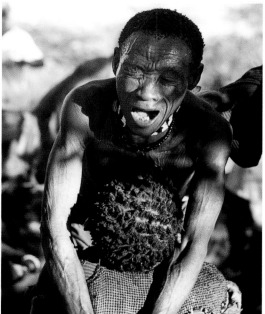

ABOVE: LEANING ON A HELPER, KXAO KASUPE SHRIEKS OUT THE KOWHEDILI, THE INTENSELY DRAMATIC CRY OF HEALING THAT EXPRESSES THE PAIN AND DIFFICULTY OF HEALING WORK.

LEFT: KAQECE (LEFT) AND GǃAQO GO (RIGHT) SUPPORT NǁAQ'U, AN INEXPERIENCED HEALER WHOSE BOILING NǀOM HAS MADE HIS LEGS RUBBERY AND BALANCE PRECARIOUS.

ing. Healers punctuate and accent their healing work with sometimes ear-shattering sounds. Their breath comes with more difficulty until they are rasping and gasping. They then howl the characteristic *kowhedili* shriek, which sounds something like "Kae-i! Kow-ha-di-di-di-di!" The kowhedili forcibly expels the sickness from the healer.

Throughout the boiling of nǀom, fear dominates; it is ultimately the fear of dying. Kxao ≠Oah describes what healers must face. "As we Juǀ'hoansi enter ǃaia, we fear death. We fear we may die and not come back!" Compared with those who keep resisting boiling nǀom, healers feel the pain and fear no less intensely; but in

transcending their fears, healers can accept the boiling nǀom and apply their ǃaia to healing. When Juǀ'hoan healers face the fact of death and willingly die, they can overcome their fear of nǀom and break through to ǃaia. They give up the familiar to enter unknown territory; they must die before they can be reborn into ǃaia.

Can this appreciation of the struggle and pain necessary for healing give strength to people in other struggles? Can the experience of meeting one's ultimate fear— the fear of dying—and learning to overcome it prepare one for the times when political decisions demand a degree of commitment and courage that is like dying to one's normal needs and wishes?

THE PATH

Finally, we consider the concept of the "path" that the healer must follow during !aia in order to turn !aia into healing actions. Along this path, healers talk about the "opening" through which they enter into the inner world of mysteries. And always the path is followed for the purposes of bringing healing and knowledge to the community. Could such a path, with its insistence that cultural mysteries be explored *in order* to serve the people, offer some guidance for effective social change?

In the summer of 1989, four healers demonstrate the continuing power of this path as they travel—as earlier

generations have—a communal journey of courage and service. There is a healing dance at ≠Oma !'Homg!ausi's camp. Besides his younger brother |Kaece, two other healers from two other camps are there: ≠Oma Djo and Tshao Matze. A little child is sick, and ≠Oma !'Homg!ausi has said there will be a healing dance and has asked for help.

The singing is strong—the women at ≠Oma !'Homg!ausi's camp are known for their passionate singing. And each of the four healers has entered !aia.

Then they begin their collaborative work. As |Kaece and Tshao Matze lie writhing on the ground, overcome with their boiling n|om, ≠Oma Djo and ≠Oma !'Homg!ausi massage and hold them, trying to cool down their boiling n|om. Eventually ≠Oma Djo lies on top of |Kaece, and ≠Oma !'Homg!ausi on top of Tshao Matze, and each massages more intensely. Then, rising up almost simultaneously, ≠Oma Djo and ≠Oma !'Homg!ausi sit astride the prone healers and begin their

HEALERS PREPARE EACH OTHER FOR THEIR PERILOUS JOURNEY OUT OF THEIR BODIES—CLIMBING THE THREADS TO GOD'S VILLAGE, THEY WILL SEEK TO RESCUE A SICK CHILD (|OMA DJO, ON THE RIGHT, LAYS ON TOP OF |OMA !'HOMG!AUSI, WHILE |KAECE, ON THE LEFT, MASSAGES A PRONE TSHAO MATZE).

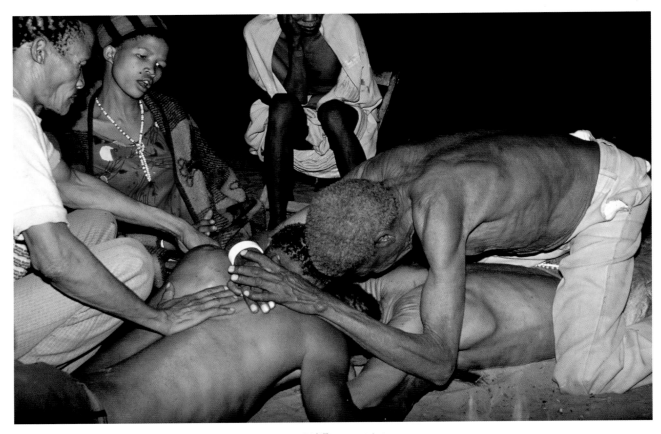

THE POLITICS OF N|OM

painfully poignant and piercing shrieks of kowhedili. All four bodies are now writhing in rhythm as, seeking to regulate each other's boiling nǀom, all are involved with healing each other. After what seems like a point beyond which their bodies can endure the painful movements of their mutual and reciprocal work, they all—again, nearly simultaneously—begin to relax into the ground.

Before the dance disperses and after the main healing work is done, we speak with each of the four healers. Independently, they tell remarkably similar stories of their healing effort.

≠Oma Djo says:

> ≠Oma !'Homgǃausi and I began to climb the threads to God's village. We traveled together, looking for that sick girl's soul. We climbed together, helping each other along the way. And we arrived in God's village, and were able to do our work. We were able to rescue that little girl's soul. And we knew she would be better.
>
> As we began climbing back down the threads, we met Tshao Matze and ǀKaece on the way. They were also trying to go to God's village to help save that little girl. We told them not to worry, that we already had done the work. We told them they could go back down now. And we all traveled back together.

As each of the four healers speaks about their efforts, the emphasis remains on their common aim: to help the sick child. ≠Oma Djo is acknowledged as a leader in that effort. It is an expression of the general respect with which he is treated throughout ǀKaeǀkae and of the fact that he was invited by ≠Oma !'Homgǃausi to help. But neither ≠Oma Djo nor any of the other three healers is given credit for the healing. As they regulate each other's boiling nǀom and guide each other's journey to God's village, these four men transform their individual healing power into a communal resource. Within the context of the healing dance, a communal path of service is dramatically created and reaffirmed.

Our experiences with a Juǀ'hoan grassroots political movement called the Nyae Nyae Farmers' Cooperative, which operates just across the border from ǀKaeǀkae in Namibia, helps us understand some of the larger ramifications of this concept of the path. We begin to see a similarity between this traditional healing path and the current political perspective on the path to community health espoused by the Juǀ'hoansi. Community health, as it always has been for the Juǀ'hoansi, is a truly holistic concept; but today it incorporates new political realities. When members of the Nyae Nyae Farmers' Cooperative speak about the health of their communities, they emphasize the recovery of Juǀ'hoan lands and livelihoods and the establishment of harmonious social relations. In its outreach to the ǀKaeǀkae people, the Farmers' Cooperative has found willing learners in the strongest ǀKaeǀkae healers.

Though there has been no overt linking by the Juǀ'hoansi between healers and political spokespersons, a large percentage of the ǀKaeǀkae people who have become active on behalf of their people's land rights and political rights are, in fact, the most powerful healers, persons who have years of experience in the demanding spiritual tradition of nǀom. Operating within their holistic concept of health, it is a natural step for the healers to move into the contemporary arena of political activity, as their healing of sick persons is always done within the general work of community healing.

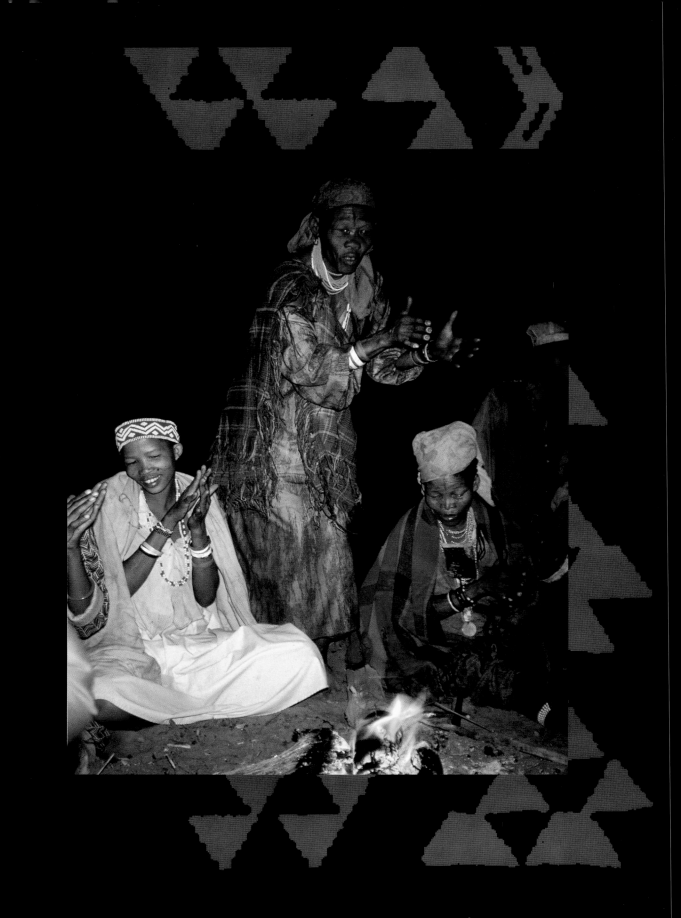

Tkaell'ae N!a'an is a tiny old woman who has lived in the vicinity of |Kae|kae all her life. Though no longer professing to have n|om herself, she nevertheless refers to the joy of healing and the very positive feelings that exist for her around drum dancing.

> Healing makes our hearts happy. When a drum sounds, my whole body, my legs here and my little arms, are lifted. Then I want to leave my house and go where the dance is. . . . I want to dance when I hear it. It grabs my stomach and grabs my legs. These days I dance right here in my blankets, because I can no longer stand up.

The drum dance coexists with the giraffe dance, which is the most common form of healing dance in the |Kae|kae region and the one usually referred to when people comment on Ju|'hoan healing. In the giraffe dance, male dancers (sometimes joined by a few women) circle behind a seated circle of clapping, singing women. In the drum dance, however, women dancers, sometimes joined by a few men, stand in a horseshoe shape with a male drummer at the mouth of the horseshoe.[1] A drum of mongongo wood (or sometimes a plastic water container) accompanies the dancers' singing and clapping.

Drum dancing has its own repertoire of songs at |Kae|kae with names like "Termite Eaters," "Springhares," and "Txaetxubi Ants." At other places, different repertoires are popular. As Tkaell'ae N!a'an explains, "People have separate n|oresi and separate ways they sing."

At the core of the drum and giraffe dances is n|om. Though men and generally women use the word *!aia* to

A SPECIAL MOMENT OF INTENSITY

BRINGS A WOMAN BACK TO HER FEET

DURING A DRUM DANCE.

9

FEMALE AND MALE APPROACHES TO N|OM

refer to the altered state resulting from boiling n|om during giraffe, women refer to their experience of !aia during the drum dance as tara. The word *tara,* which means "the action of lightning," describes the intense and rhythmic shaking, quivering, and trembling of women during their experience of !aia. But as more men, especially older healers like ≠Oma Djo, participate in drum dances in 1989, they are also beginning to use the word *tara* to describe their experiences. Women talk about how they "tremble the beads off" their skin aprons during tara. |Am explains this trembling:

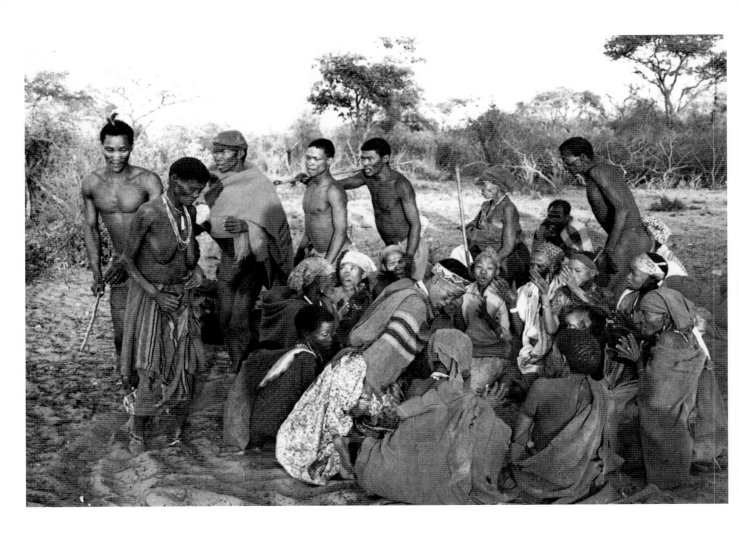

It feels like there is a hole going through your body. You tremble in rhythm, even your crotch trembles. If you reach !aia, you call out for water, because you are hot inside. Even if you don't know the songs, you can !aia. The nǀom itself tells you how to sing and dance.

Despite Tkaellʼae Nǃaʼan's disclaimers about not having nǀom, N≠aisa, wise herself in the ways of nǀom, documents Tkaellʼae Nǃaʼan's continued and intense contact with nǀom in the drum dance: "Tkaellʼae Nǃaʼan's people say she is too old. . . . They are afraid she will fall over when she tara. . . . But she can tara . . . the drum lifts her up and stands her at the dance anyway."

Julʼhoan healing dances are varied today, ranging from the horseshoe-shaped drum dance to a full com- munity healing dance of the circular form or the solitary dance, sometimes done inside a nest of blankets, of a healer concerned with one close relative. There have been substantial changes in the forms of Julʼhoan healing dances just in the last few generations, and the blending of forms is unmistakable though usually unpredictable. And so the complexity and changing conditions of women and men in the various dance forms, as described in this chapter, are the norm. Rather than seeking some preferred level of analytical clarity—for example demon- strating consistent similarities or differences between drum and giraffe dances, or offering a single version about the origin of a dance like drum—we will follow the Julʼhoan lead and try to describe the various forms of the healing dance with their inherent ambiguity and paradox intact.

One thing does seem to occur throughout the dances. Inspiration for a dance form or its revision occurs to ones who regard themselves on the cutting edge of creativity. Others do not waste much time in resistence; instead, respecting the creators, they follow their inspiration. Variety and change in the healing dances is continually nourished.

TOLERANCE OF
LOCAL DIFFERENCES

N!oresi are the subsistence territories to which Jul'hoan people are tied by kinship and knowledge of local resources. Each n!ore has a special flavor imparted to it by the individuals who live there at any given time. Jul'hoan people accept the differences among groups at different n!oresi, including local enthusiasms and current interests. This tolerance allows a great diversity of individual styles to coexist in song repertoires, in artistic approaches such as in beadwork, and in personal adornment.

Tolerance has long been one of the unifying hallmarks of Jul'hoan communities, allowing a range of approaches to almost any cultural expression. This outlook is par-

ticularly apparent to us in the area of women's and men's roles in regard to dancing and to n!om. The sexual egalitarianism we mention in chapter 1 extends markedly to individual preferences in the area of healing. At some communities and at some times, women move easily into what might be thought of as "usually male" roles and vice versa. We have been fascinated by this fluidity since the first trips to the IKaeIkae area in the late 1960s. We wanted to know if this is still the case in 1989.

We begin by asking again if there is any difference between the n!om experienced by men and that experienced by women. ≠Oma Djo, an enthusiastic participant in both giraffe and drum dances, tells us over and over that there is no difference between the n!om experienced in the two dances and no difference between the n!om experienced by women and men. Kxao Tjimburu echoes him: "The two n!om are the same. . . . It's one n!om." And Xumi N!a'an offers a variation on the same theme: "Giraffe dance and drum dance each have their own n!om, but the n!om is *one*." When we ask other people, we get the same kinds of answers.

In speaking of the n!om experienced in tara, the

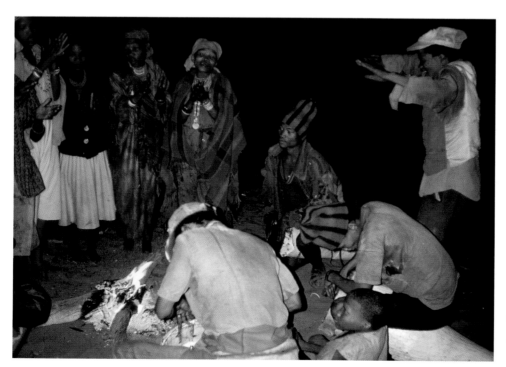

OPPOSITE: A GIRAFFE HEALING DANCE CONTINUES INTO THE DAWN, INVOLVING THE ENTIRE COMMUNITY IN ITS CIRCLE OF HEALING.

GATHERED IN A HORSESHOE SHAPE AROUND TWO DRUMS, THE INTENSITY OF THE WOMEN'S SINGING AND DANCING IN THIS DRUM DANCE IS NOT BROKEN BY THE HUMOROUS DANCING OF THE YOUNG MAN ON THE RIGHT.

FEMALE AND MALE APPROACHES TO N!OM

shaking trance associated with the drum dance, Xumi N!a'an says it is the same as that of the !aia of giraffe. As if to dispel any doubts about the relative strength of women's healing implied by our questions, Kinachau, a respected old male healer, had this to say in 1968: "It is good for women to have nǀom. If they heal, they can save you! It is the same with the men."[2] ǁUce N!a'an, a veteran of many healing dances and perhaps the only ǀKaeǀkae woman in 1989 who eagerly talks about her experiences of !aia in the giraffe dance, puts it succinctly: "There is only one nǀom, the nǀom that heals us."

Women !aia in giraffe, and men !aia in drum. N!ae, a strong singer in giraffe, talks to us about how women !aia and heal in that dance.

> When a woman in the singing circle starts to !aia, you see her singing and shivering at the same time. Her eyes might close a little and then open. When she is in !aia, that is the best singing of all. It's singing with real nǀom in it. We hear that singing and see it. She can still sing while she is in !aia. We other singers sit close to the one who is in !aia,

supporting her so that she won't fall over, but we don't rub her. We give her strength and support her so she won't fall. The men are pleased because it's all the same nǀom. . . . The healing in the singing circle is the same as the healing of the dancers.[3]

In the giraffe dance, women are more active in the singing and men in the dancing, but neither considers their own or the others' activity as the source of healing. Spirited singing or strong dancing can encourage nǀom to boil, but it is nǀom that heals, and both women and men stand equally in awe of its healing power. When asked if strong singing can cause many people to !aia at a dance, N!ae says, "When the healers fall into !aia, it is because of nǀom. We don't congratulate anyone. It is the nǀom that does it. "[4]

Only later do we realize that the dichotomy we had been pursuing is largely foreign to Juǀ'hoan thinking. Associating men more with the giraffe dance and women more with the drum dance because of the relative numbers involved reifies a gender split where for the

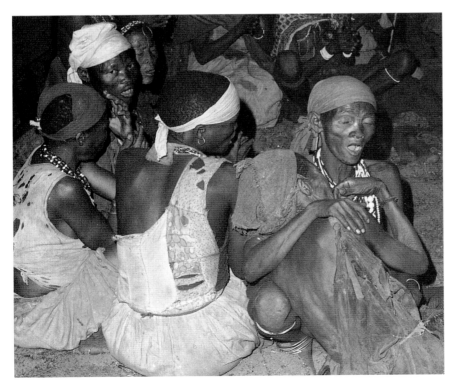

SOME WOMEN EXPERIENCE !AIA WHILE SINGING IN A GIRAFFE DANCE; OTHERS IN THE SINGING CIRCLE WILL HOLD THEM, GIVING THEM STRENGTH. HERE KXAO TJIMBURU'S MOTHER SUPPORTS ǀXOAN N!A'AN FROM ǀKAEǀKAE.

Jul'hoansi little or no dichotomy exists. For them, crossing "gender lines" in working with nǀom, we eventually learn, just is not problematic—the "lines" we thought we saw didn't exist! We had wondered about this remarkable fluidity earlier, and it applied not only to gender roles in dancing but to each individual's creativity in many areas, including the "receiving" or composing of songs, storytelling, and beadwork. The flexibility that is the rule in storytelling, for example, seems to give the Jul'hoansi great latitude for self-expression. This individualism is not a competitive one—far from it. Instead, their individualism dignifies the work of innovators, who are honored through imitation.

This honoring of others' inspiration is part and parcel of Jul'hoansi values in all their social life. Jul'hoansi accord respect to members of each sex. In their society it *works* for mutual tolerance to be the rule rather than the exception. Because social relationships are sensitive to many aspects of historical and economic change, we needed to ask whether the pressures of the last few decades might have affected an earlier balance maintained by the Jul'hoansi.

In the 1960s, for example, about one-half the adult men and about one-third of the women became healers. Strong women healers were accorded the full degree of respect that men healers received. Both men and women felt competent to initiate dances and special healings. We wonder in 1989 if the increasing sedentization and pressure from other ethnic groups and economic interests might have affected this gender egalitarianism among Jul'hoan healers.

GIRAFFE AND DRUM DANCES IN THE 1960S AND EARLY 1970S

In the late 1960s, giraffe was the most frequently performed healing dance in the ǀKaeǀkae area; it was the community's primary ritual. As the ethnographer Lorna Marshall reported, giraffe "is the one activity in !Kung [Jul'hoan] life that draws people together in groups that are of considerable size and are not shaped by family, band, or close friendship. Nothing but a [giraffe] medi-cine dance assembles all the people into a concerted activity."[5]

During the first half of the 1970s, in areas as near as twenty to thirty miles from ǀKaeǀkae, the drum dance was gaining in popularity. Most people regarded the drum dance as a more recent dance form. The drum dance also seemed to be identified in many people's minds with a new assertion of women's strength. Yet the drum dance always welcomed a few men as participants.

There is a sense in which the symbolic community relationships observable in the giraffe dance dramatize desirable male and female relationships. Men are fierce and active in lifting up healing power out of their dancing joy and artistry. Women sing and clap ardently and with finesse and beauty. Their song is regarded as a necessary vehicle of sound for !aia and soul-travel. Tshao Nǃa'an, one of the oldest active healers at ǀKaeǀkae and a man who had traveled widely performing healing dances, captured the common understanding of men's and women's contributions: "When the women sing well, when they put their hearts into it, you dance well, your nǀom is strengthened." Though the dance dramatizes desirable male-female relationships most often through men as dancers and women as singers, the more profound message is the reciprocal respect each group has for the other and the openness of each role to the other.

Many Jul'hoansi spoke of the giraffe dance as their "main" and their "strongest" dance. While drum dancing was said to have "the same" nǀom, the giraffe form clearly held Jul'hoan hearts in a deeper way. Ancient rock paintings show a dance form quite similar to today's giraffe dance, with men dancing around seated, clapping women figures (see page 53). Nothing like the drum dance's horseshoe shape can be found in those painted scenes.[6]

During the late 1960s and early 1970s, the giraffe dance was a ritual in which both women and men made important contributions; the drum dance was female dominated but could and did include men. The giraffe dance's place in the culture was more central and widespread, and thus the dance was performed more frequently. General community participation was greater in giraffe; not only was attendance at the dance open to all but so was participation. Though attendance at the drum dance was open to all, most dancers were women and the few drummers were male. For the Jul'hoansi, the giraffe dance was the "Great Dance"; they considered it an arena for helping to resolve social tensions and bring coherence to their communal lives.

Though men generally danced and women sang in the giraffe dance, these roles were not hierarchically conceived. Women praised men dancers, and men praised women singers, and both groups felt that the activity of each was vital to the whole experience of the dance. Compared with the drum dance, the gender roles in giraffe overlapped more. In drum dancing there was less overlap, and the women dancers in drum were generally accorded more status and their role more valued than men's.

Women and men both experienced !aia and healing in the giraffe dance, while in the drum dance it was the women who usually experienced !aia and who were the healers. In the giraffe dance, !aia was valued because it brought on healing, and healing was made available to all at the dance. In the drum dance, !aia was valued as an experience in itself—many women described the experience as "sweet and good." Healing was less emphasized and, when it did occur, was restricted to the female performers in the drum dance.

The giraffe dance remained the quintessential Jul'hoan dance in the late 1960s. Frequently performed and inclusive of everyone, it had areas of comfortable overlap for the activities of both women and men and stressed the availability of nlom healing for all. The balance between the sexes exemplified in the giraffe dance reflected in a sense nlom's power to unify the community. Jul'hoansi continually assert that there is only one nlom, and that it is the same for women and men. There are a few stylistic differences between the sexes in their approach to nlom, but in terms of fundamental outlook upon and work with nlom, women and men are similiar, especially so in regard to experienced healers.

It is interesting that only female healers spoke of a hole running through their bodies and out their heads during the experience of !aia. Also, women's training as healers was described as being relatively easy and brief compared with men's. Though experiencing nlom was painful for both men and women, men's training as healers was typically long and arduous, involving continual struggles with the fear of nlom.

Women's reproductive status was also explicitly tied by them to the practice of nlom, unlike men's status. Women felt it was best if nlom lay dormant during their childbearing years, since nlom was thought to be dangerous to unborn children. As a result, women generally ceased seeking nlom during their reproductive years; participation in active healing became most focused in the post-childbearing years. Men had no such connection between nlom and their status as fathers.

The contrasts between the giraffe and drum dances already were showing signs of lessening in the late 1960s and early 1970s. We could see instances where the drum dance itself was shifting toward the giraffe dance in a number of ways. For example, on one occasion a woman who had entered the death of !aia in the drum dance could not be brought back to life after her soul had left her body. The other dancers turned to the giraffe dance to bring her soul back. Two other trends were noted as well: more men were involved in the drum dance relative to earlier periods, and the singing in the drum dance was becoming more like the singing in the giraffe dance.

GIRAFFE AND DRUM DANCES IN 1989

By 1989 instances of this blurring of distinctions between the drum and giraffe dances seem to have increased. Though there are certainly numerous occasions in which a drum dance begins and ends as a drum dance, there also appear to be more times when the drum dance evolves into a giraffe dance; we have never seen the opposite occur. These evolutions of dance form were not necessarily in order to meet a specific crisis such as the woman's loss of soul described above. Often, the intensity of a particular drum dance seems to reach a certain point in which the inclusion of the entire community is not only necessary to support the emerging !aia but is a natural expression of the nǀom now boiling in the healers. This intensity often results when one or two male healers, who are not drumming, are about to !aia either in the dance or on the periphery and women in the dance, also near !aia, begin working on the men as they also work among themselves, trying to calm down the boiling nǀom that now is rising in several of them.

There has been a sharp increase in the number of drum dances at ǀKaeǀkae in 1989, in part because of the increased availability of drums. Because the Juǀ'hoan craft cooperative operating out of Maun is buying drums, a number of drum makers respond by carving drums for sale. At any one time there might be as many as three or four drums at ǀKaeǀkae. They are used until they are sold, and during certain stretches of time, we can hear drum playing almost every night in one of the camps, especially in camps where a drum is kept.[7] Such drumming often results in what could be called a minidance if not a full drum dance.

These minidances are mostly for entertainment, to hear the drum and sing together. They do not last as long as a regular drum dance—about an hour or so—and are more easily interrupted and less intense. The singing and dancing may stop and start with the arrival of visitors from other camps. At times, people who have been drinking come to these minidances seeking a night of entertainment. !Aia or healing does not seem the intention of such casual dances, and we have never seen one merge into a giraffe dance.

Sometimes people describe a dance without healing as just "play" or "playing." At one giraffe dance held during the day, only one of the healers heals as the others, including ≠Oma ǀ'Homgǀausi, !aia but do not heal. "Yes, we were playing [at that dance]," says ≠Oma ǀ'Homgǀausi. "Those of us who were nǀomkxaosi sat aside and didn't want to do nǀom that day. When nǀom wanted to take us, we stopped it. . . . Some of us feared the sun. It was a hot day, and if you ≠hoe [heal] in the sun,

nǀom will grab you too strongly." "When there's no nǀomkxaosi at a dance," ≠Oma ǀ'Homgǀausi's wife, Tiǀ'ae, adds, "sometimes we just play . . . and we play when it's only the kids dancing."

But ǀAiǀae Nǀa'an, an old man with many years of experience in drumming who can enter !aia while drumming and then leave the drum and begin to heal, cautions about assuming that a particular drum dance is just for playing around:

> There may be a person who is !aia in such a dance, but if that person fears it, they'll just go sit down. So [the dance] might look like just playing. . . . Sometimes people just play at a drum dance and sometimes it's a healing dance.

The roles of men and women in the drum dance seem to have become even more similar and more equal during the 1989 period. A number of the experienced male healers, including ≠Oma Djo, Tshao Nǀa'an, and Kxao Tjimburu, now appear to be more at ease participating in the drum dance, including experiencing !aia and healing in that dance.[8] They see themselves as having both giraffe and drum nǀom, and constantly emphasize that the two nǀoms are one and the healing work in each dance the same. Their views are very reminiscent of what we heard from women in 1968 who also experienced nǀom in the two dances; the women's two nǀoms were said "to marry," and a stronger nǀom resulted.

Not only do we frequently see experienced male healers !aia in a drum dance, but no one at the dance seems surprised when it happens. The men !aia alongside women, who are themselves either experiencing !aia, helping the men, helping each other, or often doing some combination of these roles. The horseshoe form of the drum dance often remains during these times of women and men experiencing !aia, at least at the start. All participants still stand or perhaps begin to stagger and fall into !aia, and the women and some of the men still sing while they dance. As time passes and nǀom boils more fiercely in more participants, the horseshoe shape often becomes less and less recognizable. People almost seem to dance

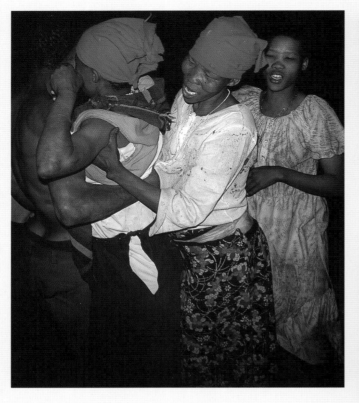

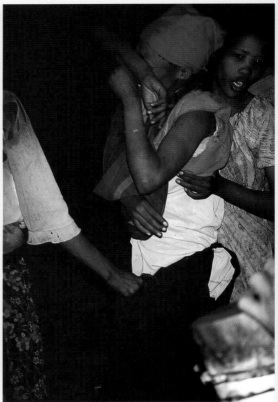

A DRUM DANCE TRANSFORMS INTO A GIRAFFE DANCE, AS AT FIRST IT IS PRIMARILY THE WOMEN WHO HELP EACH OTHER REGULATE THEIR BOILING N|OM (ABOVE, LEFT AND RIGHT), AND THEN INCREASINGLY MEN BECOME INVOLVED IN THE HEALING WORK (BELOW, LEFT AND RIGHT).

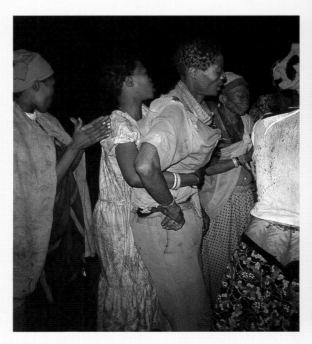

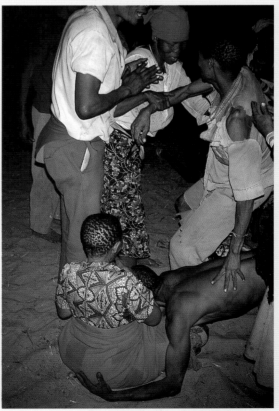

and !aia independent of a group form. The circular giraffe dance form might emerge then and bring a structure to the work of nǀom.

As of 1989 giraffe remains the "great" dance, the central arena for community healing, the ritual that invites everyone in. And now the giraffe dance seems even more ready to envelop drum—or drum seems more ready to evolve into the giraffe dance. The foundation of this interchange and erasing of boundaries remains the experience of nǀom, which women and men still constantly describe as the same—whether it occurs in a woman or a man or in the giraffe or the drum dance.

Certainly women, like men, fear the pain of boiling nǀom; in fact, because of that fear, they generally talk much less about nǀom. N!hunkxa, a woman in her thirties who experiences tara in the drum dance, describes a common set of feelings among her peers:

> [When I was younger] I just thought I'd try what I saw other people doing [i.e., dancing in the drum dance]. I liked it before I started to tara. After that I realized it was very painful. [Tara] is very painful. . . . I don't want to talk about it.

But N!hunkxa adds other common reasons why she will continue to tara. "Your body insides feel good," she says, "but your stomach and backbone hurt." Perhaps her "body insides feel good" because she knows that the eventual purpose of tara is to develop into healing. "Tara is nice," she says. "The old people would use tara in order to heal." If she could travel to her original home, !Aoan, she would be willing to try to learn to heal; she would be willing to face her fears if she were among her own people.

Koba, a young mother with one child, talks about her experience of tara, linking that experience up with the men and their descriptions of !aia:

> I went long ago to Tjum!kui and they put the arrows [of nǀom] into me. . . . [Nǀom] hurts! It grabs your front and it grabs your spine—it feels like fire and thorns. . . . It hurts and feels like arrows, the arrows they've put in you. . . . When

you tara, the stars are shimmering above you and you can't tell where anything is. The fire can be up in the sky.

Though she feels the pain of nǀom, Koba seeks it with her youthful enthusiasm: "If there is a drum, I tara. I like it."

One expression of the increased merging of the drum and giraffe dances in 1989 is that the two most respected and experienced male healers at ǀKaeǀkae, ≠Oma Djo and Tshao N!a'an, move easily between the two dances, doing their healing work in both. In the process, they are erasing the relatively more distinct role relationship that existed

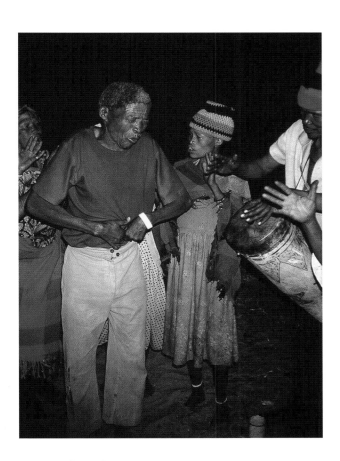

≠OMA DJO, A POWERFUL OLD MALE HEALER,

EXPERIENCING !AIA DURING A DRUM DANCE.

between the sexes in drum dances during the 1960s.

On the other hand, ≠Oma Djo and Tshao N!a'an are affirming another principle from that earlier period. With experience, differences between men and women in their work with nǀom lessen, and among the most powerful and most experienced healers, the differences become nonexistent, especially in their intimate work with nǀom. ǀAiǃae N!a'an, coming from his many years in both giraffe and drum dances, speaks succinctly: "!Aia is tara," he says, "they are the same. . . . Drum is a dance of women and also of men."

Perhaps the drum dance, as it merges more frequently with the giraffe dance, will begin to express even more fully the traditional Juǀ'hoan commitment to sexual egalitarianism. Perhaps also the long-term effects will be in a different direction. We cannot help but wonder whether these recent changes in the drum dance mark a lessening of women's control and of their opportunity to express their own particular power in the realm of healing. In that case, the direction seen in the drum dance would be consistent with a more general socioeconomic trend in which Juǀ'hoan women are becoming peripheral to areas of power in Juǀ'hoan life.[9]

AN EGALITARIAN BASELINE?

Having described the two dances, it is tempting to identify the politically and sexually egalitarian situation of the Juǀ'hoansi as part of a hunting-gathering "baseline" and to see the giraffe dance as somehow paradigmatic of a more ancient mode of group dynamics. The drum dance might then be a departure related to more recently introduced socioeconomic changes.[10]

But there is no egalitarian baseline either for all Bushman societies or for any one Bushman group over time. As to the giraffe dance, it more closely epitomizes relationships in the traditional foraging situation. In contrast, many questioned about the drum dance in the 1970s regularly made explicit reference to outside influences as a source. And we have the impression that there is a higher incidence of women's drum dancing in places where the change to a sedentary life-pattern is most com-

plete, as was the case at Gǃoci, !Aoan, and Mahopa during the early 1970s.

It is difficult to determine if the drum dance's supposed adoption and its increased frequency are related to changes in the move from foraging to the beginnings of wage labor. The form of giraffe appears to be old and well established, even though in recent decades it has taken different names and a different repertoire of songs. In contrast, a mystery surrounds the origin of the women's drum dances. We hear conflicting reports from the Juǀ'hoansi about the dance's history in the culture. We note in 1989 that many more Juǀ'hoansi seem to feel the drum dance is an ancient part of their culture, perhaps even predating the giraffe dance, whereas in the early 1970s most people felt that the drum dance was definitely introduced, usually from a vaguely northward direction. We are exploring implications of both origin explanations, as well as the likelihood that both may present part of the unfolding story, in order to understand more fully female and male approaches to nǀom.

If the drum dance has been introduced or is gaining enormously in popularity in the present transition to sedentism and a subordinate wage-based relationship with other peoples, there would seem to be a clearer case for connecting the dance to changed economic conditions. But if, as some informants suggest, the women's dance really is an "ancient thing" in Juǀ'hoan culture, we might then see it as a subtheme that provides an important element in the ongoing dynamic of their male and female relations. While the position of the drum dance is historically ambiguous, it seems reasonable to say that its assertive female emphasis represents some counterpoint statement to the more equally valued male and female contributions of the giraffe dance.[11]

REPRODUCTIVE STATUS AND FEMALE HEALING

Nǀom is usually sent into the seeker by the teacher by means of "invisible" arrows, which are felt as painful thorns or needles. Some women say that having "the arrows of nǀom" in one's belly at the time of pregnancy is

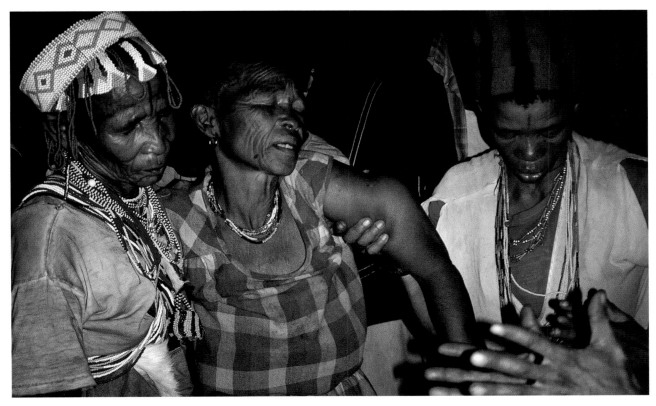

DURING THIS DRUM DANCE, IXOAN (CENTER), NOW DEEPLY INTO !AIA,

IS CARRIED AND HELD BY KXARU N!A'AN (LEFT) AND OTHER WOMEN IN THE DANCE.

dangerous for the unborn child. Others say they fear that the pain of n|om and the pain of childbirth together would be too much for them, which is why they ask for their n|om arrows to be removed when they are pregnant. Kxaru N!a'an tells us that early in life she feared this double pain too much, and therefore asked for her n|om to be removed. She "washed a lot in cold water," one way to remove the arrows, and also "walked backward on mouse burrows," closing them with her bare feet so her n|om would be trapped inside them.

Jul'hoan women often say that their reproductive status is a key consideration in decisions to seek n|om. But not all of them say this, particularly in 1989 at |Kae|kae as compared to some twenty years earlier. Tkae||'ae N!a'an, the old woman who, at the beginning of this chapter, tells how she dances in her blankets because she

can no longer stand, says she never had her n|om arrows "removed" while she was reproductively active. "I didn't do that," she says. "I wasn't afraid and gave birth just fine." When we ask why some other women were afraid to leave the n|om arrows in their stomachs when they gave birth, she replies, "Well, they just did it their own way. I myself didn't do it that way. Some people may fear childbirth, so that's why." Her positive attitude is echoed by a number of younger women. Koba, a young mother in her late teens, says, "Even if you're pregnant and have the arrows, the child will be all right."

So there is an awareness among some women that the arrows of n|om might in fact *not* interfere with gestation and birth. Learning of this awareness expands our appreciation of Jul'hoan women's traditionally active, energetic, and participatory relationship to cultural expression. Jul'hoan women healers and participants in healing dances are, like men, active in seeking to create artistic beauty and to use n!om well. Healing involves going out to do battle with the gods to rescue the sick. It involves soul-loss and daring "the death that kills us all," for women as well as for men. Facing fear is paramount in the experience of n!om for all. Both genders are equally challenged by the pain and psychic mystery of n!om.

MALE HEALERS AND THEIR WIVES

As in 1968, in 1989 we see many Jul'hoan women providing support to their husbands at dances when the men are experiencing !aia and healing. They mop their sweating brows, bring them water to drink or tobacco to smoke, and watch to make sure they do not burn themselves when kneeling near the fire to heal. At first glance, a Western observer might think of these acts as indication of a subordinate role for women. But the obvious pleasure and sense of competence with which the tasks are performed inspires us to look deeper and to ask the people about them.

Strikingly, when a male healer falls prostrate to the ground when overcome by his n!om heating up too fast or too violently, he seems invariably to fall on or near his wife. She then ministers to him and makes sure he is not

too near the fire. She can also call for water to be brought to cool him and cool down his boiling n!om or ask for other healers to help her rub his face and body so that he can again be in control of his n!om and regulate its boiling more properly.

N≠aisa, Kxao Tjimburu's wife and herself a strong singer and dancer, details some of the work she does for him: protecting him from the fire; assembling his beads, dance rattles, and dancing loincloth; and sometimes massaging and rubbing him with oil after the dance. When asked if it ever happened that Kxao Tjimburu would go to a dance but she would not be there, she replies, "No, we go together. I also want dances, and we love each other, so we go together." Kxao Tjimburu, who is sitting with N≠aisa as she talks, adds that he can hear her voice over all the other women's voices at a dance. "She works hard at singing," he says.

N≠aisa N!a'an, an older woman and the wife of ≠Oma Djo, expresses the depth of this complementarity in roles between a healer and his wife:

> When you're pregnant, your husband has to help with cooking and getting water and collecting firewood. When we dance and our husbands are healing, we stop them from getting burned. We also teach other girls who marry husbands [who are

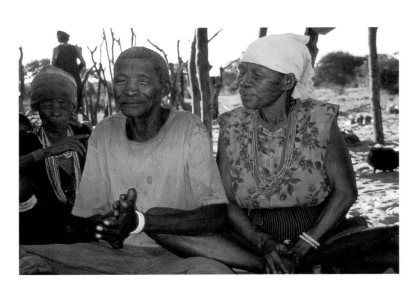

N≠AISA N!A'AN (RIGHT) AND HER HUSBAND, ≠OMA DJO, ARE BOTH STRONG IN THE WAYS OF N!OM AND HELP EACH OTHER IN THE HEALING WORK.

healers]. If you marry a man and he's doing his nlom in his blankets [i.e., singing and !aia alone at night, a common practice with experienced healers], you have to help him by singing for him, and he will then cure you when you are sleeping. You don't have to say anything.

But sometimes it's very difficult. It's those things your husband is doing. When you're asleep and "those people" [the spirits] come, your husband is crying and singing in his sleep, and you have to get up with your husband and do those things together. That makes it hard. . . . Always, when we two sleep, he's the one the spirits come to. Then he'll sing and dance for himself. I'll get up with him, and the two of us just live like that.

[Other times], I think about dancing [with him]. When you want to join in, you sing. Or when you want to, you just lie there and he himself sings. This is the thing that heals you, this singing.

[At a dance] you start to sing [for your husband] and your voice becomes sweet, so he'll dance and heal you. It's nice singing so that this guy can find a nice dance, can find good healing, and then finish.

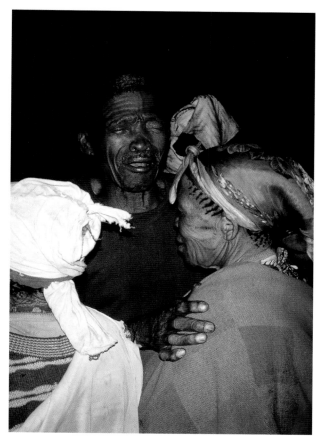

≠OMA DJO HEALING HIS WIFE, N≠AISA N!A'AN.

≠Oma Djo, who has been listening attentively to his wife, adds, "Sometimes [husbands and wives] help each other heal, too. The nlom is stronger that way. . . . And when your own wife is sick, you heal her first, then go to the other people." His wife concludes by saying she feels sorry for women who marry men who aren't healers, because the "nlomkxaosi [healers] heal you."

N≠aisa N!a'an speaks with pride about the knowledge shared between herself and her husband, ≠Oma Djo, after he comes back from a night of soul travel. "I never know when he's gone. I only hear about it in the morning. But I never tell other women," she says. "It is the secret of the two of us."

|Xoan, the wife of Tshao N!a'an, is rather more prosaic about her role. An older woman, she has always been a strong singer and trancer; her husband had a healing career at Ghanzi, where he was rewarded with goats and blankets, and now, along with ≠Oma Djo, he is consid-

ered one of the two most powerful healers at |Kae|kae. |Xoan speaks of holding her husband back from the fire when he is in !aia and of powdering him with sweet-scented *san* when he feels poorly.[12] She says that she finds things he needs and has forgotten, like his dance rattles or his loincloth. She collects his dancing skin, beads, and headband. But she is content for him to have his own secrets of what he sees when he travels out of his body at night on his healing work. "I just lie there and he goes off," she says. "It doesn't bother me."

But |Xoan did have some anxiety when she was a young bride about to enter a marriage with a healer:

I refused to marry a healer. I was afraid of nlom and didn't know yet about !aia. I just didn't know

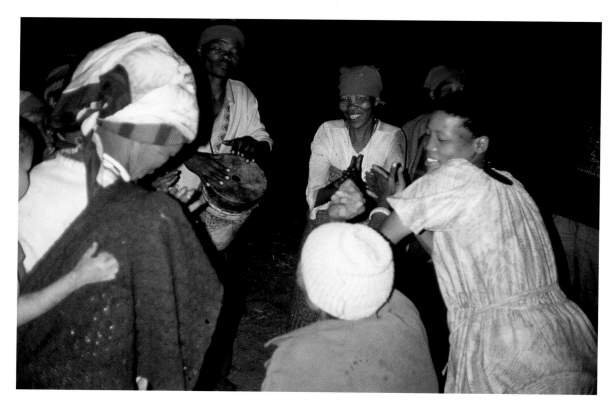

THE ENERGY THAT WOMEN BRING TO THE JUI'HOAN HEALING TRADITION

IS EVIDENCED BY THE EXPRESSIONS ON THESE SINGERS' AND DANCER'S FACES.

how to be married to a healer. But my old people told me that if I got sick he'd heal me. Then I started to fear less. I had been afraid because I had heard that a person who !aia would turn into a lion. That's why I had first refused to be married to a nǁomkxao. I thought to myself that if he did that too much we'd split up and I'd go home to my parents. . . . But now I'm glad [I'm married to a nǁomkxao].

ǀKaece China, a younger but experienced healer whose wife has died, keenly feels her absence when it comes to healing:

It's not good. I'm lacking a woman to sing for me—one of my own. [If I had a wife at the dance] she'd sit with other men's wives and sing for me to dance so my heart would be happy. When I hear other women's voices, I wish my wife was there. Women are strong things: it's because of them that we're on the earth. If you don't have a wife, your heart is full of pain. No one watches over me at the dance: that's why I don't put my heart into dancing. It's hard without a wife.

It may also be hard for Western outsiders to accept what appear to be "supporting" roles, such as those described by both women and men for healers' wives, as anything but "subordinate" roles. Yet we feel it is important to look beyond Western stereotypes of feminine power to the possibility that Juǀ'hoan women may be profiting equally with men from the *continuation* of the healing tradition. They may be sharing more and more equally in the continual re-creation and transformation of that tradition as well, as they now find their voices and try their strengths.

WOMEN AND MEN AND HEALING

In everything we have heard from Jul'hoan men and women from the 1960s to the present, there is mutual respect between the two genders with regard to nǃom. Complementarity between the roles of women and men in the context of healing still seems strong at ǀKaeǀkae. We believe that a greater percentage of women may now be healing than they once did, a change that may reflect an urgency felt by women not to be left out as their society undergoes transformations.

Yet the Jul'hoansi still say that increasing the number of nǃom practitioners increases the healing energy available to all. The increase in women's participation in drum dancing is part of the whole culture's response to new anxieties. Dynamic changes among the Jul'hoansi with regard to sex roles may still be subsumed within their cultural idiom of valuing mutual aid. Warmth and mutual encouragement for both genders are notable in all that is said about all the dance forms.

We do not want to ignore gender oppression in the ǀKaeǀkae area. But neither do we want to export expectations of it inappropriately. We think the honor shared between the genders by Jul'hoansi is yet another example of the nurturing and tolerance they extend to everyone in their society. In the last analysis, it is not our prerogative as non-Jul'hoansi to project what directions gender relationships in the Jul'hoan healing tradition might be taking. And this lack of authority should not mask the fact that, in addition, we do not know enough to make rea-

sonable predictions. The Jul'hoansi themselves are unsure of the future of their gender relationships. Some women today are more active in working with nǃom, and some are more neutral. Some more actively embrace social changes of all kinds, and some stay more neutral.

Any of "our" conclusions about women and men in regard to healing are the tentative and limited views of visitors to the Jul'hoan culture. But it does seem to us that Jul'hoan society still regards men and women as important actors in healing; ǃaia and tara are alive, and men and women use them. Both the drum and giraffe dances are seen as important. What Westerners might believe constitutes more important "activity" in dancing and healing is not necessarily the same for Jul'hoansi. We wonder whether seeing men as "participating more" in the drum dance today might not be a truer approximation to the real situation than seeing them as "gaining control" of the drum dance. Both healing dances, though they may reflect changing circumstances of many kinds, remain an important resource and outlet for all Jul'hoansi. As Diǀǀxao, a woman who can tara in drum dance and ǃaia in the giraffe dance, tells us:

> Drum dance is the dance for the Jul'hoansi. They dance also the giraffe dance, their traditional dance that they learned from their ancestors. The reason they make these [two] dances . . . is to heal a person who is sick. And if the person is getting ill we make the drum dance for her, and if she is not getting better, we will make a giraffe dance for her. Moreover, the drum dance is for both women and men. It just comes from yourself if you want to drum dance or giraffe dance.

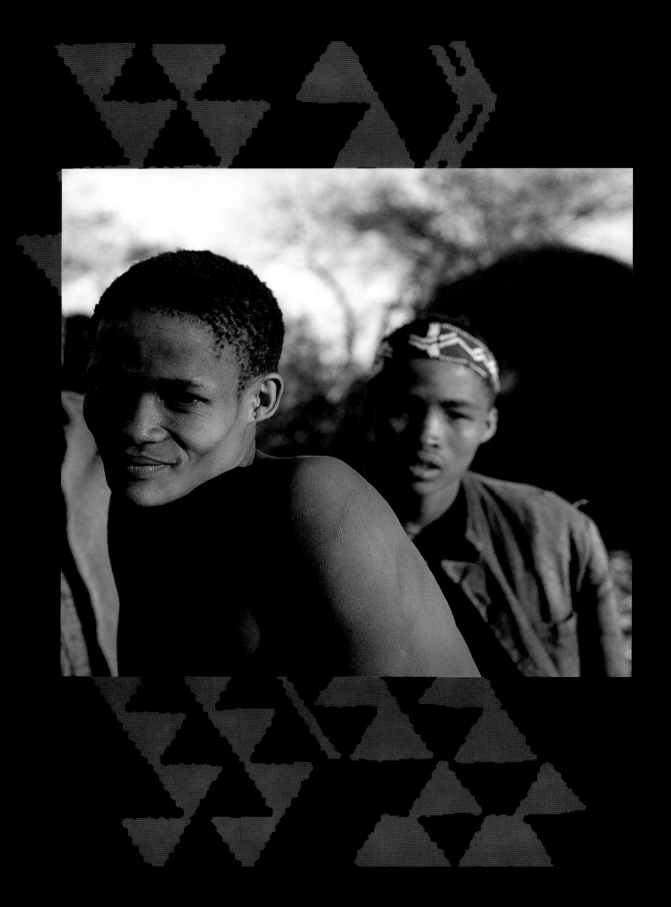

We ask ≠Oma !'Homg!ausi what will happen when the present healers are gone. He tells us:

> Our children will just stand around [and will not go forward] . . . they'll just die with no healers.

His view is a grim prospect, but it is shared by many. It is comforting, however, that ≠Oma Djo's words are also echoed by others:

> Nǀom is just the same as long ago, even though it keeps on changing. . . . The dance is still here at ǀKaeǀkae. It's doing well, and is still healing the people.

Nǀom, the profoundest expression of spiritual energy for the Juǀ'hoansi, could be linked to a humanistic and liberating outcome for their future; it may in fact become a linchpin to the evolution of their future. But in that critical and dynamic function, nǀom must rise up, boil, and heal the people within a complex set of sociopolitical forces that have their own accelerating dynamism of change, a dynamism that threatens to overwhelm the Juǀ'hoansi while ignoring their deepest needs and aspirations.

Will nǀom function as this key to liberating change? And if so, how might that be accomplished? We do not propose to answer such questions in this chapter, but in presenting some of the relevant issues and the Juǀ'hoan reflections on them, we hope to give voice to emerging Juǀ'hoan pathways into the future.

The creation of the future of the Juǀ'hoansi may be akin to the way the healing songs come into being. The

10 NǀOM AND SOCIAL CHANGE

Juǀ'hoansi believe that the great God, !Xu, puts nǀom into songs and gives them to the people. Those who receive nǀom songs pass them on freely to others, and songs move from group to group.

The process of "receiving" a nǀom song from !Xu is more than ordinary composing; there is a visionary element. Often a dream or vision occurs in which the idea or even the words are received and then transmitted to others through singing. Those who receive or create a song that carries nǀom can be profoundly moved. Lorna Marshall writes about such an experience that happened to an old Juǀ'hoan woman named Beh:

ǀKAECE (IN THE FOREGROUND)

IN 1968—A MAN STILL SEEKING

TO BECOME A HEALER.

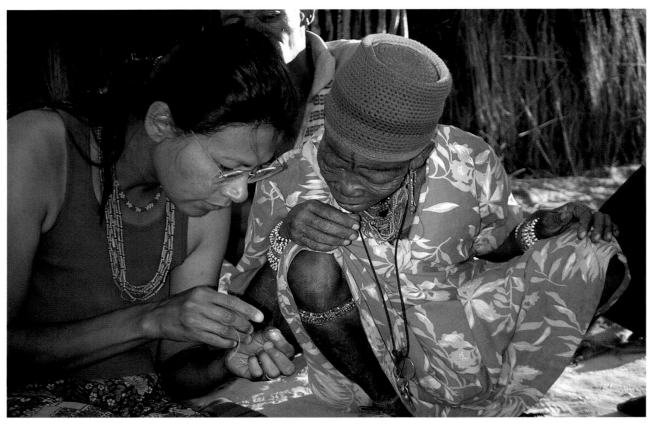

VERNA SHOWING HER FRIEND BAQ'U, AN EXPERT BEADER, HOW TO DO THE PEYOTE STITCH,

A COMMON WAY OF BEADING AMONG NATIVE PEOPLE IN NORTH AMERICA.

[God] had come to [Beh] in the days when she was young and fresh. He had appeared beside her while she was sleeping and had said, "You are crying for singing. Why do you not get up and sing!" She did get up, and she sang with him, imitating him and learning. He taught her in a kindly way and said, "Now, do not stay quiet as you used to do. Go and sing. Sing for the people as I have taught you." She was glad. When he left, she slept again. In all, he came five times to her in this way, in both the cold time and the hot time of the year."[1]

"Maybe [these songs] come from God," says ≠Oma Djo—as he teasingly stresses the "maybe"—"because later people just pass them to each other." ≠Oma Djo alludes to the widespread acceptance of songs that originally came to one person from God. These songs quickly become community property, ways to release healing to all—and the individual owner, the one originally gifted with the song, does not withhold or resent the distribution of the song but is honored through the community's use.

Tshao Matze elaborates on how this creative process ensures others can participate in its gifts.

> It's like thoughts, how you learn them; they're copies, like you make a paper. When you're setting down something, like sewing beads, and thinking how you'll do it, you might watch someone else's thoughts and later you go home and do your own, and by then the plan has grown, the thoughts are spreading.

THE POLITICS OF N!OM

When we who are men see women sewing
beads nicely, we say, "Where did you get the idea,
that you're doing such a good job?" And the person may say, "No, I'm just copying someone else."

Copying is more than mere imitation. It is also a process
of honoring. But by saying, "I'm just copying," the person
also expresses humility and a lack of personal credit
before a beautiful creation.

The primacy of spiritual knowledge and guidance in
the creative process is acknowledged, even assumed.
With such origins for artistic creations, the people simply
pass on what they have learned—they and then others
sing the song or bead the necklace until the "plan has
grown" and the "thoughts are spreading." The weaving of
the Jul'hoan future could very well spring from this spiritual source, practiced and shared by the people, so that
it becomes a community vision.

SPIRITUALITY
AND SOCIAL CHANGE

Many widely accepted models about social change focus
on a limited conception of political and/or economic
forces, ignoring the impact of psychological, ethical, spiritual, and other kinds of influences as well as their pervasive interweavings that create realities such as cultural
politics. The Jul'hoansi show us, for example, how their
spirituality lives within and on their land and its
resources. A focus on limited conceptions of political
and/or economic factors as the driving force behind
social change has proved to be an unsatisfactory explanation to many social theorists.[2]

Spirituality is increasingly looked to as a key element
in processes of social change.[3] As the Jul'hoansi survey
the many points of devastation to their culture, they still
point with assurance and pride to their healing dance.
The frequently heard statement that "we still have our
nǀom" becomes a badge of honor.

Spirituality in a culture, as is the case with the
Jul'hoansi, is often expressed with particular intensity in
its healing system. And healing systems are, in fact,
among those parts of the culture most sensitive to evolu-

tion. At the confluence of crisis, confusion, and opportunity—transitions that are the essence of culture
change—healing systems often function as the barome-
ters of and responses to such change. But there is also the
deep connection between healing systems and traditional life, and healers are often guardians of Indigenous
ways.

There are many different ways in which spirituality
has had an impact on change, including the guiding and
sometimes revolutionary role of prophets or other
divinely inspired leaders and the more often conservative
influence of organized religions. In fact, spirituality is
often reduced to religion, usually organized religion, and
then the change induced is often destructive, especially as
missionary fever is introduced.

But the Jul'hoan approach to spirituality has avoided
any of the structures such as priesthoods or formally prescribed ceremonies that typically characterize organized
religions. Jul'hoan healers, the primary guardians and
conduits of spirituality in the culture, are first and foremost individual Jul'hoansi. Like other Jul'hoansi, their
individuality is respected and supported, and that support continues into their performance as healers. There is
no proselytizing connected with the dance or with healing; rather, an open acceptance prevails. All are welcome
to join in; the different ways that others approach being
spiritual are respected. This openness gives the Jul'hoan
approach to spirituality the potential for effecting positive social change.

But the relationship between Jul'hoan spirituality as
expressed in the healing dance and social change as it
occurs in their community is not direct. Time and again
we are told that "healing is one thing, the problems with
our land and wells are another." Even when we are
reduced by our frustration to ask leading questions,
striving to connect spirituality and social change directly, they fail to budge their responses. When we ask if the
Jul'hoansi ever dance to find out solutions to the problems now facing them, ≠Oma Djo replies:

If it's something like a person who's hungry, we just
say that we're all hungry, and why is hunger perse-

cuting us? You ask each other in an ordinary way about ordinary things. You don't dance about it.

We pursue the question further by asking, "What are the things you dance about?" ≠Oma Djo's response adds clarity through its brevity: "You just dance: women sing and you dance." The dances are for healing; it was as simple as that.

"You just dance." This kind of statement, complete in itself, was to become our constant teacher as we talked with |Kae|kae healers about n|om. It was also our watchword as we teetered on the dangerous line between listening openly and asking too-leading questions.

In their own experience, the Ju|'hoansi don't waste time asking questions about the specific purpose of a dance or whether a dance causes a certain effect. Since they dance for a host of reasons at any one time, their tolerance for ambiguity and paradox prevents them from making causal connections that in the end are beyond human capacity to determine. As ≠Oma Djo says, they "just dance," and in that passionate and committed activity of the whole, they do their work of community healing.

In fact, the dance has never been unrelated to sociopolitical context. It has always been an integral part of daily life and subjected to its pressures. Historically, for example, the frequency of dances has been sensitive to the need for food and water; fewer dances were held when foraging activities were more intense. And today, the effect of alcohol consumption on the dance is never ignored, even while effective strategies of response are being developed.

We have already described in this book numerous examples of how the dance and the healing work have supported people in the past in their efforts to deal respectfully with issues of conflict and social change. A healing may focus for a time on a specific illness, but that illness is always understood in the context of, or as a reflection of, a social or cultural illness. Healing may also focus on social tensions, but they are always seen as having seeds in or repercussions on states of individual illness.

The dance as a means of helping resolve tensions within the community is well illustrated by the example of the time when the two older women, representing two sides of a divorce dispute, broke the trail of arguments going back and forth during the dance, making the heretofore broken singing circle complete, and thereby releasing healing energy to all. The work of the healers in easing and resolving tensions can be seen in the time the healer, chanting while in !aia, told the people at the dance that their disputing about cattle, a new resource in their rapidly changing world, was bringing bad feelings to the community and hence sickness to the man being healed.

On more and more occasions, healers are also becoming political spokespersons, as they are the ones who attend the meetings to discuss Ju|'hoan loss of land and culture. They are the ones who speak and are listened to. ≠Oma Djo's inescapable eloquence about the death of the Ju|'hoansi's land is but one example.

But with the new forms of change surrounding the Ju|'hoansi, and especially with the rapidily accelerating pace of that change, it seems appropriate to ask if the healing tradition is continuing—and will continue—to provide support for the people in their attempts to grapple with these changes. It is appropriate to ask, but we certainly cannot provide answers. Even if there were answers available, which seems unlikely, it is not our place to offer them. But we can, in listening to what the Ju|'hoansi are telling us, and, more important, seeing what they are showing us, offer some suggestions about how they are seeing their future.

"We still have our n|om" is an often-heard Ju|'hoan affirmation of strength, an expression of individual, community, and cultural self-esteem. "We still have our n|om" is one way of saying "We are Ju|'hoansi"; it may be the most penetrating and sensitive means to express their identity. Building on this strength of knowing who they are and what makes them quintessentially Ju|'hoan, the Ju|'hoansi can approach the challenges of social change with inner strength and conviction. Such inner resources build a foundation for an effective dialogue with and action toward the sociopolitical environment. Though

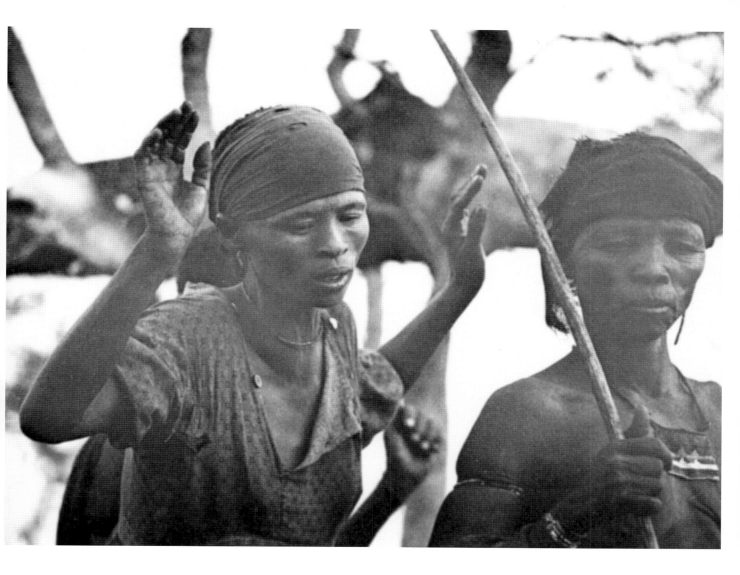

indirect, the relationship between spirituality and social change remains powerful.

We have considered some of the transformations brought about by n!om when it is activated as possible vehicles or training grounds for this inner strength and conviction. Perhaps climbing the threads to God's village or learning to "see properly" or the suffering through the pain of boiling n!om or the cultivation of heart has in the past functioned as such a vehicle—or may be functioning now or might function in the future. Certainly these transformations, which incorporate all of the individual and his or her community—body, mind, and spirit as one—offer a rich array of possibilities.

As we have seen, the dance has also in the past dealt

THE BEAUTY AND STRENGTH OF WOMEN

DANCING IN THE GIRAFFE DANCE

IS APPRECIATED BY THE ENTIRE COMMUNITY.

IIUCE (AT LEFT) MARRIED INTO KINACHAU'S GROUP.

directly with tensions within the community. There is already evidence that this function is continuing; for example, disputes over cattle, a dominant symbol of contemporary changes, have come under the purview of the dance.

As they are living out the creation of their future, the

Jul'hoansi do not seem to put a lot of energy into making what in Western analytical thinking are often assumed distinctions, for example, between social, political, cultural, and spiritual change or between the social harmony and spiritual balance that a dance can engender. Yet there are probably many good reasons for keeping the realms of the dance and politics conceptually separate. By not mixing the dance and contemporary political concerns, the Jul'hoansi can encourage the dance's distinctive function of healing and sustain a purity of purpose. No longer able to forage freely on their land, they may now be more "foragers" of consciousness, expressing through the dance traditional values such as sharing and egalitarianism as the nlom passes freely to all in attendance.

There is a promise among Jul'hoansi of what Dick has called a "renewed tradition"—change guided by sacred, spiritual traditions applied to contemporary issues and problems.[4] The introduction of the spiritual dimension into the processes of social change is not, as we mentioned, a new idea. The spiritual guidance offered through the Jul'hoan healing tradition, which demands truth of its practitioners while demanding acceptance of others, will help avoid the intolerance that historically has escalated to violence in the name of religious purity.

As guardians of a renewed tradition whose focus is the communal healing dance, the Jul'hoansi offer a particularly valuable path. In an insight picked up by many scholars, the anthropologist Roy Rappaport suggests that rituals in which we experience a transpersonal bonding are essential for the survival of humanity.[5] Only through participating in rituals like the healing dance can we overcome our separateness as individuals and accomplish the tasks essential to communal survival. In industrialized societies, individualism tends to fragment community. The transformation expressed in the dance offers an alternative to this fragmentation, stressing a transpersonal bonding within a supportive context.

Nlom could function at the core of any renewed tradition created by the Jul'hoansi. But nlom alone could not bring about desired changes, as the sociopolitical forces surrounding the Jul'hoansi are too overpowering. To understand the potential power of nlom, we must first understand more about its politics.

THE POLITICS OF NIOM

We hope this book has conveyed the depth of the Jul'hoan claim that "we still have our nlom." But equally important, we hope the book also conveys the depth of the Jul'hoan predicament—the intensity of their oppression, the pervasiveness of the devastation that eats away at their culture. The obstacles to self-determination and cultural survival Jul'hoansi face can seem overwhelming. Repeatedly we hear their observations and analyses of this terrible situation. Tshao Matze offers this perspective:

> When I think about Black people [Tswana and Hereros] and White people compared with Jul'hoansi, I want to break into tears. Today Black people are going to school and driving trucks like White people, while Jul'hoansi are still nothing. What are Jul'hoansi? We're dead. Black people don't want us to have trucks. We don't even have donkeys.
>
> Black people have their medicine and White people have theirs, and we Jul'hoansi have ours. But Black people are prejudiced and say Jul'hoansi are nothing-things and don't know anything. How is it that you people [who come to work with us] from America know we have knowledge, but those from here do not know it?

Given the bleakness of their situation, it is hard to imagine that any one factor, even something as central to their culture as the healing dance, could make a difference. But what does seem possible is that the dance, and the nlom that animates it, could act as a stimulating or organizing principle for a whole series of sociopolitical efforts toward change. Nlom could provide energy to propel the needed breakthrough, the way out of the bewildering and seemingly impenetrable net of oppression that closes tighter and tighter around the Jul'hoansi.

One example of a potential breakthrough is in the area

of Tswana and Herero attitudes toward Jul'hoansi. Much of the present oppression of Jul'hoan people is grounded in attitudes of disrespect—Jul'hoansi are seen through racist eyes as "dirty," "lazy," and "not fully human beings."

Jul'hoansi and the Tswana and Hereros presently collude in a particular interpretation about the "magic" of Jul'hoan healing. To some extent all the ethnic groups accept that Jul'hoansi possess access to mystical powers just by being "ancient people" with a long history on the land. For example, when faced with difficult cases of illness, Herero people from as far away as Ghanzi will send for Jul'hoan healers. As well, both Tswana and Herero people impute some potential for what they call "witchcraft" to the Jul'hoansi, a phenomenon known to both of their cultures but not indigenous to the Jul'hoansi. This "witchcraft," they believe, will be activated against them if they do not treat the Jul'hoansi with respect. But this is a guarded respect for the Jul'hoansi, thoroughly tinged with fear and still grounded in a generic disregard for the Jul'hoansi as a people. The Jul'hoansi, for their part, are ready to see the nǀom in other peoples' ways. They are ready to respect others when treated with respect. Can the Tswana and Herero people reciprocate?

Attitudes are one thing; land is another. Unless land once again becomes available to the Jul'hoansi, a change in attitude alone among the ruling peoples may make little difference in the actual lives of Jul'hoansi.

THE SYNERGY OF NǀOM [6]

In the traditional Jul'hoan approach to healing, nǀom is freely shared throughout the community. As it heats up, nǀom expands, bursting beyond the limits of any one person. ǀUi, who is old in the ways of healing, says, "Nǀom comes up in me and bursts open like a ripe seed pod." ǀUi waves his arms about and flicks his fingers as he describes the action of the seeds being expelled from their ripe pod. He also speaks of the sparks that leap out in every direction from a fire, especially when it is disturbed. Nǀom moves throughout the participants of a dance, bursting beyond one healer, leaping out to others. "I burst open my nǀom and give others some," said ǀUi.

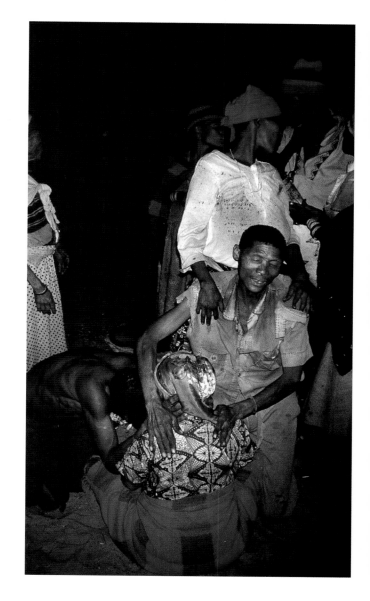

THE SYNERGISTIC EFFECT OF KXAO TJIMBURU (FACING US), HIS WIFE, N≠AISA (STANDING BEHIND HIM), AND OTHERS AT THE DANCE WORKING TOGETHER ON N≠AISA NǀA'AN GREATLY INCREASES THE HEALING NǀOM SHE RECEIVES.

Traditionally, nǀom is not in limited supply. Individuals need not compete for its healing power. The activation of nǀom in one person stimulates the activation in others. Nǀom can be infinitely divided without subtracting anything. The total healing effect of nǀom at a dance far exceeds the individual contributions toward activating that nǂom. The released healing energy binds people together in harmonious, mutually reinforcing relationships. The profound alterations of !aia are integrated into behaviors of daily life, and the two realms of experience stimulate and benefit from each other. In working with nǂom, the Jul'hoansi are simultaneously dealing with ordinary life issues and participating in a spiritual discipline. The individual enhancement of !aia is firmly lodged in a care-giving context. Healing simultaneously affirms the individual's worth and creates cultural meaning. The results can be remarkable—large numbers of persons regularly enhancing their consciousness in a way that is not only harmonious with their society but also essential to its maintenance.

This traditional Jul'hoan approach to healing, characteristic of healing in the late 1960s and still present in the late 1980s, can be called "synergistic." The term *synergy* refers to bringing phenomena together, interrelating them, and creating a new and greater whole from the disparate and seemingly conflicting parts.[7] Synergistic phenomena exist in harmony with each other, maximizing each other's potential. Two phrases capture this quality: "The whole is greater than the sum of the parts," and "What is good for one is good for all."

The Jul'hoan healing dance gains additional power because its synergy is an expression of the larger culture's general mode of adaptation and maintenance. The synergy that exists throughout traditional Jul'hoan culture resides in the collaborative use of the land and its resources. It also appears in the extensive sharing of material goods, made explicit in the way meat is distributed and in the exchange network called xaro. The network of mutually supportive relationships that maintains camp and intercamp life comes alive at the dance, providing a safe ground for the terrifying passage into !aia. The movement of healing nǂom from person to person throughout the dance reaffirms this network.

The way nǂom is activated holds the key to the healing power of the dance. Nǂom's healing power is greatest when it is received and applied synergistically. In a synergistic community, valued resources are renewable,

expanding, and accessible.[8] Traditionally, a "synergistic community" could be said to exist both within the dance and within Jul'hoan culture at large. Shared equitably with all members of the community, the whole of these resources becomes greater than the sum of the parts, and what is good for one is good for all.

Nǂom exemplifies such a valued resource. Though nǂom is seen and held by the healers, it is infinitely expandable when activated at dances. Such a phenomenon becomes difficult, perhaps impossible, to treat nonsynergistically, like trying to contain smoke in a cheesecloth bag.

Attempts to contain or hoard nǂom have occurred and continue to occur. ≠Oma Djo himself went through a period in his forties when he tried to establish the unique power of his nǂom, to get others to "pay" him for his healing efforts. He would refuse to teach others and hold back dancing directed toward reaching !aia until dawn, well past the time many women were able to continue to "raise their voices to the heavens." His behavior at this time was in sharp contrast to lUi's approach to nǂom, who spoke about wanting to be healed, for once healed he would then heal others; a benefit to him was a benefit to others:

> I need nǂom and my heart seeks it. I'm really hot
> for it. I want the youngsters to look at my shoulder
> and I want to have a taste of their nǂom. I would
> say to one of those young healers, "Hey, this shoul-
> der of mine is killing me. Let me see if you can do
> your stuff and pull something out of it." If I get a
> good taste of the nǂom, then I'll have !aia and
> [heal] others, then I'll say, "O my children, today
> you've done me properly, for now I feel myself
> again."[9]

This reciprocity and mutual enhancement now once again characterizes ≠Oma Djo's healing work as well; he has returned to the synergy of the old way.

When hoarders attempt to limit nǂom, they introduce principles of scarcity into the dance. Synergy and scarcity represent two ends of a continuum and in actual situations exist in combination.[10] A scarcity paradigm dominates Western thinking about the existence and distribution of a wide variety of resources. Also known as the zero-sum game, this paradigm assumes that valued resources are limited and that the degree of scarcity determines value. Further, it posits that individuals and communities must compete with each other to gain access to these resources and accumulate their own supply, and that sharing must be avoided. Such a paradigm of scarcity is characteristic of the capitalistic forces encroaching on Jul'hoan land and threatens Jul'hoan culture and the dance it supports.

Within a synergistic community, a resource like healing can become renewable and accessible and still remain valuable.[11] Individuals and communities function as guardians and not possessors of resources, sharing them with all members of the community. Traditional Jul'hoan education for healing ensures that nǀom will not be used for personal aggrandizement or the manipulation of others. When collaboration rather than competition is encouraged, greater amounts of the valued resource become available. Paradoxically, the more the resource is used, the more there is available. That is the life course of nǀom—as ǀUi tells us, if he gets a "good taste" of nǀom from others, he's able to return the healing effort and serve others.

But the scarcity paradigm is strong, and its grip can strangle. Even healing resources are not immune. In the Western biomedical model, healing resources are seen to be in scarce supply. People are forced to compete with each other for their share of healing.

In many cases, scarcity seems more of a function of ideology than of necessity. Though most communities in contemporary industrialized urban life function primarily within the scarcity paradigm, they nonetheless require moments of synergy in order to remain intact. The necessity of sharing is increasingly evident for the survival of the human community. Scarcity thinking helps promote actual scarcity in living, whereas an attitude of sharing could alleviate much of the scarcity that does in fact exist.

It is unrealistic to expect that nǀom and its synergistic functioning could alone change an entire way of living in which access to resources by some people stems from the disempowerment of others. We are never led to such thinking by the Jul'hoansi, who remain modest to the end about the significance of their dance. But nǀom, when functioning synergistically, does provide a living image of sharing and respect for all. Applying this image to effect concrete decisions about sociopolitical realities could allow the Jul'hoansi to benefit from resources that were always theirs to share, which would benefit all of the peoples of the region.

THE CENTRAL SIGNIFICANCE OF HEART

The concept of "heart," or *ǃka*, is very important for the Jul'hoansi. Not only does the word denote the physical heart of an animal or person and its many emotions, but it also means "inside" or "within" in a generic sense. For instance, a tuber growing deep in the sand is said to be "in the heart of the sand," or a person sitting among her kin is said to be "at their heart."

Heart is essential in the activation of nǀom and in bringing its healing effect to the people. It is the critical ingredient in a young person's desire to drink nǀom, just as it remains the critical ingredient in allowing the nǀom to boil in experienced healers. When ≠Oma Djo looks over the young people and spots one who is eager to learn healing, he comments, "That youngster will someday drink nǀom. He dances with his heart in it." ≠Oma Djo goes on to describe how he judges readiness to learn in young people:

> The guys I look for are strong dancers. . . . They are really putting their heart into dancing, they are dancing with passion. They're the guys I really want to put nǀom into. Then there is another type of guy you see dancing. He's up and down, up and down. He's in one turn, sitting at the side the next time. Even if a guy like that asked me, I would refuse.[12]

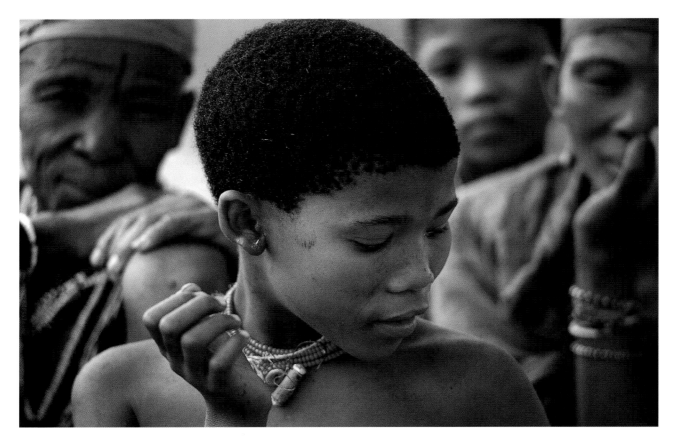

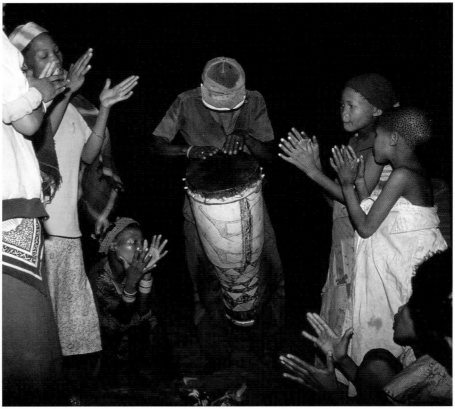

ABOVE: SURROUNDED BY THE CARING PRESENCE OF THE WOMEN WITH WHOM SHE HAS BEEN SINGING STRONGLY ALL NIGHT, A GIRL SITS PENSIVELY AT THE DANCE'S END. THEIR WORK TOGETHER MAKES THEIR HEARTS HAPPY.

THE WOMEN SING PASSIONATELY, "WITH HEART," AS THEY ORIENT TOWARD THE POWERFUL DRUM BEAT PLAYED AT THE OPENING OF THE DRUM DANCE'S HORSESHOE STRUCTURE.

THE POLITICS OF N|OM

It is not the dancing per se that matters, but heart, expressed and activated by the dancing. In his old age, ≠Oma Djo speaks on a similar theme: "I sometimes go to [a dance] and if my heart doesn't want to dance, I just watch. I sit and watch and then go home." But as an elder, ≠Oma Djo's heart always seems ready for nǀom, and he rarely just watches.

Singing must also be done with heart. When the dance is strong and boiling nǀom is imminent, women are heard to cry out to the dancers with enthusiastic teasing: "We have just begun to sing. You there, have you not yet learned to dance!" Laughing with each other, the singers continue:

> Tonight we will not move, not even to take a piss. We will stay in our places and sing and clap until dawn . . . [because] tonight is a night for our singing to climb into the skies![13]

ǀUi speaks bluntly and definitively from his more than forty years of experience with !aia:

> It's not good when the women are chattering [at the dance], because when they half sing and half talk, the music is not heavy, it is light, and the one doing nǀom has no strength behind him. But when the singing is strong and rises up toward the heaven, then the one doing nǀom, his nǀom boils hot and he can heal better.[14]

The songs call the spirits to the dance, where they seek to take the sick ones away. These songs can either encourage or prevent sickness, says N≠aisa, herself a very strong singer, depending on how they are sung.

> If people don't sing, but just lie down, the spirits will say, "What is it that these people are not singing" . . . and if you don't sing, or sing badly, these spirits will torment you.

But if the women sing passionately, that is "with heart," then, N≠aisa tells us, the spirits' "hearts will be happy," and sickness will be kept at bay.

Emotions and values connected by the Juǀ'hoansi with heart include covetousness, stinginess, and generosity; fearfulness, courage, and self-sufficiency; unhappiness and happiness; short-temperedness and patience; and judgments on whether a person acts "good" or "bad," especially in relationships with others. Ideas about what the heart and its emotions can do are strong and carry a great deal of social weight. A person whose heart is not "happy" or "at rest" is said to be prone to do damage to herself or to others. An unhappy heart comes from great sadness or envy.

Envy is an emotion of the heart that is believed to cause arrows of sickness or *xabasi* to pass from the envier into the envied.[15] Xabasi can also cause the one who feels the envy to become ill. These arrows can cause foreboding, serious illness, and even death. The sicknesses caused by disquiet hearts are preeminently those that Juǀ'hoan healers seek to cure.

Juǀ'hoan healers are specialists in matters of the heart. One of the functions they perform is to //xabe or "open up" their own hearts "so that they may feel the real feelings of their own flesh." This "opening up" in turn allows healers to open the hearts and bodies of the sick to accept healing as the healers ≠hoe or "pull the sickness from them." When healers say "healing makes our hearts happy," they are in part literally referring to the techniques for loosening their own and others' hearts so that healing and feelings of community can flow for all.

The key to singing and dancing is to have an open heart. Singing and dancing are artforms for the Juǀ'hoansi, but their expressive beauty is secondary to their power to heal. In the healing dance, one sings and dances first to activate nǀom; the pleasure of beautiful dancing and singing is a bonus. Teaching one to sing and dance with an open heart so that nǀom can boil is essentially an emotional, psychological, and spiritual teaching.

An "open heart" is the human opening to the spirits, the way in which Juǀ'hoan healers and their community can access nǀom. To have an open heart is to have courage, trust, dedication, and passion—courage to face the raging pain of boiling nǀom, trust in the community's support for the healing journey, dedication to serving the people, and passion to sustain the healer's journey despite periods of doubt and instances of "failure."

As an "open heart" allows nǀom to boil and bring the gifts of healing to the people, a "happy heart" is a resultant expression of this healing. ≠Oma Djo describes a "happy heart" this way:

> After a dance, my heart feels happy. As I walk
> across the pan, and see people, I feel good inside,
> and want to greet them. I am happy they have
> been healed at the dance.

A "happy heart" speaks of a sense of wholeness and completeness in the community, a sense of connectedness with others that ensures this community. A happy heart overflows with the joy of seeing others and seeing them well taken care of; it is a state of love for others, motivated by the desire to serve or heal them and be served or healed by them.

Contemporary political discussions have highlighted the need for heart energies that have a certain edge to them. While the healing aspects of heart remain, having a "happy" heart does not become equated with a lack of concern for or involvement with the issues of the day. !Xuma, a healer from Dobe, speaks about these energies at a political meeting in Namibia in 1991 that dealt with Julʼhoan losses and their quest for justice:

> The matters [discussed at this meeting] are matters
> of the heart. When we go to meetings like this,
> Julʼhoansi should be represented by someone
> whose heart is *not* at peace. When people talk
> together, this thing that is your heart hangs at your
> nǀǀao spot [the top of the spine where healers expel
> sickness with the kowhedili shriek]. We want people
> who really have heart to go to meetings, not just
> ordinary people who will sit there and say nothing.

As heart opens the door to nǀom, it releases synergy into the community. With heart, young Julʼhoansi could learn about healing—healing of themselves, their family, their community—even as they are surrounded by a hostile environment. Without heart, there is in fact no real learning.

CREATING THE FUTURE

Perhaps as with the healing songs, the Julʼhoan will weave some of their future from spiritually guided experiences that are shared throughout the community. The healing dance could then become a central source of change, the boiling nǀom a central energizer, helping give people the strength and confidence necessary to speak and act out for their rights.

Though the older healers may lament that too few young people are putting their heart into learning to become healers, the number of healers has never been an issue. Traditionally, those who were not inclined to "drink nǀom" because they feared the pain too much were neither criticized nor devalued. Perhaps in these times of crisis, there are still enough healers because those who pursue that aim are doing so with heart. And heart is especially needed as the threats to the dance mount; healers must be passionate and dedicated seekers of nǀom.

When some spiritual traditions have been threatened, they have moved underground, kept alive by a few passionate and dedicated practitioners. Though the flame of the spiritual practice burns low, it is never extinguished. When external oppression relaxes or ceases, that carefully tended flame burns more brightly in the open. Then the spiritual practice may flourish again.

The Native or First Nations peoples in Canada and the United States offer recent examples of this pattern of preserving a spiritual tradition through secret nurturance so it can reemerge to better serve the people. When ceremonies such as the sweat lodge and sun dance were outlawed, they were performed less frequently and more secretly deep in the bush. A few dedicated practitioners kept these ceremonies alive, and now they serve the current generations more fully. Perhaps if at least a few Julʼhoan healers continue their work with heart, they will keep the dance alive.

Julʼhoan healers, especially the older ones, are always talking about the healers of the past as having the "real" power. This deference to the past is typical of healers throughout the world. It does not, however, deny the strength of present or future practitioners. Tshao Matze in particular defers to the power of healers who have passed away. Yet today, he is one of the healers young people consider powerful. Tshao Matze has taken his place among the old ones. The young seekers of nǀom will "drink nǀom" in their own way, a way that will be different from the old ones, yet drink nǀom they will. The tradition of Juǀʼhoan healing must change if it is to live.

In addition to this reassuring presence of heart in those who already practice healing and those who seek it, there is the recent emergence of healers as political spokespersons, which has important implications for social change. There seems to be an almost inevitable movement of some of the strongest healers and supporters of the dance into positions of responsibility in regard to the Juǀʼhoansi's contemporary political and economic situation. For example, when persons from ǀKaeǀkae were invited to attend a meeting in Namibia to discuss Juǀʼhoan loss of land and resources and potential Juǀʼhoan efforts toward empowerment in the new political landscape, the majority of those who went and spoke most eloquently were healers.

The Juǀʼhoansi speak of the "path" or "road" they seek to follow in and through the dance. The dance, they say, provides an "opening" into that path. That path is a means of understanding and living the spiritual requirements of the healer's journey and the moral requirements of living in harmony with others.

The concept of a path in life—or a "path of life"—is common to cultures throughout the world, as is the requirement that the path be "straight" or approached with "straightness."[16] Among Fijians, for example, the "straight path" describes the way persons should ideally live, and healers are especially required to pursue a path that adheres to values like honesty, humility, love, and service.[17] In Buddhism, the Eightfold Path leads to nirvana, the state transcending the limitations of earthly experience and self-seeking; the Diné (Navajo) path of life stresses harmony and balance with all of nature;[18] and in the Christian tradition, the path of asceticism, contemplation, and affirmation followed by the fourth-

century desert fathers is one source of Western monasticism.[19] Among the Lakota, life is seen as a choice between the Red Road, which offers the challenge of correct living, and the Black Road;[20] and the Seven Fires of Life celebrate successive stages or levels that mark a proper transition through life for Anishinabe (Saulteaux) people.[21]

These differing manifestations of a path of life are not reducible to a single pattern, but they do share important features. The paths evolve from a relationship with a higher power or spiritual force. They are described and presented to the people by those who have learned about the path from experience and who are committed to passing on their own life experience and the ancient truths they have been taught. For Indigenous peoples, the path is simply the traditional way of life that defines what it means to be truly human; it is a series of very practical truths, as much as philosophical ideas.

Traveling along the path requires constant struggle and vigilance. It is not a clear and linear process but rather is filled with ambiguity, confusion, and temptation, leading to wrong turns on the way to understanding. Specific behaviors may be necessary to stay on the path, and along it one may pass through specific stages. But since the path presents a way of being, it is not so much an exact prescription or chronology as a guide for the way life should be lived. Critical to this way of being are fundamental values and attitudes needed to find and stay on the path, typically including respect, humility, love, sharing, and service.

The concept of a path of life is particularly strong among Indigenous peoples. As there is increasing recognition in industrialized nations, which control most of the world's resources, of the wisdom of Indigenous peoples, we hope those who control resources will listen to this wisdom in order to rekindle their own understanding of a path in their lives. If they do, they may be motivated to release the power they have accumulated—a power that is not even "theirs" to release—so that others, still denied access to that power, can take on their rightful share. As people begin to walk a straight path of life, a sharing of power becomes more possible. Those who exert inordinate control over the destiny of the Juǀʼhoansi may finally hear the Juǀʼhoansi call for the resources they deserve and the dignity they have earned. But first they must realize the Juǀʼhoansi are a "real" people and a people whose power is enlarged through their connection in the larger global context to the many, many Indigenous peoples who are also laying claim to their future. The call for spiritual guidance of human development has been particularly eloquent among Indigenous peoples who strive for the continuing life of their traditions in today's world. The Juǀʼhoansi join that call.

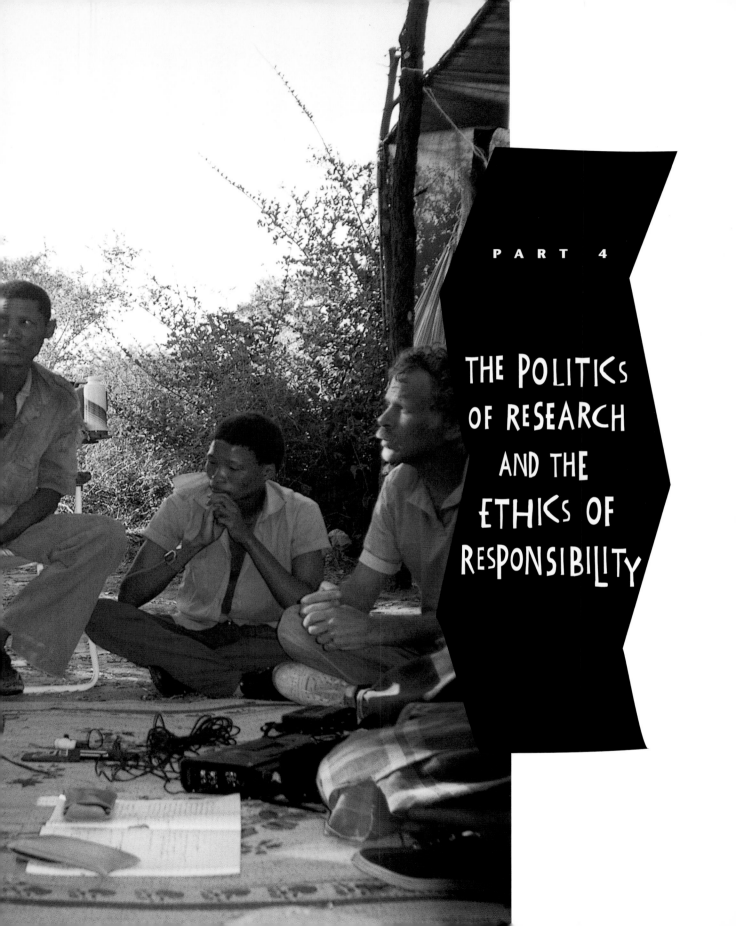

PART 4

THE POLITICS OF RESEARCH AND THE ETHICS OF RESPONSIBILITY

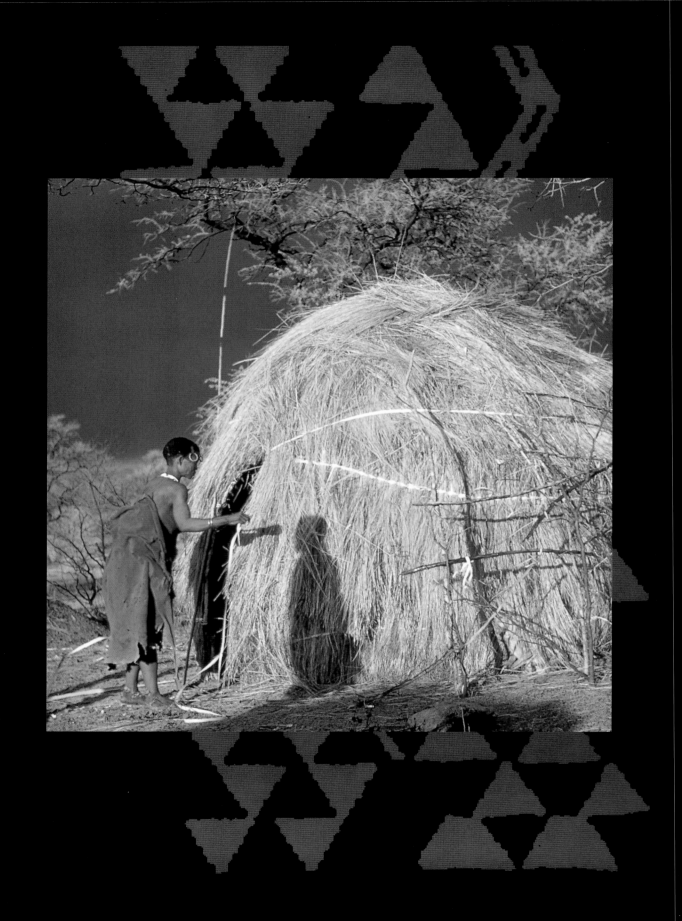

An important part of any project, especially when it is work done with another culture, is for the researchers to reflect upon and analyze critically their roles and contributions. In this and the next two chapters, we will try to touch on some of the issues that have influenced our work, whether limiting its significance and biasing its conclusions or offering a special set of insights. In appendix A, we will continue sharing our reflections, focusing more on how the relationships between the three of us as researchers added another layer of influence upon the Jul'hoan story. With this sharing we hope to illuminate further our role in interpreting the words of the Jul'hoansi.

The planning for our visit to |Kae|kae had taken two years. And even the actual trip from North America was long and arduous, especially the twelve-hour drive through unforgiving desert roads to |Kae|kae. Yet when we arrived in |Kae|kae, it seemed as if we had been teleported, so quickly and completely were we in the midst of a very different place.

When the very next morning we began talking intimately with healers about their work, Verna, who was new to |Kae|kae, began to feel that in some ways our entry into the heart of |Kae|kae life had been too easy. She wondered—given the countless examples of how Indigenous peoples have resisted the research ventures of anthropologists, at times providing superficial and even false answers just to appear polite—could the Jul'hoansi also be "resisting" this research?

On the other hand we were not your typical visitors. Two of us have long-standing and emotionally intense

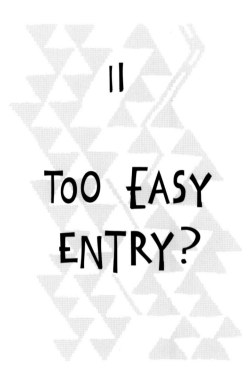

11
TOO EASY ENTRY?

connections with the |Kae|kae people. The anthropologist Richard Lee, a colleague who has worked in the area over the past thirty years, has also become active in the Jul'hoansi's efforts at self-determination. Richard enabled Dick's work with |Kae|kae healers in 1968, including translating for him. And Megan has worked in both Botswana and what is now Namibia for more than twenty-five years. She has continuing connections with Namibian Jul'hoansi and their |Kae|kae relatives, focusing on collaborative development efforts, folklore, and healing, especially among the women.

As a team, we were "old friends" to the people. In

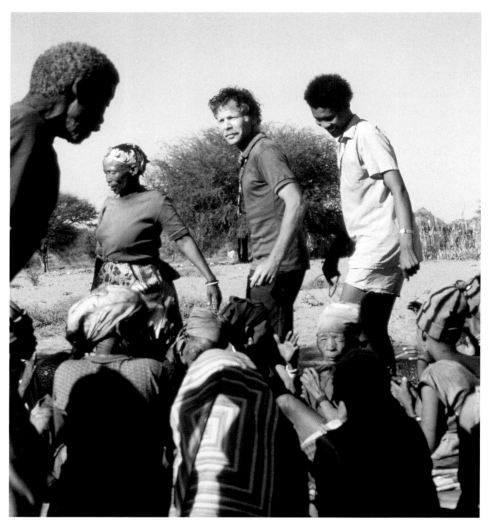

WITH ≠OMA DJO DANCING IN THE FOREGROUND, DICK RETURNS TO THE DANCE IN 1989,

FLANKED BY N≠AISA N!A'AN AND !UKXA.

addition to the joy of seeing long-absent friends, we had messages to deliver and work to do in an effort to further ongoing development projects. It is significant to note that even had we been strangers, we would likely have been well received. The Ju/'hoansi welcome most visitors with enthusiasm even without knowing them, and the healing dance is open to all. There is no need to talk with them about special procedures.

Yes, we were "old friends," but with Verna's thoughts in mind, we realized at new levels of complexity how, in addition to friendship, elements of power were at work. Verna asked us to consider, if ≠Oma Djo came to our home and decided to stay a few months, would we change our life patterns to orient ourselves around his needs to the extent he did for us? We could not deny the fact that, given his limited resources, it would be impossible for ≠Oma Djo to support such a stay, whereas our own access to research grants and personal resources made our trip to !Kae!kae possible. We all felt the implicit power, even the impertinence, that allowed us to come and go from the Kalahari at our own wish and pursue topics that fit into our own personal and professional interests.

We were not unfamiliar with how power had an impact on our relationship with the Jul'hoansi. Megan, for example, noticed during her research stay at Kauri in the early 1970s that the people were not going out into the bush on their yearly round. When she asked them why, they answered that since Megan was buying crafts from them, she had become a lucrative source of income, so why move?

The issue of inequitable power has plagued anthropological work historically.[1] Cecil King, a First Nations Odawa educator, describes consequences that result from an abuse of power:

> We, as Indian people, have welcomed strangers into our midst. We have welcomed all who came with intellectual curiosity or the guise of the informed student. We have honored those whom we have seen grow in their knowledge and understanding of our ways. But unfortunately, many times we have been betrayed. Our honored guests have shown themselves to be no more than "peeping toms," rank opportunists, interested in furthering their own careers by trading in our treasured traditions. Many of our people have felt anger at the way that our communities have been cheated, held up to ridicule, and our customs sensationalized.[2]

Floyd Westerman, a Native American artist and activist, expresses this anger and feeling of betrayal in his classic and still-relevant song "Here Come the Anthros."

And the Anthros
Still keep coming
Like death and taxes to our land.

To study their
Feathered freaks
With funded money in their hand.

Like a Sunday
at the zoo
Their cameras click away

Taking notes
And tape recordings
Of all the animals at play

Chorus:
Here come the Anthros
Better hide your past away
Here come the Anthros
On another holiday.

We too must remain suspect; though we have tried to avoid abusing our power, we must continue to examine our motives. The consequences of all our actions have to be open to question—especially what we believe are "good" actions resulting from "sincere" or "informed" motives. The thirty years of contact between the Jul'hoansi and researchers must have obligated and encouraged the Jul'hoan people to act at times like "good subjects" in order to satisfy the researchers' "needs." There must have been times when they were tired of our questions and just answered something so they could get on with their day. The ǀKaeǀkae research team's morning ritual of breakfast with several of the Jul'hoan healers was a wonderful way to visit and plan the research effort for the day; it was also an excellent breakfast for those healers.

At the same time, it's wrong to portray Jul'hoan people as powerless and always vulnerable to our needs. How have they resisted and maintained their power to endure to this day? We may never know. Clearly, if some of our Western "support machines," such as the truck and the store supply of Western food items, had broken down, we would have been dependent on the Jul'hoansi's knowledge of the land to survive. Even with these supports, we already were dependent on the Jul'hoansi to live safely on their land and cope with the heat and the presence of wild animals. And we too turned to their healing dance for sustenance.

Economic factors were an important dimension of our relationship with ǀKaeǀkae, and they always tended to put us in a position of power. Though we traveled "light," our equipment and food supplies made us extravagantly rich by ǀKaeǀkae standards. Though we participated in the local economy—buying or selling according to a fair local price plus some added dollars, we knew that we were even richer than others perceived us as most of our resources were still back home. And we were constantly pained by how stingy we could be when we stuck to fair ǀKaeǀkae prices, not wanting to be seen by others as people who "knew nothing," who were incapable of bargaining in the ǀKaeǀkae way. And how could we take comfort in the bargain prices that prevailed, knowing of the poverty of the people and our relative wealth?

Juǀ'hoansi who worked with us benefited economical-ly from their association with us and were able to pass these benefits on to their families and relatives. In addition to paying our research assistants and those we interviewed, we shared our food supplies and used our vehicle to help gather firewood and make hunting and gathering trips, an enormous boost for strenuous activities.

But these economic benefits also must have introduced tensions within the community. Traditionally, Juǀ'hoan people distribute resources such as the meat from a large kill throughout the entire community through the heads of the various families. People will complain about the fairness of any distribution; it is almost an expected way of communication. Our economic distributions were no different. In addition, by trying to recognize the efforts and services of particular people, we may have undercut the *wholesale* equitable distribution patterns of traditional Juǀ'hoan culture and so introduced new tensions. For example, we gave goods to the five healers we worked with most closely, such as

THE INFLUENCE OF WESTERN CONVENIENCES

IN OUR RESEARCHER'S CAMP

EXPRESSES OUR RELATIVE WEALTH

AT ǀKAEǀKAE.

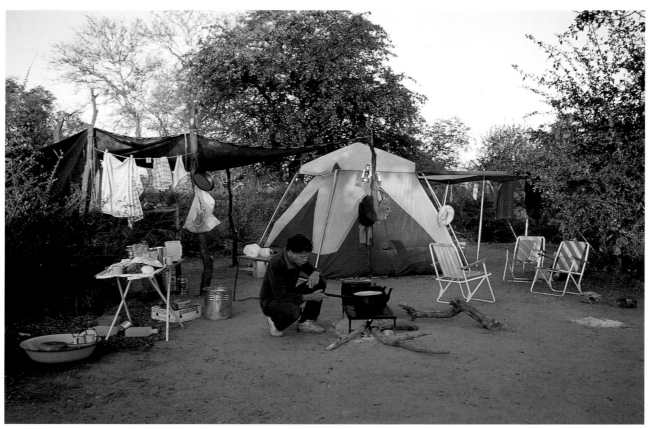

THE POLITICS OF RESEARCH

flour and tea, as well as paying them a salary as research assistants. While paying for their services, we also wished to give special honor to their work as healers. However, though we knew that these healers would distribute these goods through their own kin network, the act of singling out these five individuals, even to honor their healing work, must have created new jealousies.

We entered |Kae|kae within the context of these undeniable historical and economic factors. But we entered mostly as three human beings who came to learn—and we did learn something about how we might be of help. We hope the warmth of our everyday relationships with the people of |Kae|kae and the commitment we made to serve as their advocates justify our ease of entry.

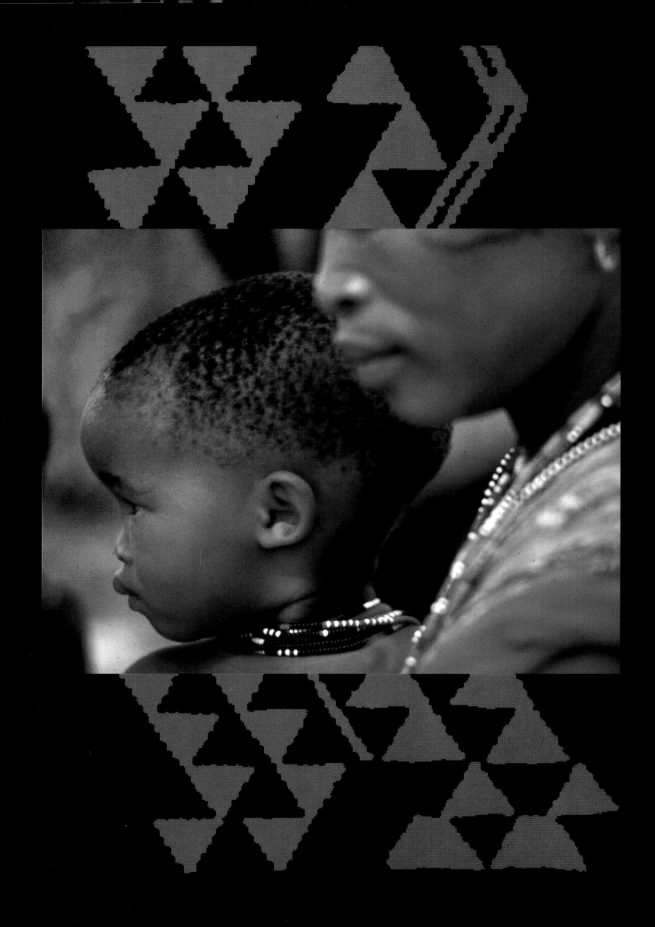

Xumi N!a'an speaks graphically of the way a moment and place in history—|Kae|kae in 1991—seem to him. In his words that follow we see his profound unease and pervasive sense that everything the Jul'hoansi possess is now to be taken from them.

> My land is the land of Botswana. Why is it that the Americans have their land, the Hambukushu have theirs—everyone has a land—but ours is taken away? We want a place called "BaSarwa" some-where. Even the Burusi [Boers] didn't pay for their land [when they settled in southern Africa], nor did the Americans. Why can't we have our own place?
>
> But the Tswana keep talking about *"tengnyana-teng."* This means "that which is deep down in the ground." This is the meaning of tengnyanateng. They mean Bushmen.
>
> Then there's another thing the Tswana say. They say *"O mang?"* [Who are you?] You say, "It's me; I want to come in." And they then say, "Don't come in!"
>
> If the Tswana are going to discriminate against us this way, we want to get together with Masire [the president of Botswana, who is a Tswana]. We want him to explain tengnyanateng and O mang to us. We'll ask him what these two things are sup-posed to mean to us. We'll see how he gets out of that one.
>
> We Jul'hoansi don't know who the government is. We all thought maybe the government was all

JUL'HOAN CHILDREN WATCH AND

PARTICIPATE IN ALL THAT OCCURS.

THEY ARE LEARNING THE WORDS AND WAYS

OF THEIR MOTHERS AND FATHERS.

12
WORDS AND VOICES

> of us. But now they say that Jul'hoansi must take care of themselves. If we'd spoke to Masire, we'd ask if we were part of the government. If not, what is the government? Why haven't we been given what other people have—land, for instance? And if he'd answer, "There's your share over there, now work for yourself," we'd say "Yes!"

Xumi N!a'an's voice is clear. He expresses a deep dis-trust for the returns on exchanges into which Jul'hoan people are being thrust—and a straightforward set of proposals for establishing equity.

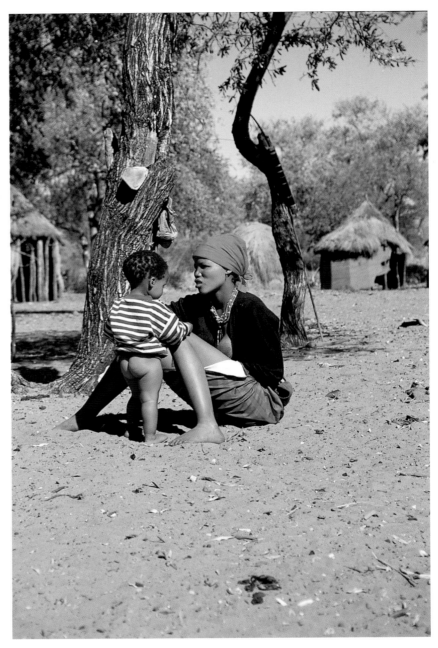

THE VAST LANDS OUTSIDE THEIR
CAMPS ARE CRUCIAL TO JUI'HOAN SUR-
VIVAL AND ARE AT GREAT RISK OF
BEING LOST TO THEM. THIS FACT IS AS
TRUE IN THE JUI'HOAN AREA OF
NAMIBIA, WHERE THIS PHOTOGRAPH
WAS TAKEN, AS IT IS IN BOTSWANA.

Cultural translators such as ourselves face a substantial challenge. Not only do we have to command enough of the people's language to get the basic translations correct, but also we must try to understand and convey the nuances and metaphors involved. This is especially important and difficult when Indigenous peoples are actively seeking to get past barriers of language and nonliteracy in order for their truths to be heard. But perhaps the hardest challenge for translators is to resist the temptation to construct their own messages out of the raw material of people's voices as projection occurs insidiously.

One way to think through these problems is to regard sophisticated media and tools of literacy as just that—tools—but tools that are made to be shared, to be loaned.

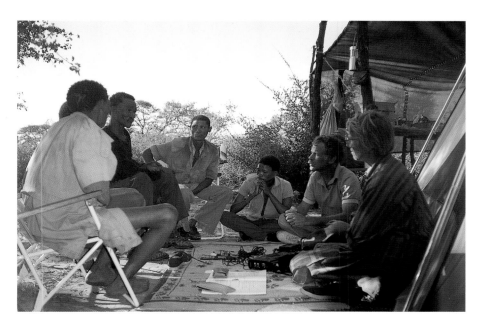

DICK AND MEGAN INTERVIEWING THE HEALERS—(FROM LEFT TO RIGHT) ≠OMA !'HOMG!AUSI, ≠OMA DJO (NOT VISIBLE IN PHOTO), TSHAO MATZE AND KXAO TJIMBURU—WITH THE TRANSLATING HELP OF TSHAO XUMI (SITTING NEXT TO DICK), ANOTHER MEMBER OF THE RESEARCH TEAM.

They are special tools in that others are meant to be taught to use them. Being used in fresh and new ways by new users, these tools become better. Increasingly, Jul'hoansi are requesting tools of literacy from outsiders because they find themselves in a situation where they need immediately tools that are still unfamiliar to them. Though many young Jul'hoansi are already learning the literacy skills they require, the need to communicate on their own behalf is already before them. While they are learning, the Jul'hoansi are asking researchers like us and development workers to assist them in getting their message across. And if this assistance is given in the right way and freely shared without "strings attached," the Jul'hoansi learning of literacy skills will be even more dramatically encouraged.

When Jul'hoan leaders from the soon to be independent Namibia spoke to the ǀKaeǀkae people about their own new success in political organizing with their Farmers' Cooperative, they emphasized communication. Tsamkxao ≠Oma expressed the sentiment of those Namibian Jul'hoansi:

> [One big thing] is radio-telephones. As we sit here today, Namibia is becoming independent, but talking together is still hard because not all of us can speak each other's languages. This is a problem when we try to work for land rights.
>
> We work with the Farmers' Cooperative, which isn't even government, but in fact even our speech is capable of going onto a cassette. Tape recorders don't refuse it. We're doing it in a small way; we're just at the beginning. But people have told us this way of speaking is powerful; it has nǀom.

Receiving the messages Jul'hoansi want to send—about the loss of land and access to food resources and the difficulties they have in finding political representation—requires a careful listening. It also involves a willingness to listen while things are being worked on and worked out, forgoing the expectation that only polished statements and conclusions will emerge.

In doing the careful listening that has resulted in this book, we offered Jul'hoan people a chance to express themselves in the unfamiliar forum of our interviews. This opportunity had of course a dual potential; being unfamiliar, it could have either forced them to respond in artificial and limited ways or encouraged them to respond in more creative, perhaps more reflective ways. It is likely that both occurred and in differing degrees with different people. On the whole, the Jul'hoansi seemed to welcome the chance to explore with us during the interviews what they wanted to do and what they could do to make their lives meaningful and enjoyable despite unsettling new challenges. People looked forward to the interviews and never seemed to tire of talking about their concerns and aspirations. Those who were not the specific focus of an interview might join in the discussions or merely sit with us, listening to one of the healers speak.

However, though much sincere friendliness prevailed, it was necessary for us to keep in mind the inequities inherent in the interview situation. Using the tools of literacy to facilitate communication between the Jul'hoansi and others involved us in many issues of exchange and power. Cultural "brokering" or cultural translation provides by its very nature a privileged grasp on other people's reality, which may have critical implications for them in the wider world. When, for example, something is broadcast over radio or TV or is published, many middlepersons profit from the transaction and may change the meaning of the message.

In the end, whose words and whose voice comes across? Who profits from the words of the people? Are the people even informed about the journeys their words take? The irony is that the Jul'hoansi do not hoard their knowledge; in offering it freely to those who need it or are interested in it, they are defying profit structures. But when these structures scoop up their words, it is only right that the rewards accrue to them. The possibilities for corrupt communication are even more pervasive than those for economic corruption.

What does it mean that we outsiders envisioned our research project and the messages it produced as important priorities for the Jul'hoansi? If we had not come to |Kae|kae in 1989 with a grant for that project, Jul'hoan people who spent time with us would have been occupied in other ways. What would be the proper balance between conducting our "research" and heeding what might be for them more pressing concerns?

But when Tshao Matze invited us to become "paper people," he was helping to create that balance by inviting

but not demanding our research to move toward becoming work on "pressing concerns." When he spoke to us *as* paper people, Tshao Matze talked about the perennial need of his community for the water and food that come from having clear access to land. But he was also talking about wider issues of communication and power, the frustrations of illiteracy, and the tasks an Indigenous community could reasonably ask of outsiders schooled in the tools of literacy.

Part of the story we have to tell involves the interplay in contemporary Jul'hoan tradition of expectation and observation, of conservative ideology and creative symbolism. It is a story of history—both past and present— told by a "committee" of Jul'hoan people. The voice of this book is not one person but a medley of voices. It is a story of differing authorities, of deference and tolerance. A story where truth lies—if it exists—in verbal communication. And most arrestingly, from our perspective as concerned outsiders, it is a story of the dialogue of question and answer and how that dialogue may create a new understanding that is both mutual and useful to the Jul'hoansi.

Given the holistic ethic of the Jul'hoansi, we expected that their healing tradition would be directly and explicitly related to contemporary social changes, but we found a far more complex and subtle relationship. Ours became a long and conscientious job of listening and being open. To hear how healing and social change were actually related for the Jul'hoansi, we had to ruthlessly abandon our presuppositions.

We struggled with a series of questions, many of them expressing problems both imponderable and insoluble: What is the usefulness of a document prepared "about" others, even though both parties collaborate closely in its preparation? What is the best way to ensure real collabo-

CHILDREN AND ADULTS ALIKE LOVE THE DELICIOUS

KALAHARI "ORANGE," N!OH, A FRUIT THAT HAS BECOME

MORE AND MORE SCARCE EACH YEAR.

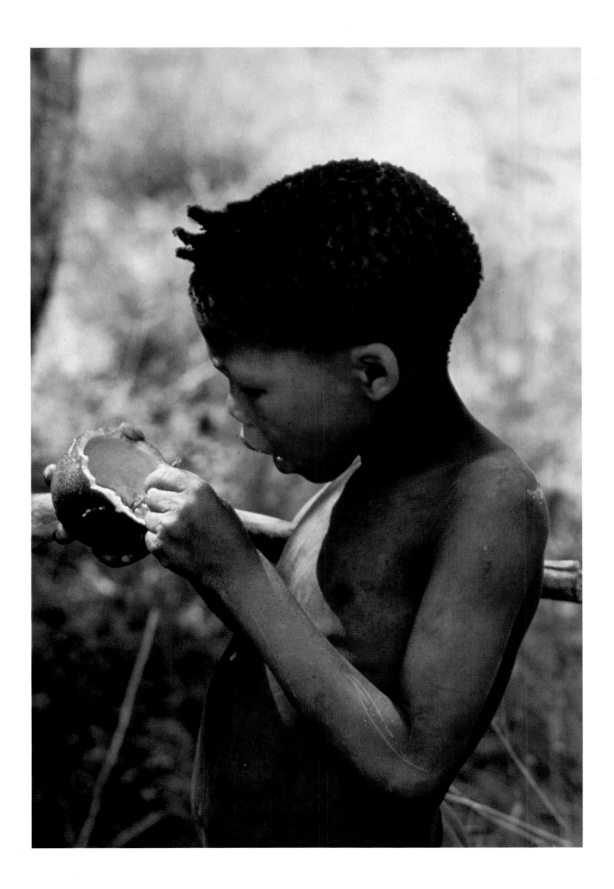

ration on that document? And in the final analysis, is there a way a book about a cultural tradition, upheld by a people whose livelihood is in jeopardy, can help them achieve more of what they need from an oppressive situation? These were questions each of us already had in mind through our ongoing work as "paper people" for various Indigenous peoples: Megan considers these questions in her work as documentarian for the Nyae Nyae Farmers' Cooperative; Verna in her work with Indigenous education; and Dick in his work with Indigenous spiritual healing systems.

Verna was able to be uniquely interactive with the

Jul'hoansi because so many of her people's experiences paralleled their own. Thus, she was especially helpful in moving us toward more effective responses to the above questions. She also made the other two of us, each in our own way, more aware of the subversive complexity of several classic pitfalls. The first is the so-called pornography of the poor, where humble details of the lives of dignified and economically oppressed people are given a lurid and false portrayal in the "high relief" of the media without showing their true place in either history or power relations. A second pitfall is that of portraying people as voiceless and "acted-upon" rather than as actors and creators of their situation. And a third pitfall is the need to avoid coming to conclusions from a "scientific" perspective that has neither interest for nor bearing on the problems of the people whose tradition is being discussed.

The issue of mutuality in the creation of a meaningful cultural document has been the subject of debate for us

AFTER THE DANCE, THE WOMEN AND GIRLS, WHO HAVE

SUNG TOGETHER ALL NIGHT, ENJOY THE STRENGTH

OF THEIR CONNECTEDNESS.

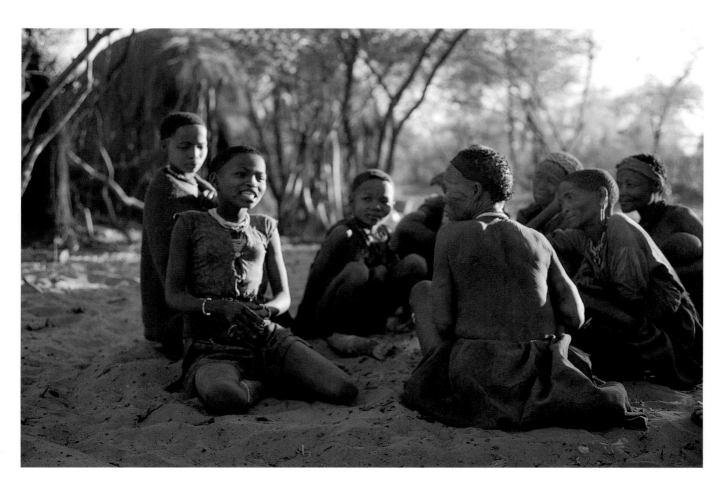

as well. It is all too easy for literate and privileged out-siders to come up with an ambitious plan for how to design a communication project or to present words in a book and then carry the project along with insensitive enthusiasm, missing the fact that the local collaborators' nod of agreement may be one of bemusement or con-ventional politeness. Working on this book has brought up such issues, since we three authors have had different access to enabling education, to leadership roles, and to gender and ethnic privileges. Struggling with such issues, we "authors" have also tried to make this book a fair col-laboration not only among ourselves but, more impor-tant, with the entire community we spoke to and lived with at ǀKaeǀkae.

Many discussions surrounded the intense communi-cations that occurred among the three of us and between us and the ǀKaeǀkae people while we were working in the Kalahari together in 1989. Especially since 1989, we three have been speaking with each other regularly through round-robin discussions and conference calls between Saskatoon, Saskatchewan, where Dick and Verna live, and Austin, Texas, where Megan lives when not in Africa. We considered the concept of a "book without authors," and settled on the ambitious practice of collaboration. We have written chapters or sections of chapters most close-ly identified with our particular experience, but each of these sections has been creatively transformed by addi-tions from the other two.

Making the book a real collaboration with the Juǀ'hoan people has always been our primary aim. While in the Kalahari, this collaboration was worked on direct-ly and continuously. In the writing, we included a feed-back process to help maintain the connection. Because Megan travels regularly to the Juǀ'hoan area, she has been able to check back with some of the healers on questions that have come up during the writing and to hear their continuing expressions of support for the project and the way it is unfolding. As well, she carefully went through the entire manuscript with Kxao ǁOǀOo, checking with him on the accuracy and sensitivity of the material to the pressing concerns of the people.

This process of collaborative writing has not been without difficulties. There are many questions about the representation of other people's realities and about the distortion of media portraits that have troubled us and caused us, on more than one occasion, to doubt ourselves and the worth of the endeavor. Literate and relatively privileged people must become more and more aware of the power implications of "inscription"—the written representation of oral, kinetic, or other nonwritten man-ifestations of cultural reality. Articulateness can itself be a misrepresentation. An outsider can so overstate the case for the "plight" of "disappearing" peoples that the gen-uine contemporary efforts of such peoples can go unno-ticed. Many "vanishing" or even "vanished" people thrive today as they re-create their traditional wisdom.

As with the persisting balance between Juǀ'hoan women and men held together in a valued complemen-tarity, Juǀ'hoan young and old continue to relate with mutual respect. The energies of today remain grounded in the wisdom of the past. Despite their new aspirations, young people still routinely defer to their elders in many graceful ways. Older people allow younger ones their say, much as they have always tolerantly allowed any individ-uals their say. Views expressed by all are for the most part modest and unassuming.

A teenager, for example, would normally answer a question put to her in the presence of an older person by saying, "I'm still a child and have not yet learned the wis-dom of the old people." Or a young hunter, asked about his success when he comes back from hunting, should say, "I didn't see anything." This holds whether he in fact saw nothing or he has put a poisoned arrow into a huge antelope and is waiting for the next day to go back and track it.

Juǀ'hoan humility, in fact, amounts to a way of being that permeates their social lives. Juǀ'hoansi routinely speak in idioms of community rather than of individual self-aggrandizement. We were thoroughly challenged by the task of rendering these modest and modulated Juǀ'hoan ways of speech, knowing full well that readers raised in a more individualistic, competitive culture

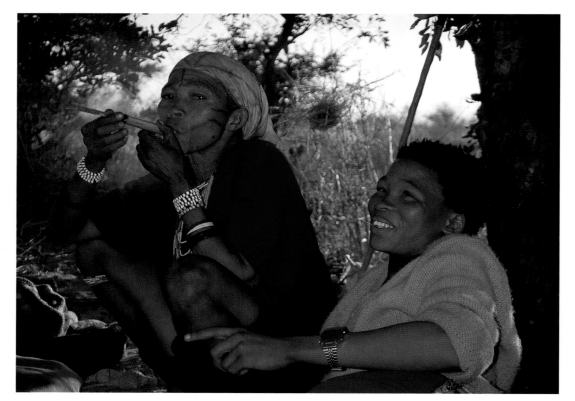

TIMES OF RELAXED VISITING INVIGORATE. HERE TI!'AE, WIFE OF THE HEALER ≠OMA !'HOMG!AUSI, HAS A SMOKE IN A BUSH CAMP, AS TSHAO XUMI RECLINES NEARBY.

might miss both the actual existence as well as the meaning of Jul'hoan humility.

While questions of how to present material confronted us at every turn, the larger issue of how we might be taking Jul'hoan knowledge out of its context preoccupied us during our writing despite the fact we were requested to "tell the Jul'hoan story."

We also discovered how much difficult judgment would be necessary as we made decisions about what to include in the book and what to leave out. We tried to follow the lead of our Jul'hoan collaborators, instituting specific suggestions they made and in general acting in harmony with their attitudes and wishes. Our Jul'hoan collaborators were courageous for working with us because they live all the time on the front line. Not only do they have to face the questions the book raises about changes in their society, but they have to face the political consequences of raising them. Therefore we tried to exclude material that would lead to negative consequences, such as a Jul'hoan criticism of Tswana leaders that might lead to recriminations or backlash. But since

the Tswana treatment of the Jul'hoansi and their concerns is so pervasively unjust, it was impossible to omit all criticism without severely distorting the situation.

We also omitted material that seemed like an invasion of personal privacy, such as mentioning the names of persons abusing alcohol. But here also problems emerged because we cannot tell if material that we did choose to include might in the future prove to have revealed too much, to be embarrassing to a new generation, or even to have some negative political repercussions. The same dilemma existed about presenting the political views of particular Jul'hoansi. In all cases, we always erred on the side of caution, believing that respect for the Jul'hoansi dictated omitting material whenever there seemed a danger of revealing too much about their lives. The entire process entailed great responsibility for bringing the book into being. Since we did not have the information to make decisions about future consequences of material presented in the book and since it was not really our sole responsibility, we relied heavily on the Jul'hoansi themselves. In an ethical sense, they were the ultimate judges.

THE POLITICS OF RESEARCH

The Jul'hoan people have here an opportunity for a degree of self-presentation, which they asked us to help them communicate. We decided the best way to do this would be to tape and translate as much of their own speech as possible and to call on them to speak for themselves as often as we could in writing this book. Thus, with the permission and eager support of the Jul'hoansi, we recorded many hours of tape during our stay in the Kalahari, tapes of meetings, conversations, and general talk as well as our long, open-ended interviews with healers and their spouses. Megan spent over a year translating these tapes into English.

The translations alone, however, could not communicate the complex and rich reality of healing with nlom at lKaelkae today. The contextualizations—including descriptions of the dance and personal histories of the healers—were largely up to us. And they needed to be as good as we could make them. If this background work was adequate, the quoted material would sing on its own. We wanted to include many of the spontaneous words we heard, as well as those that came in response to our questions. And we decided that words spoken with enthusiasm or earnestness would be our guide to what the Jul'hoansi truly cared to convey.

Whether the topic be individual health or the health of the land, enthusiasm for the old or interest in the new, Jul'hoan words and voices reflect an enduring vitality. Neglecting this vitality and painting a picture of hopelessness can be a great disservice to a people as well as to truth. Great care must be used in showing that people are endangered so as not to endanger them further. But "endangerment" itself is a romantic stereotype we wish to avoid.

The Jul'hoansi's vitality allows sadness, pessimism, frustration, and anger to exist, but it doesn't feed images of endangerment. The vibrant statements of the Jul'hoansi filled the air, giving negativity and pessimism room to exist without becoming overpowering, as evident in the words of Dillxao ≠Oma, a woman from lAotcha, Namibia:

What is a government that can say we have none? When someone says, "You Bushmen have no government," we'll say that our old, old people long ago had a government, and it was a glowing coal from the fire where we last lived, which we used to light the fire at the new place where we were going to stay . . . so I say, "Don't hold us back. We want to go forward. We have our own talk. "

A similar enthusiasm lit ≠Oma Djo's features when he described the pleasurable feeling of llxabe or "unwinding" that healers seek during !aia:

I want to llxabe so I can feel myself again. When I llxabe, I feel my body and my flesh properly. I unwind and unfold myself; I open myself up in the dance. I feel lousy when there is no dancing. The singing and the nlom let you llxabe yourself. I want to pull [heal] myself so that I can llxabe myself.[1]

!U'u N!a'an, many times a grandmother, talked of how she felt about abundance and good health.

For us, when we're feeling truly alive, maybe when a lot of rain has fallen, our hearts leap upward and we say, "A-a-ah! That cloud sitting up there in the sky!" Then you're a "real person" and you feel like clearing and chopping out a field. Next you get seeds to plant, and you plant them and cry out, "Oh! I wish I could hurry and plant more with this good rain! I wish I were even stronger!"

Descriptions of the joy of discovering and receiving nlom shared this kind of enthusiasm and vitality. Kommtsa N!a'an told us:

Many men came to me to help my father [give me nlom]. They gathered around me and helped me dance, and it made me happy. . . . When I heard nlom stories, I asked myself if nlom were a good or bad thing. I said it must be a life-thing to help heal the people. When people jumped up to cure others, I saw their strength.

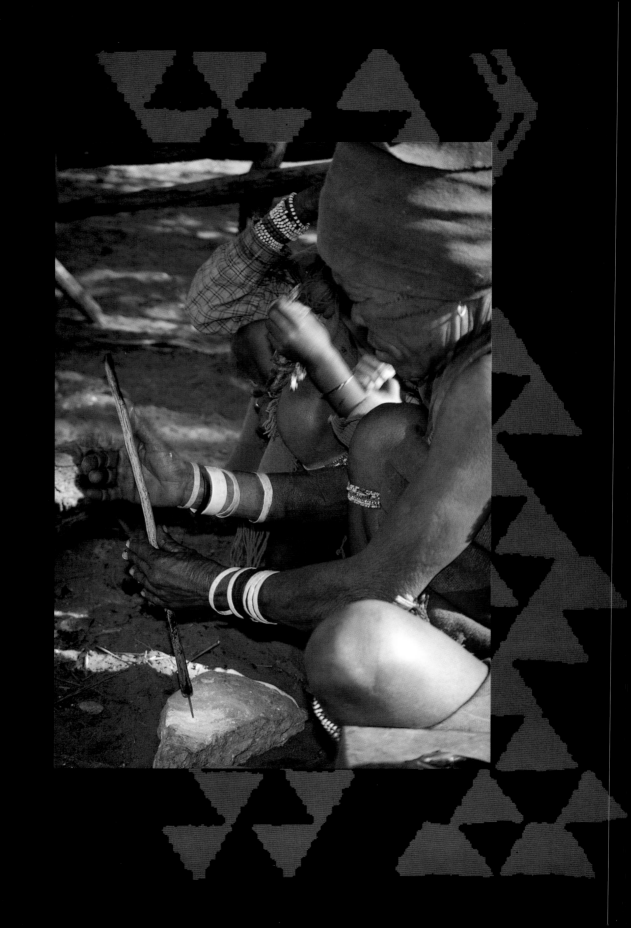

In this chapter, I (Verna) want to tell the story of an experience I shared with the Juǀ'hoansi as a North American Indigenous person. During our ongoing discussions with the people of ǀKaeǀkae about their political situation, I would mention similar experiences from First Nations or Indigenous peoples in Canada. As a Cree/Metis woman who does research on the historical and contemporary struggles of First Nations peoples, I spoke from both a personal and scholarly perspective. This was a rare opportunity for those at ǀKaeǀkae to hear firsthand about other Indigenous peoples in a different part of the world, and they were deeply intrigued. First Nations peoples seemed familiar to them, like relatives. But Canada, whose snow was practically impossible to describe in the heat of the Kalahari, remained a distant, even exotic land in their minds, and so in part did the First Nations peoples I talked about.

Many at ǀKaeǀkae wanted to hear more. We set up a meeting for me to talk at length about First Nations peoples; everyone was invited, with a special effort extended to the healers we worked with and their spouses. I was excited about the opportunity we would have during that meeting to highlight the struggle we shared as Indigenous peoples, and that thought gave me strength and hope.

With the time of the meeting approaching, I thought about ways to connect concretely with the Juǀ'hoansi so that I could really convey what I saw as our common experiences. Knowing that First Nations peoples in Canada shared a powerful history with Juǀ'hoansi as hunters and gatherers and participants in the trading of hides and furs, I took out a pair of beaded moccasins,

ǁUCE NǃAʼAN, A STRONG SINGER AND WIFE OF THE HEALER TSHAO MATZE, PREPARES PIECES OF OSTRICH EGG SHELL FOR A NECKLACE—AN IMPORTANT JUǀʼHOAN CRAFT.

some beaded earrings, and a tape of powwow music I had brought from home. Maybe these items of my culture would help them hear my words.

As the Juǀ'hoansi gathered in our camp, I saw that most of them were elders. I thought to myself, "Who am I, as a child, to address these elders?" Yet I was excited they had come.

"Just as you have lived here in the Kalahari long before others arrived," I began, "so did my ancestors live in North America long before the Europeans came. And just as you live as hunters and gatherers so too have my people." I talked about the animals we hunted, how all parts

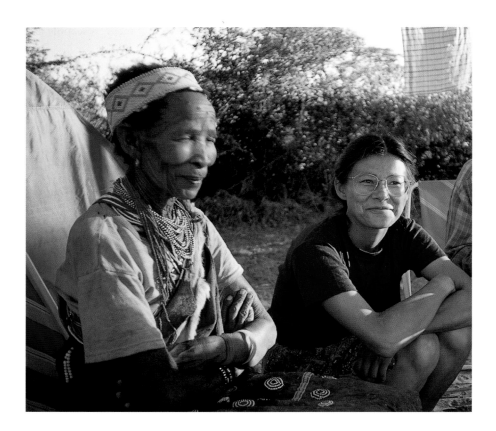

VERNA INTERVIEWING THE
EXPERIENCED AND RESPECTED
FEMALE HEALER KXARU N!A'AN.

of the animals were used, and the respect given the animals. Then I took out the moccasins and described their construction from pieces of hide and sinew. "This was one way we used the animals," I said.

People leaned forward to examine the moccasins as they were passed around the group. They fingered the stitching, carefully tracing its pattern. Murmurs spread through the group, expressing a collective appreciation and a specific admiration for the actual "fingers that sewed" those moccasins. A new level of interest had emerged throughout the group; First Nations peoples in Canada became alive.

Xumi N!a'an was the first to speak. "Oh, can it be," he exclaimed excitedly, "that there are people, even in Canada, that are like us?!"

"The sinew used to sew these moccasins was taken from along the spine of large animals, like the moose," I added. That brought further enthusiastic comments because sinew among the Jul'hoansi is obtained from a

similar source, the long back sinews of antelopes. "You also have warm-blooded animals, with skins like our animals, even in that cold place where you live?" several Jul'hoansi asked at once.

The discussion about sinew raised further meanings into our gathering because Jul'hoansi feel that sinew is quintessential to their culture, serving as a metaphor for what it is that connects people, holds the fabric of life together, and makes us human. At this moment the Jul'hoansi saw themselves as related to First Nations peoples, who seemed at first so far away.

Then, turning to the beaded earrings, which I passed around, I spoke about the arrival of Europeans in Canada and how they exchanged beads for furs. I detailed the oppressive trading relationship that was established and the eventual colonization of First Nations land. Then I touched on ways in which First Nations peoples have resisted this physical and spiritual invasion.

The Juǀʼhoansi remained very involved in the discussion. But now I had a fear. While realizing that what I was saying was true, would others, especially the Botswana government, interpret my words as "inciting" people? Knowing how difficult it was for any kind of political change to occur among Indigenous peoples, I also became concerned about raising expectations unrealistically. But I continued on.

I talked more about the sociopolitical history of First Nations peoples, emphasizing their struggles and their aspirations. For example, I described the "pass system," which regulated the movement and economic activity of First Nations peoples up to the 1950s, as well the numerous hunting and fishing restrictions now in place; and we made a connection to the hunting licenses and other restrictions that have recently come to ǀKaeǀkae. I detailed the changes that residential schools and Christian missionaries wrought, robbing the people of their language, their culture, their identities; and here we talked about the plans for a residential school for the ǀKaeǀkae children. And the Juǀʼhoansi listened, their faces showing the depth of their gratitude. I felt humbled by the commitment and fullness of their response.

They were hearing "their story"; they were learning of their brothers and sisters in Canada, of the common struggle of Indigenous peoples. The parallels in the history of our two peoples were striking but not really remarkable. The oppression at the hands of those who came to our respective places, seizing our lands, exploiting our resources, such as furs and hides, and attempting to "civilize" us through church and schools, was eerily similar.

While I spoke, people nodded in agreement, offering at times descriptions of their own history to cement the solidarity of experience. It was sad to hear once again of the suffering of Indigenous people.

Toward the end of our gathering, I spoke more about the emotional effects of the residential schools and how they separated children from their mothers and fathers, causing untold pain and the resulting breakdown of families, and how the widespread use of corporal punish-

ment in schools left deep emotional scars. Xumi N!aʼan, a strong supporter of the ǀKaeǀkae school, nevertheless expressed passionately his displeasure with the school's use of corporal punishment, which exists in stark contrast to the tolerant and more nurturant Juǀʼhoan style of discipline.

I also spent some time on the problems that have resulted from alcohol abuse among First Nations peoples in Canada and throughout the world. This was not an easy task, as I realized ǀKaeǀkae people were still in the early stages of dealing with alcohol consumption; drinking was still considered largely a problem that certain individuals had, and at times not even a "problem" but "their way of behaving." Yet knowing there was also an awareness that these "ways of behaving" caused problems in the community—"alcohol makes us fight," Juǀʼhoansi say—I described the awareness in First Nations communities of alcoholism as a political and community problem and not just a personal tragedy. Hoping to give people some practical examples of positive actions, I emphasized the important function that women have in ending the cycle of alcohol abuse in their roles as mothers, sisters, and wives.

The last topic I wanted to cover was the growing realization among First Nations peoples of the importance of our languages, healing traditions, and community ceremonies in reclaiming our culture and our land. To provide a concrete example of similarities in our ceremonies, I played some powwow music from back home, hoping ǀKaeǀkae people would hear themselves in a new form.

At first, people sat totally still, transfixed by the intensely spiritual tone of the lead male singer and the strong, chantlike singing of the rest of the drum group that was playing the powwow songs. Then excited conversations broke out as people remarked on how much this sounded like their own healing dance. They were really appreciative of the connection. Xumi N!aʼan, one of ǀKaeǀkae's best drum makers, put some of this excitement into words: "These [First Nations] people hunt; we already know that. Now we see they also have a spiritual dance and they're passionate about it. These people [singing] are working, working really hard. There is strength in that music. It's different from ours . . . but it's also like our healing music."

I felt good, knowing that a deep connection had been made as we moved surely and swiftly beyond a superficial display of cultural artifacts. The moccasins, beadwork, and now the powwow music took on real political and spiritual meaning because they were shown to a people who knew similar items as essential parts of their lives. And then I wished to myself that these ǀKaeǀkae people could meet other Indigenous people in the world, whom they could both be inspired by and inspire.

My final words at the meeting were about specific political and legal ways in which First Nations peoples were reclaiming their land and insisting upon political and legal representation at all levels of government. I wanted to end on a positive and, I hoped, a helpful note.

As the gathering was about to disperse, an older, usually quiet man, gained the group's attention. He spoke about his attempt to better himself and his family by raising goats and farming, and how difficult it was to keep the traditional Jul'hoan sharing ethic alive with these "new" subsistence activities. A woman, who liked what he said and how he spoke, wished to affirm his thoughts. "What Kodinyau just said is true," she offered, using the man's Herero name. Many Jul'hoansi are given Herero names when they work for the Hereros and those names tend to stick with the person. Kodinyau looked at her, reflected for a moment, and then without rancor but with great pride said, "Call me by my Jul'hoan name. Call me Kxao, not by my Herero name."

What we call ourselves is very much who we are. "We are Jul'hoansi," the people say, "we are only people, we are real people." That statement is overwhelming in its simplicity; it humbly presents the facts and nothing more.

Yet there are countless and continuous examples of people in power giving names to other people whom they are trying to control, and those names usually have a painfully derogatory and dehumanizing connotation. Indigenous peoples in particular have suffered this manipulation by naming. For example, Lakota people were named "Sioux" by the White colonizers, a corruption of a word used by one of the Lakota's local enemies that originally meant "snake," a highly unflattering label. Inuit people were named "Eskimo" by the European colonizers, a corruption of a word used by the Inuit's First Nations neighbors that originally meant "raw fish eaters"—those First Nations people always cooked their meat and fish thoroughly and considered any other way of eating such foods as "primitive."

Jul'hoan people have been called "Bushmen" by the Afrikaners to signify their "primitive" or bushlike nature, though there is also the connotation in that name that by surviving in the bush the Jul'hoan people have demonstrated their strength and independence, their resistance of efforts to "civilize" or control them. In fact, some young Jul'hoansi, emphasizing this connotation of resistance, strength, and independence in the term "Bushmen," have sought to ennoble it as one of their self-chosen names.

Names are still very important for Indigenous people, their meanings rich and varied. Special names are often given in "naming ceremonies" that connect one to the spirit world. Names are earned, recognizing one's strengths and celebrating one's struggles. As well, ordinary names remain important in kinship, telling us who we are by telling us how we relate to each other.

Reclaiming our names is an act of cultural and personal affirmation and political liberation. The ability to name oneself is an indicator of power, the power to determine how one is represented to oneself and to the world.

In Canada, so-called Indian reserves are reclaiming their identity as they reclaim their names, dropping the names instituted by the Department of Indian Affairs and reinstituting their original self-established names. For example, what had been called the Sandy Lake Reserve is now called Athapkakoop First Nation, and the James Smith Reserve is now called the Muskoday First Nation. These reclaimed names are used at first by people on the reserve and increasingly by others who have historically controlled their destinies.

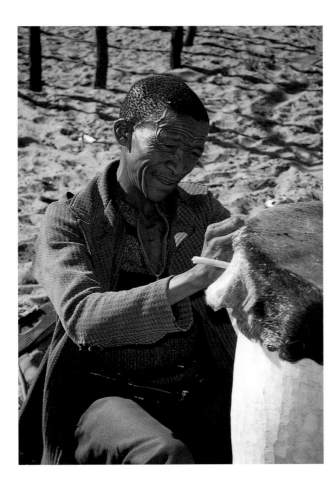

places, those aboriginal homes, that the industrialized world seeks to exploit, tearing out the land from its roots, which are embedded in the people who first live there. As land feeds culture, the lack of land and the lack of the ability to feed and care for oneself can lead to the creation of the urban poor, the increasing condition of many Indigenous peoples.

Education would certainly be another issue on people's minds and hearts at such a meeting of Indigenous peoples, particularly the colonizing structure of European schooling, with the painful and devastating effects of residential schools and the pernicious efforts of European schooling to eradicate Indigenous languages. As the land is our life, language breathes life into our culture. I know there would be some difficult conversations about how to combine respectfully in the schools traditional and contemporary knowledge, two ways of knowing that at times seem so contradictory.

And then there is the resistance, the revitalization, and the political struggle toward self-determination and self-government that must be discussed. Ju|'hoan people from |Kae|kae already know of the small though significant successes experienced by their relatives across the border in Namibia; they would hear of larger victories elsewhere and perhaps become strengthened in their own resolve.

In the end, I believe the exchange would turn to what Indigenous peoples throughout the world believe is their most valued resource: their spiritual teachings. The spiritual basis of life is what connects everything and everybody; it is what can fuel the sociopolitical and educational struggles into a truly liberating effort, a struggle guided by the vision of the elders, a struggle toward

Later that day, I reflected further on the old man's request: "Call me by my Ju|'hoan name." He was connecting himself and his people to the worldwide struggle of Indigenous peoples for their lands, their culture, their spiritual lives. I thought again about how wonderful it would be if |Kae|kae Ju|'hoansi could meet other Indigenous people, and strengthen their own determination in sharing their stories. And I knew such meetings were inevitable.

Having been at various international meetings of Indigenous peoples, I could hear some of the exchange that would probably occur. The land would remain the foundation of that exchange. "Our land is our life"—throughout the world, this is the fundamental vision of Indigenous peoples. Their struggle for self-determination is deeply rooted in their sense of place, and it is those

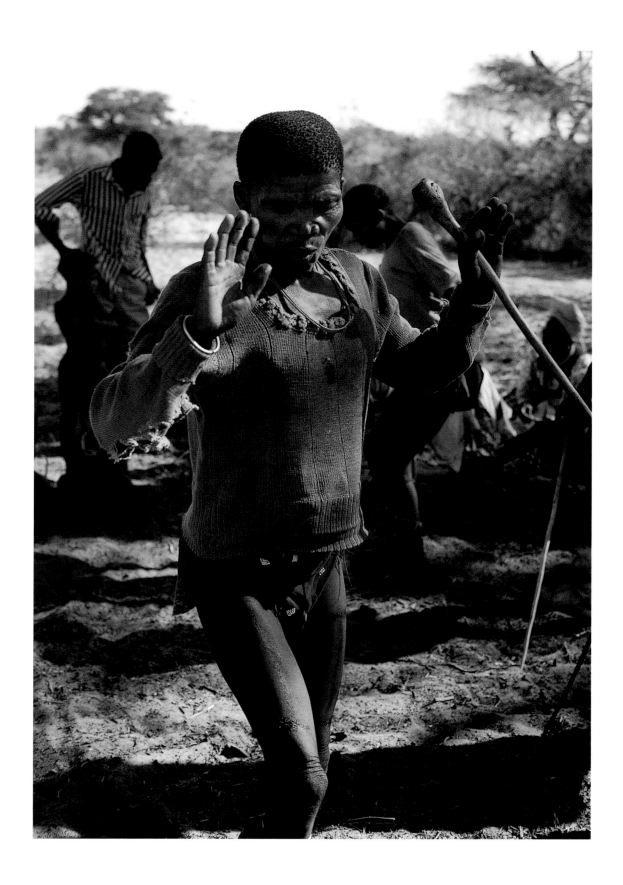

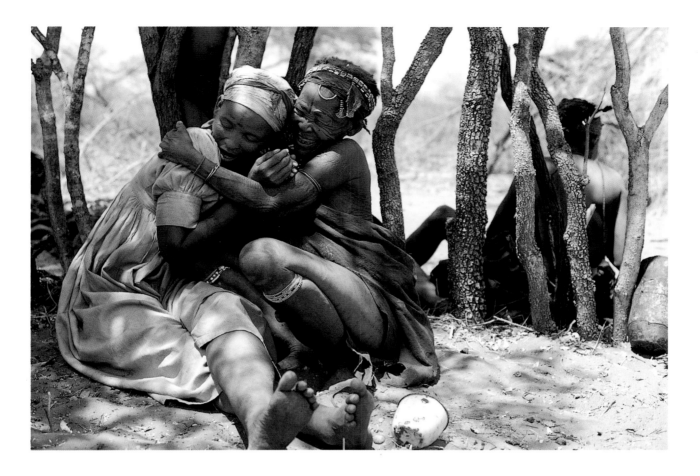

JUǀ'HOAN PEOPLE ARE ALWAYS IN CLOSE PHYSICAL CONTACT AROUND THE CAMP, SITTING NEXT TO EACH OTHER, BODIES TOUCHING, SUPPORTING EACH OTHER. HERE ǀXOAN (LEFT) AND TCUǃXO ENJOY A GOOD LAUGH TOGETHER.

OPPOSITE: KINACHAU, AN EXPERIENCED AND RESPECTED HEALER, DANCES WITH HIS CHARACTERISTIC INTENSITY DURING A GIRAFFE DANCE IN 1968.

spiritual integrity and harmonious relations.

I know other Indigenous people would listen intently and respectfully to the story of the Juǀ'hoan healing dance. Remaining for Juǀ'hoan people a powerful com-munal source of spiritual strength, that dance is a rare gift in a rapidly changing world, which is constantly sucking out the spiritual life from healing ceremonies. Telling the story of their dance to the wider community of Indigenous peoples could only help Juǀ'hoan people endure and remember who they are.

The Juǀ'hoansi are part of the global movement of Indigenous peoples toward self-determination. As their connections with others increase, their dedication to their own journey intensifies. The bond of common struggle feeds. As with all Indigenous peoples, they realize their journey is more than their own and that they struggle for others as well. The healing dance brings the people a "happy heart," which expands into the principle that we all care for each other.

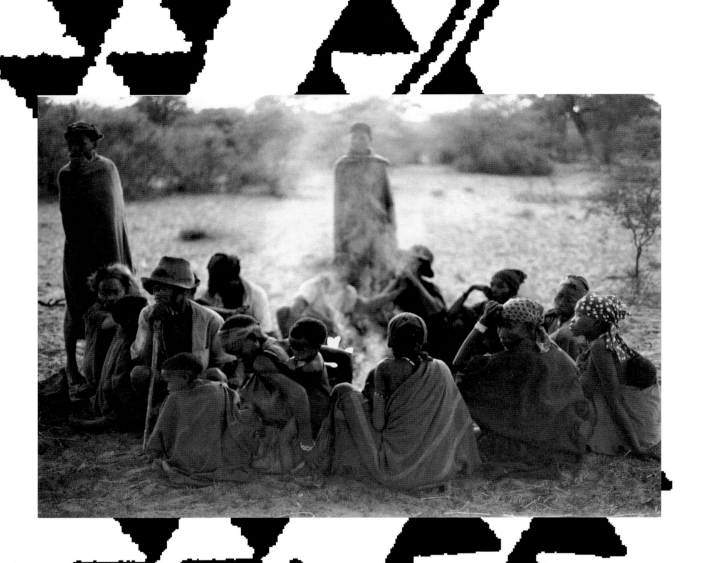

EPILOGUE

AFTER WE LEAVE ǀKAEǀKAE in 1989, some time goes by without much news for us from there. Then it is July 1992. A truck carrying Tshao Matze and Xumi N!a'an, as well as others from northwest Botswana (Ngamiland), is heading toward eastern Botswana. There they will attend a preliminary meeting to plan for a larger international gathering to be held in the capital city of Gaborone in October. At this larger gathering, Juǀ'hoansi from Botswana and Namibia will meet with each other, with development organizations, and with government officials from both countries. The people will be able to describe the difficulties of their situation and to present their ideas for a more promising future. It will be one of the first real opportunities for ǀKaeǀkae Juǀ'hoansi to make their voices heard by the Botswana government and to gain the special strength that comes from being with and exchanging ideas with so many other Indigenous peoples.

THOSE WHO HAVE MADE THE INTENSE JOURNEY
TOGETHER THROUGHOUT THE LONG NIGHT OF THE
HEALING DANCE SAVOUR THEIR SENSE OF COMMUNITY
WITH EACH OTHER AT THE DANCE'S END.

Tshao Matze, the experienced and powerful healer, and Xumi N!a'an, the fervent supporter of the healing dance and ardent drummer in the drum dance, are two of the most respected residents of ǀKaeǀkae. They are also two of the most insightful at analyzing the contemporary Juǀ'hoan sociopolitical condition and most articulate in offering life-enhancing visions for the future.

The two men, as well as the others at ǀKaeǀkae, have waited decades for this chance to speak about their community. Now, on the edge of their new voice, the ǀKaeǀkae people meet one more tragic obstacle. There is an accident; the truck is hit by a tractor. Tshao Matze and Xumi N!a'an are both killed. No alternates are sought. The preliminary meeting and then the international gathering in Gaborone are held, but with no representation from ǀKaeǀkae or the larger Dobe area. The deaths of Tshao Matze and Xumi N!a'an go unnoticed at the meeting.

In a small village like ǀKaeǀkae, this tragic loss of life is especially devastating. Yet the larger struggle of Indigenous peoples for land and a dignified way of living remains affirmed. The meeting in Gaborone is a historic occasion—and ǀKaeǀkae will eventually feel its effects.

Another of the respected ǀKaeǀkae healers we worked with in 1989 was ≠Oma !'Homg!ausi, also a forceful advocate of Juǀ'hoan identity and rights. He succumbed to tuberculosis in 1993. The opening for new voices in ǀKaeǀkae, especially among the young, is ever more pressing.

Perhaps the wisdom of old ≠Oma Djo can be an inspiration. As a young man he ran down eland on foot in the traditional manner; his more than eighty years span the more traditional and contemporary Juǀ'hoan cultures. As an old man he is the one other healers turn to for help; his long, dedicated, and highly respected work as a healer opens the door to Juǀ'hoan healing knowledge. ≠Oma Djo lives at the spiritual heart of his people.

The summer rains of 1994 are near. ≠Oma Djo goes to the bush with his ax to strip bark for lashing down the thatching to his house so the rain and wind will not tear it off. He stays gone so long that the people become worried. They begin to follow his tracks. They follow them

SICK LITTLE ≠OMA IS HEALED BY ≠OMA DJO AS HE IS GENTLY HELD AND CRADLED
BY HIS GRANDFATHER, ≠OMA !'HOMG!AUSI (WEARING THE HAT).
≠OMA DJO WORKS ON THE BOY, STANDING UP, KNEELING DOWN, LYING DOWN,
BACK AND FORTH, WHEREVER HIS BOILING NǀOM LEADS HIM. BY LAYING HANDS
ON THE BOY, AS WELL HOLDING HIM AND RUBBING HIS HEAD AGAINST HIM,
≠OMA DJO PUTS NǀOM INTO THE BOY AND TAKES OUT SICKNESS. THE
GRANDFATHER, HIMSELF A POWERFUL HEALER, BECOMES AN ACTIVE PART OF THE
HEALING EFFORT AS HE HOLDS THE BOY.

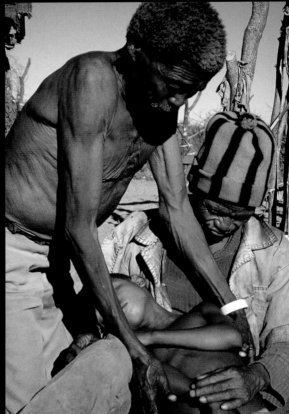

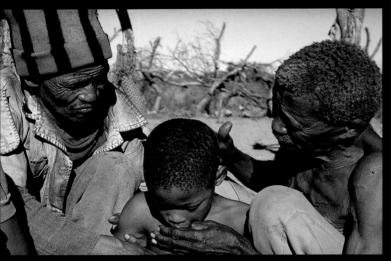

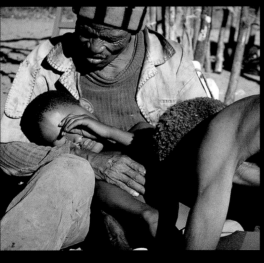

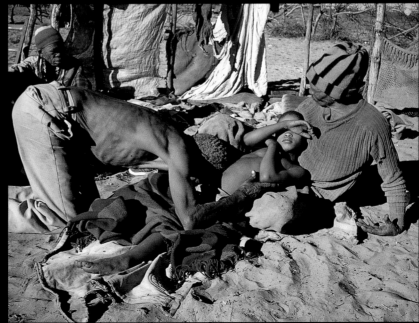

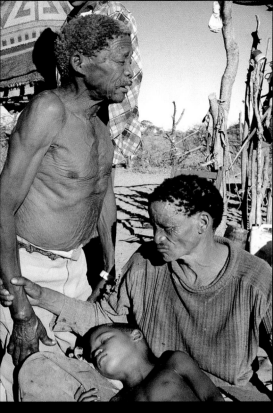

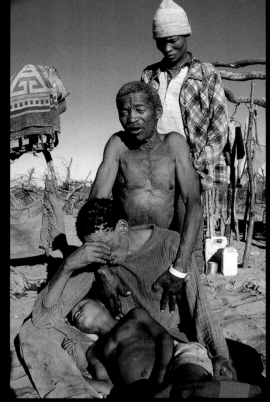

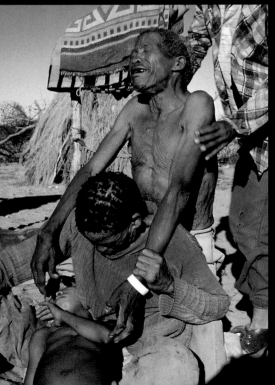

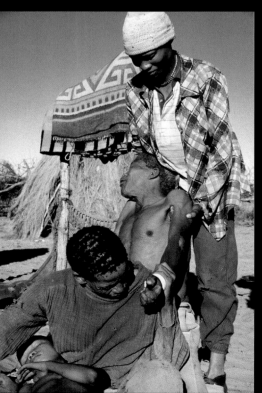

COMMUNITY AND CONTINUITY ARE ENHANCED AS BOILING N!OM SPREADS AND SYNERGY INCREASES. AS ≠OMA DJO'S N!OM BOILS MORE FIERCELY, HIS HEALING WORK ON LITTLE ≠OMA INTENSIFIES, AND THE HEALING EFFORT ITSELF ENLARGES, AS THE N!OM ALSO BEGINS TO BOIL MORE STRONGLY IN THE BOY'S GRANDFATHER, ≠OMA !'HOMG!AUSI . THE YOUNG MAN ≠OMA (TOP RIGHT), ≠OMA DJO'S GRANDSON, COMES TO LEND HIS SUPPORT, STANDING BEHIND HIS GRANDFATHER, READY TO HOLD HIM. AS ≠OMA DJO COLLAPSES IN THE AGONY OF HIS !AIA, SO DOES ≠OMA !'HOMG!AUSI. THE FOUR ≠OMAS, DEEPLY CONNECTED IN KINSHIP AS NAMESAKES, FORM A CIRCLE OF HEALING, AS THE BOILING N!OM WHICH MOVES BETWEEN THEM ERASES BOUNDARIES BETWEEN HEALER, HEALEE, AND HELPER, THEREBY INCREASING ITS POTENCY.

into a thicket and then cannot find where the tracks lead beyond that point. The tracks go into the thicket and just disappear. The whole ǀKaeǀkae community, joined by the government police, continues trying to locate ≠Oma Djo throughout an extensive area. They never find him—or his ax.

Before he left, ≠Oma Djo told others that he did not want his children to come to ǀKaeǀkae and "be sad about me." People are in fact very sad. But there is a recognition that ≠Oma Djo must have known when his end was near, that he planned his departure, and that his "disappearance" was in keeping with the life he lived as a powerful and much loved healer.

≠Oma Djo's death has clearly left a deep impression on the young, many of whom are becoming aware that they have choice in the matter of retaining their healing tradition along with the "new things" they are learning in school and elsewhere. And the young Juǀʼhoansi are emerging to claim their voice. Still respectful of their elders, in the traditional Juǀʼhoan manner they do not speak first and then only briefly when in a group of mixed ages. But alone, they express their views at length.

ǃXam is an adolescent of the village. He hunts with the men and also has his own cow. Though he has not thus far succeeded at school, he is determined to complete Standard 6, and has returned to that class even though, being in his late teens, he is several years older than his classmates. ǃXam is ≠Oma Djo's grandson and is already a strong seeker of nǀom. "I want to be a healer," he says in 1989, "so that when my grandfather dies, I'll take over."

ǃXam also sees the bleakness of the Juǀʼhoansi's present economic situation: "I don't know how everyone at ǀKaeǀkae—[Juǀʼhoansi, Tswana, and Hereros]—will manage to live together. What will they eat?" He is especially rueful about the heavy drinking he sees around him.

> When there was no beer, and someone like ≠Oma ǃʼHomgǃausi would kill a kudu or tell people to go kill a kudu for him, he'd set a dance. Then we'd spend the night dancing and everyone would eat.
>
> [Today, with all the meat that has come in] there

is a lot of drinking. I don't know why they're now selling meat to buy beer. They're "drinking the meat."

> Beer is not good. It makes people fight. If two people have been drinking, and one asks the other for something, the reply may be: "Don't you have money to buy your own?" And the other one says: "Why are you not sharing with me?" So anger rises in both of them. And they fight.

We ask ǃXam about drinking just a cup or two of beer, which others had told us might not obstruct one's work with nǀom.

> No, even if I drank two cups of beer, I'd still fear nǀom, as if I hadn't drunk anything. Nǀom grabs in your stomach, that's what they say.
>
> Drinking beer makes me tired quickly at the dance, and then I get weak. If I take two cups, I won't do nǀom because it would make me crazy, so I wouldn't see what's going on and wouldn't pay attention to the person who was teaching me.

The group of school-educated young Juǀʼhoansi offer yet another view into the future. As their employment opportunities often arise away from their home village, the transvillage perspective fostered by their schooling is reinforced. Certainly as a group they represent a striking resource of potential leadership.

Among these formally educated youth, Kxao ǀOǀOo has been especially articulate and successful in securing employment. His grandfather was the powerful and blind healer Kxao ≠Oah, but being in school so much prevented Kxao ǀOǀOo from keeping an intense commitment to learning how to heal. Yet he respects the dance and sees its contribution to contemporary life. "I think children should do both things," he says, "learn the things of the old days *and* the new things." Once called Royal, Kxao ǀOǀOo is returning to the use of his traditional Juǀʼhoan name.

One May afternoon in 1995, Megan sits down with Kxao ǀOǀOo and goes over this book, still in manuscript form, page by page to ask for his reactions. It is one effort in our commitment to be sure the book gives the Jul'hoansi their voice and does not contain material that would be antithetical to their aims. While pointing out two sections that need to be revised, Kxao |O|Oo is in general very pleased with the book. Most important, he is inspired to get together with other Jul'hoansi and write a book about the developments in Namibia over the past few years that have given strong support to Jul'hoan aspirations. The request that has guided so much of our work—"Tell our story to your people"—would then take on a new, more powerful meaning.

Since this book went to press, the situation facing the Ju/'hoansi and their neighbors in Western Ngamiland, where /Kae/kae is located, has become very grave. Because of an outbreak of lung sickness (bovine pleuropneumonia), 400,000 head of cattle had to be killed, thus undercutting the local economy. There are now government plans to turn a significant portion of Ju/'hoan land into commercial cattle ranches that will be leased out to wealthy livestock owners, most of them from outside the region. Large syndicates of Herero and Tswana ranchers from the eastern part of Botswana will thus claim land around /Kae/kae in every direction based on cattle ownership, a criterion which can be met

by virtually none of the Ju/'hoan inhabitants and few of their neighbors. The Botswana government has also stopped issuing game licenses for subsistence hunting, and many new fences have been constructed that are adversely affecting game movements. People are suffering increasingly, and in a very real way they are, in the words of a Ju/'hoan leader, Tsamkxao =Oma, "cut off from their own food."

These recent events bring into sharp focus the situation of local peoples, whatever their ethnicities, as they face the effects of an increasingly globalizing economy. Many Ju/'hoan people feel that to call attention to these painful effects they must speak out. As /'Angn!ao /'Un expresses it:

> We say that if you have problems you should solve them, not hide from them. If you hide from them, it means you still have the problems, the problems of your heart, because they lie within your burning heart. But if you take these problems to the midst of people and speak of them openly, if you bring this pain to others and ask for their help, all of you together will find a way.

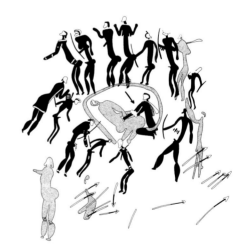

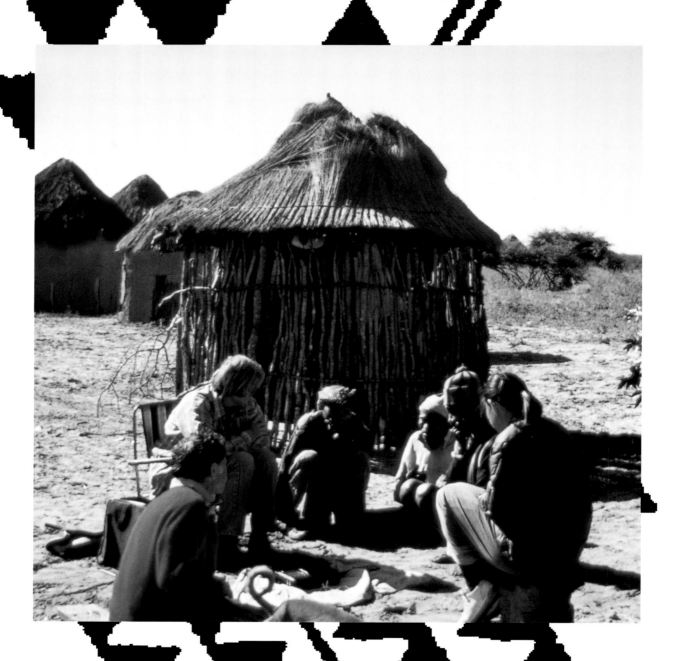

REFLECTIONS ON AIMS AND OUTCOMES

Throughout this book, we have tried to work with and through the one voice of the editorial "we." We have worked on and with our differences, trying to preserve those differences that highlighted important insights. This consensus approach has helped to pool our resources and synthesize our insights. And in assuming a single authorial perspective, we hope we've made the material more accessible and in that provided a clearer voice to the Jul'hoansi.

In this appendix we offer some final reflections on our project, separating each voice out before coming together again. We wish to highlight the complexity that consensus can mask if it is only seen as an end product. Forsaking the editorial "we," this appendix assumes a dialogical structure. We hope that stressing the variety of ideas that springs from our diverse backgrounds and experiences, while emphasizing the importance of viewpoint in determining the nature of truth, will ultimately enrich the book.

What follows is an edited transcript of three-way telephone conversations we had in February 1995.

Dick We wanted to use this opportunity of our talking together as a kind of "looking back" over the whole project—reflecting on our work in the community and with each other, and on the meaning of issues of help and helping. Each of us comes from a different place in terms of experience, skill, understanding, and commitments. I think it's important for our readers to know the kinds of questions that we raised with each other and with the project.

Verna I continue to be anxious about doing research on

IN THE STILL PERVADING COLD OF AN EARLY JUNE MORNING, A DIALOGUE ABOUT HEALING BEGINS WITH DICK, MEGAN, VERNA, AND THREE OF THE HEARLERS WHO ARE PART OF THE RESEARCH TEAM—(FROM LEFT TO RIGHT) KXAO TJIMBURU, ≠OMA DJO, AND TSHAO N!A'AN.

what has been called "the other." I'm concerned about the exchange, really the lack of exchange, that characterizes the whole history of writing about other people. I was just talking to a new graduate student who had done a lot of work in West Africa. On this side of the ocean, her university group is quite pleased with themselves because they've been very "productive," meaning they've published a lot on their research findings. But on the other side of the ocean, the people being "studied" don't see what's come of all of this, particularly in terms of their own lives.

As I was telling this graduate student about my involvement in our Kalahari project, I wondered to myself if it would have been better if we had used all the money we got in research grants to do something concrete for the people, like securing a big chunk of land for them. I know that option is probably unrealistic, but I continually struggle with the idea of whether we could have used that research money for something of more tangible benefit to the people.

Megan That question of jumping between research and securing land is the kind of thinking that must go on for anybody of conscience. The whole research enterprise has this possibility of skimming off the cream of people's cultures and giving nothing back. I think we're still, even today, struggling with that. I would be struggling even more if I didn't have the years of development work behind me. I've been able to start thinking that any information I have gathered or been able to understand about Jul'hoan people is part of that development effort—part of me. A lot of what I do is the handing over of tools of communication—people are asking me to perform practical communication tasks, and I've tried to help in that way. And the more that I know and understand about the people, the more that helping has been facilitated.

I agree with Verna that a great deal of the postmodern critique raises enormous questions of conscience and power, of exchange and use. If there is not a way for us to actualize our mission of committed scholarship, then our research and writing is still empty rhetoric. And I think the questions that you, Verna, just now asked are perhaps the most powerful ones that unite the three of us, coming as we do from such different backgrounds.

Dick   The way Verna stated the question is very important because she not only raises the critical issues of power and control, respect and exchange, in a generic way, but also, by discussing the money we were given to support our research and considering its actual and potential uses, she raises these issues in a concrete and thereby less comfortable and less distant way.

Even though ours was a relatively low-budget project, how does one begin to understand or even justify the spending of that money for our trip as compared to what it could buy for the Jul'hoansi—whether it be spent for land or education or other resources?

Certainly we did the research and are doing the book in hopes of stimulating a larger effect, an effect that, in raising consciousness and feeding a people's empowerment, goes beyond a mere dollar amount. And through royalties accumulated by this book, we also hope to earn money that will be given directly to the Jul'hoansi. But still we can never dismiss the question of what is the best way to have spent the money behind the project. Yes, I believe the more concrete we make our discussion of issues of power and control, the more unsettling and powerful that discussion becomes.

Verna   I feel that of the three of us I will be judged the most harshly about the value and validity of our book because I'm an Indigenous person and therefore "should know better." Because the topic of the book deals with who I am . . ., I mean, it's what my life is about. People will expect a special understanding because of that, and so I feel anxious that we "get it right" with this book—and I'm not sure we have. I was always uncomfortable with the power we had as researchers—especially as researchers from the First World—to just walk into the Jul'hoan community and begin our work; that power of privilege made me feel in some ways no different from the missionaries and all the other government agencies that have arrived in my own community and home.

Megan   "To get it right," yes, I agree. And to be sensitive

to those cues that indicate areas of discomfort or insensitivity in your own experiences, Verna, with our project.

Verna   Throughout the whole project, I kept wondering "What am I doing here?"—and still I wonder!

Dick   Each of us has deep reservations about the inequities of power and exchange in our project, but Verna's reservations, enriched by the understandings of her own life experience as an Indigenous person, are especially important. I feel grateful she has struggled to stay within the project. And each of us may always feel our reservations, no matter how far the book goes. They will not be resolved simply by talking about them.

Megan   I truly believe it's important to bring messages from Indigenous peoples to my people, and therefore I can't keep hedging around and saying that the reason I am doing this work is everything but that idea of "bringing messages." There are a lot of other reasons, but bringing these messages is one of them.

Dick   That's very important. I've worked with Indigenous people, especially healers, at different times and in different places, and on several occasions I've been asked to "tell our story to your people." At first I was unsure about how to fulfill that request, unsure about my qualifications, unclear about the form in which to tell the story. These feelings were appropriate and necessary. But soon I began to listen more seriously to what people actually were asking me to do. Taking their instructions as my guide, I must now just do what they asked, trusting their judgment that I'm fit to do so.

In this book, Jul'hoan people asked us to tell their story. I've tried to do that according to their wishes. It's not just a story of healing, though that in itself is important to tell, and can impact the lives of Jul'hoansi and many other people. But the story we are now telling goes more directly into the political substance of people's everyday lives and seeks direct action links to improving the quality of that everyday realm.

Megan   I try to imagine what "tell our story" would mean if people who ask that of us had knowledge of all of the powerful media that are at our disposal. And I believe that facilitating their access to those media, getting their voices on those media, is part of the process of "telling the story." This communication aim is one aspect of our project that I feel extremely positive about.

Verna   When I think of the many tapes we've collected, with interviews and discussion, I want to be sure they are made available to Jul'hoan people in Botswana. The tapes provide a record of their history, a record of their old people's wisdom.

Megan   Absolutely, and that is something that can easily be done and should be done. By the end of l992, I had completed more than two hundred tapes of the Nyae Nyae Farmers' Cooperative. I had them all duplicated and labeled and gave one entire set back to the Farmers' Cooperative. They now have an archive of their own, which they're very pleased with.

In connection with the tapes and the translating, I wanted to mention something that's been on my mind for quite some time. I listen to National Public Radio a lot, and I've been hearing a number of Indigenous groups speaking out on various programs. I'm faintly disturbed by the format into which they get put on the radio. I began to realize all these Indigenous groups were sounding exactly the same. Part of it is that the issues these groups face are very similar all over the world. But there's also something about the way that languages lose their individuality in translation, and the way that individuality of expression gets lost as a result of the relationships that get established between the various foundations supporting the Indigenous people and the people themselves.

I feel our book has tried to remedy that situation with accurate and direct translations. Some of the Jul'hoan quotes in the book are quite startling—maybe not what one would expect. There are very colloquial expressions used. Maintaining the freshness of the language has been primary in our minds as we have tried to do translating. I like doing a workman-like job of being a good technician, specifically in this case of being a good translator.

Dick   This discussion about translating touches on the importance of Jul'hoan voices in the book and the validity of that source of knowledge. We've chosen to avoid the formal academic mode with its many references to the "relevant literature," and its emphasis on theory-building and comparative analysis as legitimating features. Instead we want the book to speak more in the mode of an oral communication, to be accessible to many people. Our book is filled with Jul'hoan discussions about land, water, food, and healing—fundamental facts of Jul'hoan life—and it is through these facts that they make known their needs and aspirations, their beliefs and values. The book rests on a strong foundation of empirical data and experienced analysis, essential to any scientific enterprise. And to the extent the book succeeds in letting the Jul'hoan story be told fully and accurately, to that extent I believe the book is truly and deeply scientific.

Verna   I want to say something about another possible reaction to our book in terms of the debate going on now in anthropology about self-reflexivity. There are those who say "Oh no, we don't want to hear again about the struggles of the researcher. Who cares about that? Why does that now become the main story?" I don't want our book—especially considering an appendix like this dialogical one—to be dismissed by such persons. We have to talk about ourselves in a way that adds to the book's content.

Dick   I want to return to Megan's idea of the translator as a good technician. The best translator, either in the specific act of translating someone else's words or in the more general act of telling someone else's story, has to be a good technician, a person who works effectively and cuts down on the noise level—getting him- or herself out of the way so the story can emerge. Elders I work with in the Cree and Saulteaux nations describe the work of the good traditional storyteller in a similar manner. Such storytellers don't let their own personality interfere with the story; they don't create their own version of the story, but instead try to relate the story as accurately as possible, as they themselves heard it. Creative storytelling then becomes accurate storytelling; truth is more important than originality. Only then can the real message or spiritual teaching of the story emerge.

Verna   That makes me think that part of my reservations about our book deals with who we have in mind as our audience. For me, I think first and foremost about Indigenous people as my audience and then the writing becomes much harder. Because we are writing about their lives, it's much more of a challenge to write well for them—to write sensitively, respectfully, and truthfully.

Dick   I agree with Verna—and I also feel our first audience is the Jul'hoansi. But this idea of audience also raises another of my reservations. Sometimes when I give a talk about Indigenous spiritual healing traditions I've worked in, I find there is the possibility, even the probability, of misunderstanding. For example, in my book on Fijian spiritual healing, *The Straight Path,* I described how my teacher of Fijian healing emphasized that spiritual work must be done carefully, slowly, and patiently, and that healing rituals cannot simply be taken from an Indigenous culture to be used by a Western psychotherapist. Yet a person who read the book, who in his own spiritual work is neither careful nor patient and who has appropriated Indigenous rituals into his own therapy, felt affirmed by my teacher's words. I worry our book may have some of these unintended, and I believe unproductive, consequences.

Megan That's a good point, Dick. We don't want to make it easier for Jul'hoan culture to be appropriated, and yet we also want to let people know the important things about it. So we're really caught in quite a dilemma here.

Dick Another part of this idea of really hearing what the Jul'hoansi say and not misdirecting or misinterpreting its meaning deals with the money we're trying to raise on their behalf. We want to follow their lead in deciding how that money is spent. We have to listen to them. But I know that some people who may want to give money will also have ideas about how that money should be spent, ideas about "good" development projects or "healthy" alternatives to support. They might already have an idea of what it means to be "helpful," even being convinced they know what the Jul'hoansi "need." But from a Jul'hoan point of view, the proposed project may not be so "good" or "healthy."

I believe we have to listen to the Jul'hoansi and follow their lead, not blindly, but respectfully. We have to respect their ability to know what they need, what is "good" for them.

Verna One way I've turned the project into something I could consider "productive" or useful is to think about how the book might facilitate the connecting of Indigenous peoples throughout the world. I remember thinking how important it would be if some ǀKaeǀkae Jul'hoansi could meet other Indigenous people and know that they are not alone in their struggle.

Megan There was an example of that recently. In late 1993, Aboriginal people from Norway and Australia visited some Jul'hoansi people in Namibia; it was a very revealing meeting and successful for all parties. Under the sponsorship of the Swedish and Norwegian governments, the people came to Namibia for two weeks. Their hosts were Jul'hoansi from the Nyae Nyae Farmers' Cooperative. The Jul'hoansi were able to talk about their success in starting a community development cooperative.

In the global multicultural village of today, I believe that the voices of Indigenous peoples can be seen as the voices of elders in a community meeting. These voices are being heard today because of the new communications technology and new political ideologies that are sweeping the world. I have recently begun discussions with computer experts involved in a "Planet Keepers" project about how Indigenous peoples may be enabled to carry their ideas to others around the world by connecting them to the Internet by satellite—no electricity, telephones, or even radio telephones would be needed. And so I believe we are performing a valuable job in connecting Jul'hoan people with this global network.

When I think more directly about the contributions of our project, I turn immediately to the Jul'hoan tradition of healing. The project has given me an overwhelming sense of the reliability of their healing methods. These methods are reliable not because they are magic but because they are socially effective, reassuring, and validating. And the efficacy of the dance is fostered by many things—the sensations at the dance as well as the community participation and mutuality in the dance. The people place their faith in the healing dance, and their faith is rewarded.

I also believe our project makes a contribution by placing the healing dance in *particular* points in history. So much of anthropological documentation takes place in a kind of ethnographic never-never land, without the concreteness of specific dates. It then becomes harder for the reader to realize the actuality of the people being described as living, breathing human beings.

It's hard to estimate the degree to which we may have supported the local Jul'hoan healing tradition, but I believe there is a germ of truth in the idea that our interest in and respect for that tradition has helped the Jul'hoansi bring it up in front of their own eyes once again and reevaluate its meaning.

Dick   Might our project contribute to the strengthening of the Jul'hoan healing tradition? I want to emphasize that the primary contribution comes from the Jul'hoansi themselves; it is their tradition, their lives, and without their own affirmation of their healing work, nothing we could do would have much impact. The Jul'hoansi were constantly demonstrating in their dances their respect for and support of their own healing work. They underscored these affirming actions with a constant refrain, further articulating their pride and confidence in their healing: "But we still have our nlom." Building on this foundation of self-affirmation, I believe our project, with its deep respect for Jul'hoan values and healing, could have a positive influence. And that is my deepest hope.

Certainly the primary function of the Jul'hoan healing tradition is to keep the Jul'hoansi "alive"—as so many told us, they would "die without nlom." But the Jul'hoan healing tradition also has so much to teach others throughout the world about spirituality and healing, especially considering the bankruptcy of models of social change that focus exclusively on political or economic variables. But critical to any contribution our project may or may not make is the fact that we also have tried to stress the concreteness of the Jul'hoan sociopolitical context, and its devastating effects. Certainly the Jul'hoansi never let the importance of their dance blind them to the even more important realities of everyday subsistence.

In the end, however, we don't really know what effects our project will have—if any—on the Jul'hoansi, or the larger community. All we can say is that we struggled, with all our hearts, to "do it right." And then we must trust in what we were continually shown—the strengths and wisdom of the Jul'hoansi.

Verna   Once again I feel like I want to go along with you both, but my heels are dug in. There is something that has been on my mind from the very beginning, and now it comes up again after hearing what you are both saying.

I think we have to acknowledge a very potent presumption: we are saying that we have the power to legitimize a tradition in another part of the world. Because we from the outside believe the Jul'hoan healing tradition is important and should be supported, therefore the Jul'hoansi will continue to value that tradition. This presumption is based primarily on the unequal power relationship between nations of predominantly White people and nations of people of color, an inequality that is supported by and supports racism, including internal racism.

At the same time, I also agree with you both that it is important for us to validate Jul'hoan healing traditions. Anything we can do to encourage strength among the Jul'hoansi is important, considering the enormous pressures they must face. We must also acknowledge the presumption that underlies our efforts to validate, even though we try not to be party to the racism that fuels that presumption.

Dick   Perhaps one way to continue to deflate the power of that presumption is to stress even more the Jul'hoansi's own affirmation of their healing work.

I'm also reminded of what Ratu Noa told me after I had worked with him for two years, studying Fijian healing traditions. He said I must write a book about Fijian healing because at certain points in history an outsider who understands the story of that healing must tell it. He went on to explain the reason: those who must hear that story, the doubters about Fijian healing, would be more receptive to an outsider's voice, especially one from the West whose values they seek to emulate—these doubters would include government officials who can affect the destiny of the healing traditions as well as ordinary Fijians who have forgotten traditional knowledge. Maybe we're also at such a point in Jul'hoan history, and therefore our efforts may have a certain value.

But I want to end by again saying that Verna's point about our presumptions based on historical power inequities is the primary one. It deserves a straightforward acknowledgment and acceptance, and I don't mean to undercut it by some of the things I've just said.

As a team we have worked hard at working together, and I believe we stand strongly together in our approach to this book and our various contributions to it. We've had our differences, but they didn't evolve into interpersonal tensions. Rather, I think we ended up educating each other and in that way reaching resolutions. Verna challenged me to more fully realize the depth of my sense of entitlement as a White person by working in a less ego-filled and more honest way. Her ability to discuss matters in a simple and concrete manner as a way to raise meaningful and profound issues and her sense of justice were invaluable. And

Megan offered an extraordinary depth of knowledge about the particular situation in the Kalahari and her desire to explore things from a spiritual perspective. Her highly skilled translation of the Ju/'hoan texts and interviews was essential. Megan, you raised the act of translating to the act of honoring others.

Verna   I know that Dick cares deeply about all these issues and concerns I've raised. But I also know that just because he is a White person, others may not know that about him. At the same time, there's a difference between being Indigenous and non-Indigenous that can never be overlooked. And in regard to you, Megan, I've always appreciated your ability to do the translating and also the attention you have paid to "getting it right." This development work and research is not something that you are just doing for a couple of years—it has become an ongoing part of your life. This brings a sense of credibility to the work you've done that is very important to me.

Megan   I think the occasional dissonances between our voices has ultimately kept the inquiry open and kept us aware of the questions that we started with and are now ending up with. I also have a sense we were a little family. Not the usual sort of family, but when we were doing the fieldwork, for example, it was important in some almost undefinable way that the three of us were there. For example, it was very important to me that there was another woman in the project. I haven't been privileged to work with women in the field as often as I have with men, and I found it very personally validating.

But Verna's participation in the project challenged me, as a White person and as a long-time and close research collaborator of Dick's. But every one of my fears has been replaced by a recognition of the richness that Verna's presence has brought to our work. Everything I write in connection with the book, I ask myself, "Well, what is this going to sound like to Verna?"

And as far as working with Dick, I've always appreciated that steady light of the larger, spiritual dimensions that Dick has kept on everything that we have done together. In all the years of our productive collaboration I have been aware of Dick's tendency to keep after a question until you get to the bottom of it. As his translator in the field, I sometimes found it hard to sustain the patience needed to translate the question one more time a slightly different

way. Yet I believe such an approach has a positive outcome in that it forces us as researchers, along with the people who are being interviewed, to look at things from many different angles.

Dick   I'm also reminded of what our young Ju/'hoan research associates told us when we asked them about our project. /Ukxa, Kxao /O/Oo, and Tshao Xumi, all of whom have achieved advanced educational status, were deeply involved in the interviews with healers, translating for us and also helping to formulate questions. They all talked about learning new things about n/om and the dance from participating in the interviews. And all said they were grateful for that opportunity. I got the strong impression that this new knowledge was more than a surface accumulation of facts. /Ukxa, for example, when learning how healers climb the threads to God's village—new information for him—changed his outlook on n/om and its functions, developing a new admiration for the skill and courage of the healers. Whether this new information would lead to /Ukxa or others actually becoming healers is unclear, but it does seem that information could lead to a new and enhanced respect for healers' work. Maybe one of our project's strongest contributions will be among these young, educated Ju/'hoansi.

Verna   That is one final point I wish to raise. For too long anthropology has been describing culture as a static, homogenous entity, with clear boundaries; as a corollary to that, there is the assumption that there is a "pure" or at least "purer" or more "traditional" form of that culture, and it always exists sometime "in the past." I want us to avoid that kind of thinking; it isn't a correct description of culture, which in fact is constantly changing and has great variety within. This dynamic concept of culture is important because it allows for younger Ju/'hoansi to develop their own self-respect and identity. I don't want our book to present the picture, for example to Kxao /O/Oo's children, that the "real" Ju/'hoan culture was "in the past," that the "real" healers were his grandparents or great-grandparents. If our book is to make a valuable contribution, we can't contribute to a closing down of possibilities for the future, a devaluing of contemporary and future Ju/'hoan efforts. We can't present the current young people as "less than" the prior generations; they are doing what they can to forge their future and we must respect that.

THE RESEARCH TEAM

The early morning sun's warmth is just beginning to make inroads on the night's chill. The breakfast fire in our camp has already put forth its friendly heat for those of us still clad in clothes better suited to a New England fall, and now the water for tea is boiling and the hot porridge is ready. Various members of our research team have drifted quietly into the camp, and amid visiting and joking the tea and porridge are served. Slowly and gently, our informal research meeting begins and we plan the activities for the day.

This is a near-daily occurrence at our camp, which is an ample circular space surrounded by a "fence" of thorn bushes to keep out the cattle in the manner of many |Kae|kae living spaces. Inside the fence are three tents. A cooking grate placed over the fire, some pots and pans, a set of dishwashing bowls, and two food trunks sitting under a plastic tarp constitute the kitchen area. Several chairs, two thirty-gallon water drums, and clotheslines that sometimes double as places to hang meat to dry fill out the camp area. Outside is parked our Toyota Land Cruiser, which except for another Land Cruiser owned by a Herero man is the only vehicle permanently at |Kae|kae. Government vehicles, connected with the school, clinic, or other government programs, only pass through for various periods of time.

Though we live simply by Western standards, we are incomparably rich in |Kae|kae, and this material disparity makes the power differential we struggle even to acknowledge fully all the more difficult to ignore. Although our living space is smaller and so much better equipped than other Jul'hoan camps, it fits in with our neighbors, whose camps lie several hundred yards away in a large arc to the north. We are living in a place chosen for us by the Jul'hoansi of |Kae|kae, who have sought through fictive kinship to include us in their extended family.

Though our research team is neither firmly bounded nor formally constituted, there is a group of people we work with most closely. Not only do they assist us in the design and logistics of the overall research process, they are also the ones we primarily interview. It is also the group of people we spend the most time with visiting and sharing; work and play go togther. Among the team's central members are five of the most respected and experienced healers at |Kae|kae and their wives. By name, these members are ≠Oma Djo and his wife, N≠aisa N!a'an, Tshao N!a'an and |Xoan, ≠Oma !'Homg!ausi and Ti!'ae, Tshao Matze and ||Uce N!a'an, and Kxao Tjimburu and N≠aisa. All five of the wives are centrally involved as singers in the healing dances, and |Xoan also experiences !aia and is a healer.

Also central to our team are three young Jul'hoan men who are among the few Jul'hoansi who have passed their Junior Certificate, a high school diploma roughly equivalent to completion of the American eleventh grade: |Ukxa, Kxao |O|Oo, and Tshao Xumi. Having learned English in school, they serve as excellent translators. Finally, there is Florence Molebatsi, a Tswana university student from the Botswana capital of Gaborone who is especially helpful in interviews with such Tswana officials living at |Kae|kae as the schoolteachers and the nurse.

In 1989 Verna and Dick live in the camp from May through August, joined for a month by Megan while she is on leave from her ongoing work in Namibia, and also for a month by Florence. |Ukxa and Tshao Xumi, both living in |Kae|kae, are with us the entire time, and |Ukxa lives for a time at the camp. Taking time off from his job in Maun, Kxao |O|Oo spends several weeks with us. We all try to live in a way that is harmonious with |Kae|kae life and engage in a wide variety of Jul'hoan activities, including hunting, gathering, and dancing.

We also conduct more than sixty open-ended interviews of about an hour's duration with a wide range of Jul'hoan women and men, focusing on healers and those involved in the healing dance, as well as several interviews with various Tswana and Herero officials whose jobs impact on Jul'hoan life, including schoolteachers, health providers, and the village headman. In addition we attend nearly forty dances—a number of them drum dances, the remainder giraffe dances—sing and dance with the others, and help when we are called upon.

Often during our morning gatherings we get advice from team members as to whom to interview, what questions to ask, when dances are going to be held and why, and the general direction our project is taking. Certainly we have come to the Kalahari with a research plan and an orientation toward questions. But these are loosely held and the day-to-day research tasks often change in response to advice.

≠Oma Djo and Kxao Tjimburu, who are both healers, and ǀUkxa and Tshao Xumi, who serve as translators, are the ones we spend the most time with, the ones who most frequently offer advice. When we go to an interview, we are usually accompanied by some or all of these men, and the interview at times becomes a lively group discussion as ≠Oma Djo and Kxao Tjimburu offer their opinions or suggest new lines of questioning. Our interviews become a dynamic process of exchange, an unfolding talk rather than a prearranged schedule of questions and answers.

Megan has a special role in the work of translation. During her time at ǀKaeǀkae she both translates the interviews and helps train ǀUkxa and Tshao Xumi in translating skills. As well, she and Verna do some interviewing alone with some of the women. The interviews are taped, and Megan subsequently listens to all of them, translating them into English or correcting and refining the translations made by others in the field. We all realize that translation is at best imperfect. But as Megan's knowledge of the Juǀ'hoan language is rare among English speakers and her understanding of Juǀ'hoan culture and healing, in particular, is profound, we believe the words spoken to us by the Juǀ'hoansi are at least at the first stage of being heard—they are as accurately as possible translated into English.

Our research in 1989 sits within a much larger context of experience and research among a network of researchers and scholars who over the years have worked with Juǀ'hoan and other Bushman peoples. In the bibliography, we have indicated others whose research serves as a foundation for our work.

Unfortunately, our bibliography contains nothing from Juǀ'hoan scholars, as no works are yet in print. Yet Kxao ǀOǀOo and some others intend to change that state soon. More and more, work like we have undertaken must take into account a new readership—that of newly literate Juǀ'hoan people who will scrutinize such work to see if they recognize their own people's true voices in the writing.

WRITING THE JU|'HOAN LANGUAGE: SOME POLITICAL CONSIDERATIONS

Until 1991 a number of different orthographies or "ways to write language" were used for Jul'hoan Bushmen by scholars and linguists. The language as used by Jul'hoan people themselves was unwritten. In the late 1980s, a grass-roots people's organization, the Nyae Nyae Farmers' Cooperative located in what was then still South West Africa, just across the international fence from |Kae|kae in Botswana, began a move to establish an educational project in their own language. Through a nongovernmental organization called (starting in 1991) the Nyae Nyae Development Foundation of Namibia, a linguist and an anthropologist were employed—Patrick Dickens and Megan Biesele, respectively—to help them in this work. In 1991 the new orthography of the people's cooperative was formally adopted by the Namibian government as its orthography for the Jul'hoan language. It is now being used in Namibia for the first three grades of schooling. In 1994 the orthography was recognized at the International Conference on Khoisan Linguistics and Ethnohistory held in Munich, Germany.

Interest has also been shown by officials of the Botswana Ministry of Education in eventually using the orthography and curriculum materials in the Jul'hoan language developed in Namibia. Our book has adopted the spellings of the new orthography in the interests of clarity, secure replicability, and democratic communication among newly literate Jul'hoan people, who mandated its creation for their own educational efforts. The orthography was published by Patrick Dickens in 1991. An English-Jul'hoan and Jul'hoan-English dictionary by Dickens was later published in 1994.

IMPLICATIONS OF THE NEW JU|'HOAN ORTHOGRAPHY AND DICTIONARY

Before Patrick Dickens's linguistic work for the Nyae Nyae Farmers' Cooperative, scholarly materials on Jul'hoan language existed mainly in Afrikaans. By the time of Namibian independence, the Jul'hoansi were like many other Namibians in wanting to discard the language of their for-

mer oppressor. English was made the national language at that time. Dickens and the Jul'hoansi agreed that materials previously available in Afrikaans such as Jan Snyman's *Zu/'hoasi Fonologie and Woordeboek* (1975) should be made available in English as well as augmented by new material.

An existing orthography, also by Jan Snyman, was revised and streamlined for practical use by both native speakers and scholars. Dickens also wrote a practical grammar of Jul'hoan (in press) and created numerous curriculum materials at several levels for teaching Jul'hoan. He used all these materials to teach both adult learners and the first sixteen young people who would become the teachers of Jul'hoan primary students.

This work, done collaboratively with the Jul'hoan community, has already had a profound effect on both Jul'hoan educational opportunities and politics. An educational program for and with the people in their own language was launched in 1991. Not only has this program made a dignified entry for the Jul'hoansi into Namibian national education possible, but it is being used as a model for other Indigenous peoples' educational efforts such as those being made in the former Western Bushmanland of Namibia by Vasekela Bushmen and in Ghanzi, Botswana, by Nharo Bushman groups. More than that, it has made possible the entry of the Jul'hoansi into the political life of their new nation—using their own voices and more frequently on their own terms.

There is in fact a very close connection between the community linguistic work undertaken by the Jul'hoansi in recent years and the creative survival and future development of this minority and their language. There are parallel efforts and issues in other parts of the world, such as the Oaxaca Native Literacy Project in Mexico begun by Russell Bernard and others in Ecuador and Cameroon.[1] It is particularly true of the Jul'hoan case, however, that making the Jul'hoan language visible, and its use practical in Namibia at the time of national independence, had the effect of improving the people's chances to retain their land-base and argue for fair political representation.

While the linguistic and curriculum materials were being developed, Jul'hoan community members of all ages were continuously involved. Thus, it has been a triumph of the people's own plan for their literacy—and of many years of linguistic and textual work going hand-in-hand with development efforts—that has brought educational efforts to such fruition for the Namibian Jul'hoansi. Their new orthography has been the one of choice in the political arena, too: the Jul'hoan people's representations—verbal and in writing—have attracted national attention in Namibia, first at the historic Land Conference in 1991 and since then at many national and international meetings of Bushmen and other Indigenous peoples.

In October 1993 such a meeting was held in Gaborone, Botswana, and one of the main items on the agenda was the Bushman peoples' right to primary education in their own language. The educational program of the Nyae Nyae Farmers' Cooperative was held up at that meeting as an inspiring example. After the meeting, there was talk of the curriculum being extended into the Jul'hoan area of Botswana, should Botswana educational policies move toward the received opinion of early childhood educators around the world. It is generally agreed that the skills of literacy and critical thinking are best learned in the first three or four years of schooling in the mother tongue. These skills then can be generalized to whatever lingua franca—such as English—is politically appropriate.

For scholars, the realization that the Jul'hoansi have had a hand in developing what may be called "self-literacy" has profound implications. The Namibian Jul'hoansi themselves are the ones choosing what they want to come out of the verbal realm into print. And the day will come when they will critique the many miles of print that have been written about their own culture.

At present, young Jul'hoan people are using tape recorders to learn how to transcribe their own language. Within their educational program, young people are interviewing and taping older people and writing down their old ways and knowledge for posterity. In-depth cultural knowledge can expand exponentially, and reflexive self-awareness of change and educational processes can be carried out by the people themselves.

Language recognition and cultural recognition, in short, are important parts of political empowerment for Indigenous peoples. It is appropriate that scholars and other outsiders to their culture honor the local linguistic and educational efforts of Jul'hoansi and other Indigenous peoples by using their own adopted orthographies whenever possible. Our use of the new Jul'hoan spellings and other orthographical conventions in this book is an attempt to reflect the respect we have for the efforts the peoples are making on behalf of their future.

THE QUESTION OF NOMENCLATURE

Readers familiar to some extent with the anthropological literature may find themselves in some confusion over what the Jul'hoan people and Bushman peoples in general have been called. We will attempt to clarify some areas of nomenclature in regard to an overarching term both for Kalahari foraging peoples and for specific linguistic groups.

Some scholars in recent years have advocated the use of *San* to avoid the pejorative connotations of *Bushman* as used by Afrikaner and English-speaking settlers of Southern Africa. But both labels that refer to a group of many foraging and recently foraging societies are the subjects of ongoing debate among these peoples as well as by scholars and development workers. At present, some leaders of grassroots movements advocate "ennobling" the previously negative term *Bushman*. This book follows their lead, especially since at several recent meetings of different groups in both Botswana and Namibia, no consensus on the matter of a group appellation could be reached. No group recognized *San* as its choice, either, and there is some feeling that this label, coming from the Nama language, may be even more pejorative.

In Botswana these societies are collectively referred to as "BaSarwa" by the Tswana ruling majority. This term has also with use come to have pejorative connotations. For most Tswana, the term implies "people without cattle," which is to these proud pastoralists derogatory in itself. But many Bushman peoples have tried to ennoble this term as well in Botswana, bowing to the inevitability of a SeTswana language term being used for them.

Jul'hoan, meaning "real" or "ordinary people," is the name the people previously called !Kung in anthropological literature use for themselves. Previous spellings included Zhultwa, Zul'hoa, and Julwa.

A CHRONOLOGY OF
RECENT JU|'HOAN HISTORY

Note that when independence came to South West Africa in 1990, it was renamed Namibia. When independence came to the British Protectorate of Bechuanaland in 1966, it was renamed Botswana. The modern country names will appear in this chronology once these independence dates have occurred. Until that time, the colonial names will be used in order to properly attribute the responsibility for actions to the regime actually in power at the time, for example the apartheid policies of the government of South West Africa.

1850s   First recorded contacts between Jul'hoansi and Black and White peoples occurs in South West Africa.

1860   Commercial elephant hunting begins in South West Africa.

1860s   Herero pastoralists expand into the Nyae Nyae area of South West Africa when guns become available.

1870   Tswana people first come to the Dobe area.

1874–77   Afrikaner Hendrik van Zyl decimates the elephant population north of Nyae Nyae.

1880s   A German colony in South West Africa and a British protectorate in Bechuanaland are established.

1885–95   The Ghanzi Farm Block in Bechuanaland is settled by Afrikaner farmers, dispossessing Bushman groups.

1896–97   A rinderpest epidemic of wild and domestic ungulates (hooved mammals).

1900   Tswana loan earliest "mafisa" cattle to Jul'hoansi.

1904–7   Nama uprising against Germans occurs in South West Africa.

1908   Diamonds are discovered in South West Africa.

1910–31   Stock theft by Bushmen leads to anti-Bushmen patrols in South West Africa.

1915   Germany surrenders South West Africa to South Africa.

1917   Tswana from Lake Ngami are given permission by Tswana tribal authorities to graze in Jul'hoan area of South West Africa, leading to resistance by some Jul'hoansi and police reprisals.

1900–1920   Tobacco becomes available through trading.

1920   The establishment of vagrancy and stock theft proclamations against Bushmen in South West Africa.

1920s   Investigations into Jul'hoan slavery and other human rights violations in Bechuanaland are conducted by the League of Nations and the International Labor Organization.

1927   A government act in South West Africa makes bows and arrows illegal.

1927   A government act in South West Africa reduces the allowable limit for Bushman families squatting on farms to five persons.

1928   The South West African administration takes chiefs' power into its own hands and allows its administrator to recognize anyone it wants as chief.

1928–34   Herero pastoralists begin settling on Jul'hoan lands in Nyae Nyae and on the natural water pans of Bechuanaland.

1930s   Central District of Bechuanaland investigates beating deaths of Bushmen at the hands of neighboring pastoralists.

1935   Hereros are evicted by Bechuanaland police.

1936   Slavery is abolished in Bechuanaland.

1930s, 1940s   Border beacons and a road are built between South West Africa and Bechuanaland. Attempts are made to involve Jul'hoansi in Bechuanaland in agriculture, road work, and problem animal control.

1948   Isak Utugile, a Tswana, is appointed headman of the Dobe area.

1949   "Native affairs" in South West Africa are put under the South African Parliament.

1950   The first visit of the Marshall family to Jul'hoan areas of Bechuanaland and South West Africa, beginning a series of their anthropological expeditions.

1951–54 The Schoeman Commission recommends the establishment of a Bushman homeland in South West Africa.

1954 A major influx of Hereros from Makakung in Bechuanaland to Nyae Nyae in South West Africa.

1954–60 Jul'hoan resistance, sometimes assisted by South West African police, to Herero settlement.

1959–60 The start of administration of Bushmen by South West Africa rather than South Africa; a Bushman Affairs Commissioner is appointed in Tjum!kui in the Nyae Nyae area.

1959–60 A twenty-year ban is instituted on ethnographic observation of Bushmen in South West Africa, and Bushmen are encouraged to move to the Tjum!kui administrative center.

1961 A mission is established in Tjum!kui by Dutch Reformed Church at the same time that a trading store opens there.

1963 The Odendaal Commission in South West Africa recommends setting aside two areas for Bushmen that are a fraction of the former Nyae Nyae territory.

1963 Richard Lee and Irven DeVore conduct a survey in Bechuanaland to prepare for future anthropological work by themselves and other researchers, including Megan Biesele and Dick Katz.

1965 Publication in Bechuanaland of the Bushman survey report by George Silberbauer.

1965 The erection of a border fence between South West Africa and Bechuanaland. The Jul'hoansi retain unspoken permission to cross using stiles.

1966 Bechuanaland, henceforth known as Botswana, achieves independence from Great Britain.

1966 The United Nations revokes South Africa's mandate over South West Africa; the South West Africa Peoples' Organization (SWAPO) begins a military liberation offensive after South Africa refuses to comply.

1967 The first store opens at !Aoan in western Ngamiland, Botswana.

1969 A "homeland" for Bushmen in South West Africa is declared, modeled along lines recommended by the Odendaal Commission.

1970s, 1980s Jul'hoansi in South West Africa leave their land and are settled further west in Tjum!kui.

1970s, 1980s Jul'hoansi on both sides of the border between South West Africa and Botswana are recruited by the South African Defense Force to fight against SWAPO; police in South West Africa establish border posts manned by Jul'hoan Bushmen to "watch for SWAPO."

1970s, 1980s Dependency on imported foods becomes noticeable.

1973 Kalahari Peoples' Fund (KPF) is established.

1973 A government school opens at !Aoan, Botswana; it is later partially supported by KPF efforts.

1974 A mobile clinic begins visits to |Kae|kae.

1974 Bushman Battalion 31 is established by the South African Defense Force.

1975 Tribal Grazing Land Policy (TGLP) is announced in Botswana, constituting a major step toward eventual commercialization of ranching. The progressive dispossession of non–cattle holders, such as the Jul'hoansi, results.

1975–76 The first KPF project is initiated: Megan Biesele works in Botswana as research-liaison person for the new Bushman Development Office, helping to inform and aid Jul'hoan people in taking advantage of their citizens' rights.

1975–76 Jul'hoan people in Botswana attempt to register wells and garden lands under TGLP.

Mid 1970s KPF supports agricultural demonstrator Leonard Mathlare to work in the Dobe area and assists this and other Botswana Jul'hoan communities with hand-dug wells.

1976 Bushmanland in South West Africa is declared a nature conservation area and Bushman people are evicted.

1976 A government school opens at |Kae|kae.

1978 A drought symposium held in Botswana draws attention to the plight of rural peoples, but litigation statements avoid the issue of whether Bushmen have a legal right to access to land.

Late 1970s Village Development Committees are set up in Botswana, but Bushmen are included only in a token manner.

1980s Bushmen in South West Africa start a back-to-the-land movement in three communities.

1981 Ju|wa Bushman Development Foundation (JBDF)

is started in South West Africa by John Marshall and Claire Ritchie to aid Jul'hoan communities with cattle and boreholes; this group becomes the Nyae Nyae Development Foundation of Namibia (NNDFN) in 1991.

1986   Julwa Farmers' Union (JFU) is started by Jul'hoansi in South West Africa.

1988   The number of back-to-the-land communities in South West Africa grows to twelve.

1989   United Nations Resolution 435 is put into effect in South West Africa; Jul'hoansi begin widespread information-dissemination and democratization processes.

1990   South West Africa, henceforth known as Namibia, achieves independence from South Africa.

1991   Namibian Jul'hoansi take part in the National Conference on Land Reform and the Land Question.

1992   Botswana and Namibian Bushmen meet with other Bushman peoples at an international conference in Windhoek, Namibia, and discuss their mutual concerns.

1993   The number of back-to-the-land communities in Namibia grows to thirty-five; the Nyae Nyae Farmers' Cooperative (NNFC), formerly the Julwa Farmers' Union (JFU), is diversified and reorganized.

1993   Botswana is increasingly accused by other nations of human rights abuses against Bushmen, including government violence, murders, forced resettlement, and land dispossession.

1993   A second international conference for Botswana and Namibian Bushmen to discuss mutual concerns is held in Gaborone, Botswana. After many years of waiting to have their voices heard, |Kaelkae-area Jul'hoansi have no representatives present. The two delegates from |Kaelkae, Xumi N!a'an and Tshao Matze, are accidentally killed on the way to Gaborone.

APPENDIX E

CONCRETE CHALLENGES
FOR DEVELOPMENT WORKERS

"Undertaking for another," as Ralph Waldo Emerson called it, is always a doomed enterprise. I (Megan) have found this statement a helpful guide. Over the decades of researcher involvement with the Jul'hoansi, there has been much debate and trial and error about the best way to be of help to someone or a group without compromising that group's dignity and initiative. With Indigenous voices speaking for themselves more and more often in recent years, this issue is now openly contested in anthropological and development circles. Today there is the stark question of whether peoples such as the Jul'hoansi even want outsiders' help, since in the past such help has sometimes come with strings attached or has caused more problems than it has solved.

There are many ways of giving, some less problematic than others. All three of us have been active in development, advocacy, or educational work in various ways, and we felt this book would not be complete without a discussion of some of the practical issues involved in offering help to others. I present here some concrete examples of work I have been involved in to illustrate possibilities, particularly as they have been tried in the Jul'hoan areas of Botswana and Namibia.

Before presenting these examples, I want to offer certain cautions. First, the fact that these examples will be drawn largely from the work of someone trained as an anthropologist does not mean that this discipline is uniquely or even specially qualified to do development work. Certainly the results of the efforts we will describe have been mixed. But my familiarity with the particular development efforts described gives me a chance to present relevant details of the actual work involved and insights about its actual functioing.

Second, most of the examples are directed toward facilitating Jul'hoan access to mainstream resources and facilitating their assumption of positions of empowerment in the sociopolitical system with which they are confronted. The task of building development projects on the foundation of traditional values and culture, so that they continue to

express these values, remains largely undone. For example, I will not be describing projects built upon the reality and functioning of nlom in Jul'hoan life or even projects that take healing as their central or organizing principle.

The fact that the development examples described are all presented from the viewpoint of the development workers—themselves outsiders to Jul'hoan culture—is a third caution. This appendix is geared to prospective development workers and their actions, feelings, capacities, and strengths. Generally missing is the voice of the Jul'hoan people about specifically what "help," if any, they see ensuing from any project. But I can say that Jul'hoansi either initiated or requested help in initiating most of the projects described and have not rejected any because of their ensuing results. However, it is becoming clear very recently that Jul'hoan people are resisting anything that reminds them of paternalism, and in some cases this resistance has brought previously accepted development projects into question. There is now a growing literature from recipients of development projects all over the world, mostly from Third and Fourth World peoples and Indigenous peoples, telling development workers what in fact is helpful and what is not. This literature, sometimes from oral transcription from aid recipients but increasingly self-written, provides vitally important documentation of both the obstacles to accepting "top-down" development and the substantial internal dynamism of so-called traditional societies. As the Jul'hoansi are adding their voices to the dialogue, we hope this book joins that literature in an accurate and compelling manner.

Fourth, I want to point out that evaluating outcomes of development projects is one of the hardest tasks associated with them. Outcomes are hard to judge because of both varying time frames and points of view. For example, projects that may seem to have short-term benefits can prove to have a long-term negative impact and vice versa. And whether a project is deemed helpful or not often depends on who you speak to and their relationship to the project. Also, all of the projects described are relatively young—

their long-terms effects are still to come. Because of these ambiguities, we are focusing here on intentions and emerging realizations from approaches and situations well known to us, without presenting judgments as to the effectiveness of certain programs.

Finally, the examples given highlight work by individuals and the small nongovernmental organizations (NGOs). These small-scale efforts must be seen in the wider context of development philosophies and approaches of the two countries involved, Botswana and Namibia. In 1974, Botswana inaugurated within its central government an office for Bushman development, which later was institutionalized as a national Remote Areas Development Program (RADP). Many of RADP's effects have been quite positive, particularly in drawing attention to the special needs of "Remote Area Dwellers" (RADs), most of whom are foragers or ex-foragers and almost none of whom have cattle, which form the national economic mainstay of Botswana. The thrust of projects aimed at Jul'hoansi and other Bushmen, however, encouraged them to "settle down" and leave their nomadic ways because nomadism was seen as "uncivilized." The long-term sustainable land-use patterns of the Kalahari were not taken into account. It was also unrealistic to expect that foraging people, without either capital or training in the care of cattle, could suddenly become pastoralists like other Botswana citizens. Recently, policies of "settlement of nomads" have even been used as a tool to dispossess Bushmen of lands. These policies have also provided entry for other citizens of these two countries to take over services available at the settlements, under the protection of a government rhetoric of "equal opportunity."

Equally unrealistic was a land allocation policy that based land use on cattle ownership yet contained no provision for "indigent" persons to obtain cattle. The Botswana government has maintained over the years that it has "no Indigenous population," that all citizens were alike and should receive equal treatment under law. Yet the rich got richer and the Jul'hoansi and other poor, cattleless peoples got poorer. Hunting and gathering sustained the Jul'hoansi for centuries but was not recognized as a legitimate form of land use. Jul'hoan foraging territories were steadily encroached upon as borehole technology was improved and cattle-owning peoples like the Tswana and Hereros moved into Jul'hoan areas with their herds.

A recognition of the catch-22 nature of cattle ownership for the Jul'hoansi and its effects on their shrinking land-base

caused several groups of outsiders during the early 1970s to call for time and strategic help for BaSarwa—the Bushmen—to make these transitions. Outsiders who had some effect in buying time for the Jul'hoansi of the Dobe area included an advocacy group called the Kalahari Peoples' Fund (KPF) started by anthropologists who had worked in the area, including myself and Dick Katz. By the mid-1970s, KPF had joined forces with Botswana government efforts to create a pilot experimental program that eventuated in several so-called Remote Area Development projects.

It is generally accepted by government workers and NGOs alike that smaller, local organizations can often function more effectively than large-scale government projects when feasible. The literature on these kinds of projects is extensive and beyond the scope of this appendix. But it may be informative to look at the efforts of some of the individuals involved and to learn from experiences of the action groups they formed. In the next several pages, I want to describe my role as anthropologist and development worker in more than twenty years of work in Botswana and Namibia and how that role has changed in response to lessons given me by the Jul'hoan people. Because personal decisions about concrete ways to be active on behalf of the Jul'hoansi are at issue here, I will concentrate on my own experiences and decision making. I am highly aware of my colleagues' contributions and plan to discuss the story of our intertwined efforts in another place.

My own career as a development anthropologist could be described briefly as turning from an advocate into a hired (but, I hope, still objective) documentarian. Steps along the way included what some of us called committed research, political engagement, mentoring, translation, and other forms of facilitating communication, and acting as a direct consultant to a people's organization. In trying out these formulations of my role and in observing their practical consequences, I was offered many invaluable lessons by the Jul'hoan people.

In anthropology in the 1960s and 1970s, there was lots of discussion about "participant observation" as a field research method. I learned from my participation in both observation and action with the Jul'hoansi some truths about their society that I believe can only be known through close involvement. Learning these truths has thus resulted, I believe, in my being able to offer both better practical help and better anthropological documentation.

Or, put better, it has brought these two aims together and made them inseparable. The key to the identity between the two aims is understanding that women and men of *any* society create that society every day by living it through their daily choices.

In practical terms, the approaches and roles I tried in relationship to the Jul'hoansi and their struggle for self-determination were closely connected to both historical events and governmental and nongovernmental institutions connected with their lives. In 1973 those of us who were part of the Harvard Kalahari Research Group of anthropologists started, with help from associates, the Kalahari Peoples' Fund (KPF). Casting around for a rationale and description for our as-yet ill-formed intention to be helpful to the Jul'hoansi, we styled it an advocacy group.

The intent of this group was to provide a funded non-profit entity for the strategic support of local development initiatives. Its purpose was also to publicize the needs of the Kalahari peoples in a manner informed by the anthropological and other research done by KPF members. The members shared a feeling of indebtedness and concern. They formed KPF out of a desire to explore ways they could help meet the Jul'hoansi's real needs rather than merely make careers from research on the Jul'hoansi's lives. Several anthropologists associated with KPF became involved in concrete ways with Jul'hoan groups, particularly during repeat visits after their first fieldwork. Their assistance can be grouped under a number of headings, including transport, communication, organization, and facilitation.

In 1975 I returned to Botswana to work closely with the new government BaSarwa Development Office. Private gifts to KPF allowed me to work in Botswana for eighteen months as a Research/Liaison Officer for the Northwest District, an experimental position then being tried by the BaSarwa Development Office for possible expansion to other districts. My work consisted of informing Jul'hoan people of their rights and duties as citizens of the young, democratizing country, especially in terms of their rights to land and resources under the then new Tribal Grazing Land Policy (TGLP). The TGLP provided that groups of Botswana citizens could organize to establish rights to garden lands and water sources improved by themselves, along with land within a certain radius around them for grazing purposes. I traveled extensively in the Jul'hoan area of western Ngamiland, Botswana, to let communities know about and help them take advantage of these rights.

I thought of this work as advocacy and political activism. I and many of my colleagues justified the "special pleading" we did for the Jul'hoansi as an effort to help them gain time to make the changes that seemed inevitable if they were to determine their own future from a position of any strength.

Much of my actual work took the form of community liaison and facilitation, as well as communication and cultural translation for agencies of the Botswana government. With KPF funding, I also arranged for Leonard Mathlare, a Botswana citizen, to be hired as an Agricultural Demonstrator especially for the Jul'hoan communities. Leonard assisted in the Northwest District for many years in providing training, seeds, and subsidized plows for new Jul'hoan farmers who wished to supplement their increasingly circumscribed foraging. Other activities of the liaison work included the promotion of crafts development, health and sanitary awareness, and political participation on a local community level.

Another facet of my work supported by KPF was to provide assistance to two new schools—one established first at !Aoan, and the other at ǀKaeǀkae—in areas of parent-teacher liaison, pupil transport and school feeding, and cultural trouble-shooting. Providing better water systems and promoting fuller Jul'hoan participation in the Botswana Land Board system were two other aspects of my job.

Taken as a whole, my years of development work in Botswana could be characterized as a time of transition. A researcher in social anthropology, I took some fumbling, first few steps toward a transformed role of being an activist, advocate, and facilitator. These years and these newly formulated roles were not easy, nor were they satisfying in terms of apparent effectiveness.

I did not really begin to find the balance that felt completely respectful and reasonably effective to me until I had the chance to work with a Jul'hoan people's organization. This became possible only on the Namibian side of Jul'hoan territory, where the apartheid government of then South West Africa had so oppressed people like the Jul'hoansi that their politicization had proceeded far beyond that of their relatives in Botswana.

In 1981 a foundation conceived as a sister organization to KPF was begun in South West Africa by filmmakers John Marshall and Claire Ritchie. I became its Project Director in 1988 and later went on to become Foundation Director.

This organization, established in Windhoek under South West African laws, continues to be active today under the independent Namibian government as a registered "welfare organization." Known at first informally as "The Cattle Fund," this nongovernmental organization (NGO) eventually came to be called first the JuǀWa (Juǀ'hoan) Bushman Development Foundation (JBDF), and later the Nyae Nyae Development Foundation of Namibia (NNDFN).

Through NNDFN and the grassroots people's organization it partnered in 1986—the Nyae Nyae Farmers' Cooperative—I was closely involved in community organization work. This work was geared to helping the Juǀ'hoan community prepare to participate actively in the transition from apartheid rule to democracy that took place in Namibia in 1990.

NNDFN's program was built around the concept of integrated rural development, a holistic approach to establishing economic self-sufficiency along with secure land tenure and meaningful training and education for the future. I acted as both an advocate and a mentor, my work consisting of institutional development with the Nyae Nyae Farmers' Cooperative, which was eventually to take over all aspects of the NNDFN program. My tasks included daily attention to internal and external communications about a complex, integrated rural development program; fund-raising and donor education about the special needs of the communities; training and leadership education facilitation for the new jobs and capabilities that were now necessary for the Juǀ'hoansi; and informed communication on a national and international level about land rights issues, economic development concerns, and cultural continuity challenges facing the Juǀ'hoan community.

Since 1991 I have worked with other linguists and educators to provide a community-based education program to the Juǀ'hoansi of Nyae Nyae. This program has involved documenting a new orthography of the Juǀ'hoan language (the one used in this book), as well as developing a dictionary and grammar of the language and curriculum materials. It has paved the way for a dignified bridge for the Juǀ'hoansi to the new national education system, which uses English instead of the former Afrikaans. It also has promoted awareness of and some of the means for cultural and linguistic continuity for the Juǀ'hoan community. It has given people choices for their future, ones that need no longer be mutually exclusive.

These language developments have promoted cultural pride, which has been used by the Juǀ'hoansi to good advantage in communications regarding their land needs in Namibia. As well, the ownership of authoritative knowledge of their environment and sustainable lifeways are beginning to be foregrounded effectively by the Juǀ'hoansi in both local and international forums.

My own relationship to these processes of self-representation and assertion of intellectual property rights has been one that started in observation and mild exhortation and is now at a point of withdrawal to a respectful distance as Juǀ'hoan activism takes over. More and more, I think of myself as being hired by the people's organization, which I am proud to serve, to do specific tasks they see as necessary. One of these is documentation and another is translating—which is becoming less and less necessary as Juǀ'hoan translators receive training.

In 1991 I was asked by the Farmers' Cooperative to work as a documentarian of their recent political history. Since then I have been translating and transcribing a series of tape recordings made of their internal and external meetings between the years 1987 and 1993. I continue to write articles and books covering this history; and several projects now in hand will be coauthored with Juǀ'hoan people whose education I helped to facilitate. All such work comes, for me, under the heading of helping Juǀ'hoan voices to be heard.

Chief among the challenges of outsiders' involvement with Indigenous peoples is the important task of facilitating representation so that local voices reach the venues where decisions affecting those communities are made. A related and equally important goal is that of ascertaining "what the people want" and what they genuinely see as a logical next step for themselves in their situation. Sometimes this task involves helping people to communicate with each other in new ways or in unfamiliar forums to explore creative solutions to new problems.

Often such work involves not so much living by high-minded political rhetoric but quiet, dogged, behind-the-scenes, and very mundane labor—work like documenting conversations and agreements; helping people keep records; training people in accountancy or other skills they need to run an organization; providing a focus for discussion of community issues ranging from public health issues to alcohol-related violence; writing or transcribing letters; carrying messages to government entities; raising funds;

writing proposals and press releases; and helping people get access to public services.

Such work often entails developing a philosophy and practice that may not be immediately understood by all involved; this is perhaps one of its hardest aspects. Explaining why available money cannot be used to generate handouts for the few at the expense of more substantial assistance for many—explaining often not just to local people but to funding agencies themselves—is one of many tasks requiring steady courage. Mediating competing ideas and interests both within and around a developing community is another big challenge. Typically both the ideological grounds and the physical grounds—the land rights—of an Indigenous community within a nation-state are contested terrain, often hotly disputed by many parties. Staying responsibly active in such charged situations requires developing clear, flexible approaches and agendas. These tasks are often a difficult charge for conscientious individuals.

It is also necessary to keep a firm grasp on the economic and political realities of the people's situation. In development and advocacy work, it is too easy to prove that "the road to hell is paved with good intentions." Any development may—and usually does—bring mixed blessings. One example was seen at ǀKaeǀkae when the income resulting from a crafts development project was used to buy alcohol instead of food and clothing. Informed, judicious help requires constant vigilance about the consequences of one's actions, con-stant reevaluation of distance and closeness of involvement, and constant awareness of one's own ultimate outsider status. Ultimately, we as outsiders cannot assume that the "good" aim or value in our "good intentions" is in fact a "good" aim or value for the people. We have been very lucky; when the Juǀ'hoansi have asked us to help them, they have usually also told us how to help in no uncertain terms.

Development projects all go through periods of confusion and dissension precisely because so much belief about "the nature of human nature" is involved. They call forth both the best—altruism and wide vision—and the worst—personal neediness and ideological rigidity—in those who would help. Everything known and believed about human interchange is drawn upon and sometimes drained dry by efforts at intercultural mediation and amelioration. In the end, most conscientious workers arrive at a humble position of offering their labor as functionaries or technicians. If they are fortunate to be working with an Indigenous group that is organized well enough to be able to say effectively what they want, they are in a position to help promote those people's autonomy further. If not, they can work quietly toward encouraging self-empowerment. The best outcome of all for an outsider in development work, of course, is to work oneself out of a job. If that happens, the whole situation may turn out to have been beneficial for everyone concerned—going far beyond what is truly a rare learning privilege for the outsider.

ENDNOTES

PREFACE

1. The Jul'hoansi are a specific people existing in a certain place at a certain time in history; it should not be assumed that they provide a living picture of the Paleolithic. Nevertheless, there are some lessons we can learn from their example of solving certain fundamental human problems of living with a social technology that was once widespread. Archaeologists and social anthropologists estimate that for 99 percent of human history all our ancestors lived as hunter-gatherers by foraging on their areas' wild produce. We are fortunate to have a chance to learn about foraging from the few remaining societies that, like the Jul'hoansi, have retained the social traits and organization to allow them to use hunting and gathering for at least part of their subsistence today. For a more extended discussion of the historical and archaeological relevance of contemporary foragers, see Kelly 1995, Solway and Lee 1990, and Woodburn 1980.

2. Ennoblement of a name like "Bushman" is a conscious political decision to reverse a usage that has been stigmatized by negative attitudes. The process can involve many layers of irony. In the present case, it involves among other things revitalizing the positive valuation of a Bushman, based on the Afrikaner derivation of the word, as an "independent" and "nonconforming" person, one who cannot be controlled by the central authorities. Since this book went to press, however, the Namibian Bushmen agreed to the general term "San" for themselves.

3. Linguists differ on the classification of various Bushmen language groups, but they generally agree that Jul'hoan is one of the so-called Northern Khoisan languages spoken by Bushmen; that other Northern languages include !Xu or !O!Kung of Angola and ≠Aullei of Western Botswana; that the Central languages include Khoe or "Hottentot," Haill'om, and Kwadi; and that the Southern languages include Ta'a, !Wi, and lXam of the South African Cape (Barnard 1992).

4. The very effective but slow poison, which comes from bettle larvae activated by the juice of wild asparagus roots, is rubbed on the arrow shafts.

5. Around Ghanzi, Botswana, is one area in which Bushmen encounter a dominant Afrikaner presence. Most Afrikaners there have been and continue to be cattle farmers. *Boer* is the Afrikaans word for *farmer,* and the Jul'hoansi refer to Ghanzi-area Afrikaners as *Barusi,* a corruption of the word *Boer.* It must always be kept in mind that the economic and social situations of different Bushman communities across southern Africa vary greatly according to differences in their environments, geography, and local history.

6. Renato Rosaldo (1993) is one of a growing number of anthropologists and cultural studies scholars who challenge static and neatly bounded definitions of culture and cultural traditions. He points out how such descriptions are often generated by Western writers and applied to cultures distant from the West, perpetuating both a romanticization and a colonization of those cultures.

7. The process of colonization has established a hierarchy of nations and peoples in terms of economic and political power and access to resources. The colonizing nations, who still dominate power and access, assign themselves to the status of First World nations, and others to the status of Third and Fourth World peoples.

8. Because we centered our work on a return to lKaelkae, *Healing Makes Our Hearts Happy* deals mainly with that community and its surrounding area (see map on p. 33). lKaelkae is fairly representative of the situations of Jul'hoan and other Bushman peoples of the western Kalahari.

9. The Nyae Nyae Residents' Council formerly called itself the Nyae Nyae Farmers' Cooperative. The name was changed because the Namibian government will not recognize this peoples' group as a "cooperative"; the new name allows the group to have legal relationships with the government.

MEETING AND TALKING WITH THE PEOPLE

1. Some Jul'hoan names are followed by the father's name. However, our use of a double-naming system for the

Jul'hoan people mentioned in this book is inconsistent because of changes in naming conventions that were occurring during the course of our fieldwork.

A WORD OF CAUTION

1. Taussig 1987, p. xviii.
2. Pastoralists—like the Hereros and also the Tswana (who as agriculturalists also rely on cultivating crops)—base their livelihood on the care of stock like cattle, sheep, or goats. The way of life of pastoralists and agriculturalists involves more centralized authority and more division of labor than the foraging on which people like the Jul'hoansi have depended.

PROLOGUE

1. Quote appears in Katz 1982a, p. 42.
2. The preceding dialogue appears in Katz 1982a, p. 116.
3. There are strong links between *Boiling Energy* and *Healing Makes Our Hearts Happy*, describing as they do largely the same places and persons over a twenty-year period. For readers already familiar with *Boiling Energy* or for those who wish to read this detailed account of Jul'hoan healing in the late 1960s, it may help to connect a few of the persons and places in the two books, because different ways of writing the Jul'hoan language are used in each. *Boiling Energy* focuses on the *Zhu/twa* people of */Xai/xai*, now spelled the *Ju/'hoan* people of */Kae/kae* in *Healing Makes Our Hearts Happy*. Central figures in the earlier book who reappear in the later one include */Toma Zho*, now spelled ≠*Oma Djo*; *K"au Dwa*, now spelled *Kxao ≠Oah*; and */Wa N!a*, now spelled */Xoan N!a'an*. *Boiling Energy* also talks about healing activities in the villages of *!Kangwa*, now spelled *!Aoan* in *Healing Makes Our Hearts Happy*; *!Goshe*, now spelled *G!oci*; and *Chum!kwe*, now spelled *Tjum!kui*.
4. Working in other cultures, including two years in Fiji, I have always tried not to abuse the power and privilege that inhered in my situation. On the contrary, I tried to live simply. Participating in the ongoing life in the village, I've opened myself to many of the same physical, psychological, and spiritual vulnerabilities the people experience. But my camp is far better equipped and stocked than others' in the Kalahari—and back in my middle-class North American context, I am rich in material possessions far beyond the Jul'hoansi's experience. Most important, I have *chosen* to live simply and know I can and will be leaving—so the vulnerability is often muted and a power differential remains.

CHAPTER 1

1. By using the phrase "I gave birth to my children," ≠Oma Djo is emphasizing the important role men played in caregiving within a hunting-gathering context as the people relied on resources from the bush for babies to be born and to grow.
2. In the dry environment of the Kalahari, arable agriculture is even more risky than raising stock.
3. Lee 1979.
4. Lee 1979, p. 159.
5. Lee 1979, p. 205.
6. Early in the season these marula nuts are covered with chartreuse fruit that quickly ferments in the sun and makes the elephants who eat them drunk.
7. A pan is a shallow depression in the Kalahari that holds water during the rainy season.
8. Marshall 1976, p. 140.
9. Ordinarily there is no stealing from someone else's wild vegetable patch.
10. Quote appears in Lee 1993, p. 103.
11. This section on Jul'hoan healing is adapted from Katz 1982d. For a more complete description and discussion of the Jul'hoan approach to healing, see the book-length treatment by Katz (1982a) and articles and sections in books by Biesele (1993), Guenther (1975b, 1986), Lee (1967, 1993), Thomas (1988), L. Marshall (1969), Shostak (1983), and the film by J. Marshall (1965).
12. *Djxani tcxai*, or "to dance a song," is how Jul'hoansi refer to the whole event of a healing dance. They also use the word *tcxai* (song) to refer metaphorically to a dance.
13. The following discussion of n!om is adapted from Katz 1982a, pp. 93–94, and Lee 1993, p. 115.
14. Quote appears in Katz 1982a, p. 42.
15. The cry of the healing work has been referred to by anthropologists as "kowhedili." During that cry, healers are expelling sickness from themselves. An aspect of !aia, the healing cry expresses the great pain healers feel as the boiling n!om works inside them; it is accompanied by an equally dramatic set of shuddering and convulsive behaviors. "Kowhedili," then, is merely an anthropological rendering—and only a reductive approximation at that—of a very intense, complex, and variable sound. The healer's expulsion of breath, which is followed by a rhythmic thumping sound, has been rendered by anthropologists as "hididididi."

16. Quote appears in Katz 1982a, p. 216.

17. Marshall 1961, p. 234.

18. !Xu, who is seen as the captain of the spirits of the dead, has a wife, whose name is Koba. Koba is known as "the mother of the bees."

19. Quote appears in Katz 1982a, p. 45.

20. See chapter 14 in Katz 1982a for the data substantiating these findings.

CHAPTER 2

1. Cattle and cattle owners compete with the Jul'hoansi for the very bush foods and game forage on which they have traditionally depended. Cattle compete with the Jul'hoansi for the water they drink and for the water their wild game needs in order to survive. The hooves of the cattle, not delicately adapted to moving through the Kalahari sands like the hooves of indigenous antelopes, break the soil surface and cause erosion even as they trample over and kill the leaves and stems aboveground that identify the edible bush roots below.

2. Changes in hunting laws as well as hunting by outsiders have reduced the efficiency with which Jul'hoansi have always been able to hunt. This leads to their feelings of substantial deprivation. Some younger Jul'hoansi have not learned to hunt or gather because of the devaluation of these skills through the implicit teachings in the new school and other cultural pressures. The loss of this knowledge removes one option on which older people knew they could rely. Fences erected around parts of their hunting areas have interfered with game migrations—one result being reduced access to water—and drastically lowered the available game. The border fence on the west (in 1965), the Kuke fence on the south (in 1958), and the more recent fencing of the western side of the Okavango swamp to keep wild game and their diseases separate from the cattle in the drier reaches of northwestern Botswana have profoundly affected game densities in the western Kalahari.

3. A borehole is a mechanically drilled well. It is usually equipped with a mechanism to bring water to the surface for use.

4. A personal communication from Patricia Draper in May 1995 helped clarify the historical point about Jul'hoan relationships with Tswana and Herero cattle owners.

5. Hitchcock 1992.

6. The condition of slavery for Bushmen took many tragic forms, including long hours, no wages, payment only in unwanted food and clothing, lack of shelter and sanitation, no land rights where they were living, no legal recourse of any kind, emotional subjugation, physical punishment, and even uninvestigated murder.

7. The Twsana ethnic majority allied itself with British protectorate policies in the establishment of Tswana "headmen" for remote areas, even those which previously had few Tswana residents.

8. In the midst of the destructive effects of Jul'hoan alcohol use and abuse, there was one positive side effect—bonds were sometimes established with the Tswana and Herero, which sometimes facilitated getting cattle at reasonable prices from them. Personal communication, Polly Wiessner, May 1995.

9. The deleterious effects of excessive sugar and other refined carbohydrates, such as alcohol, in diets are becoming well known in the industrialized world (Sudah Shaheb, M.D., personal communication, 1992 and see Abrahamson and Pezet 1951, Duffy 1975, and Mintz 1986). Tragically, this information is much less widespread among Indigenous peoples, who in seeking newly available "modern" foods may be trading the healthy, natural foods they have grown up with for empty calories and chronic nutritional problems.

10. Borehole syndicates are groups of cooperating ranchers who organize to drill and utilize borehole water resources, an expensive proposition. In practice, therefore, only wealthy cattlemen can provide watering points for stock, and thus acquire land leases.

11. See Constitution of the Republic of Botswana, Section 14(3)(c); Tribal Grazing Land Policy, 1975.

12. Quote appears in Lee 1993, p. 166.

13. So-called Remote Area Dwellers (RAD) are those who have the least material resources, and who live far from urban centers. This group includes mostly Bushman and Kgalagadi peoples, both of whom, as non–cattle owners, have low status in Botswana's largely pastoral society. The RAD Program was created in the 1970s to address the needs of these "rural poor," whose residences in remote areas made the provision of government services, such as schools and clinics, very difficult.

CHAPTER 3

1. Quote appears in the film *N!ai: The Story of a !Kung Woman* by John Marshall. See also Volkman 1982, a study guide written to accompany the film.

2. Quotations appear in field note translations by M.

Biesele of the 1991 Namibian National Conference on Land Rights and the Land Question. Some of the quotations also appear in the video made for the conference, entitled *Voices from the Land,* by Richard Pakleppa, New Dawn Video/Government of the Republic of Namibia, 1991.

3. Marshall 1961.

4. Lewis-Williams and Dowson 1989. The comprehensive body of research generated by Lewis-Williams and Dowson demonstrates that the rock art is narrative only in a restricted way; its details are in fact rich with visual metaphors referring to the transformation of consciousness in healing.

5. Arbousset 1846.

6. Quote appears in Katz 1982a, pp. 152–53.

7. Quote appears in Katz 1982a, p. 119.

CHAPTER 4

1. Quote appears in Biesele and Weinberg 1990, p. 13.

2. At times the government was not passing out food and stated that food relief programs were to be discontinued. Consequently, there has been uneven compliance with government settlement efforts, resulting in confusion.

3. See endnote 9 for chapter 2.

4. Along with the destructive effects of sedentization, settlement and the attendant public health measures have sometimes increased the stature and fertility of formerly seminomadic people. Though some have seen these as two positive outcomes of this sedentization process, the issue is more complex than that.

CHAPTER 5

1. Discussion of the ǀKaeǀkae school during Mr. Seelapilu's tenure, including the early successes of the ǀUihaba dance troupe, draws heavily upon personal communications with Richard Lee and the discussion in Lee 1993, pp. 177–81.

2. While publicly emphasizing that the widely dispersed nature of the Juǀ'hoansi makes residential schools a compelling alternative, the government privately emphasizes the need for the cultural "re-education" provided at such schools. The misleading nature of their public comments is evidenced by their wish to send ǀKaeǀkae children to a residential school—even though ǀKaeǀkae already has a school of its own.

CHAPTER 6

1. Quote appears in Katz 1982a, p. 220.

2. Quote appears in Katz 1982a, p. 56.

3. Katz 1993.

4. In their adherence to a classical biomedical approach, the bureaucrats would be committed to a top-down health-care system in which power and expertise reside in a few highly trained individuals. See Davis-Floyd (1992) for a discussion of this top-down approach as it relates to birth in many North American hospitals.

5. See Katz 1993, Katz and Rolde 1981.

6. Adapted from a quote in Lee 1993, p. 122.

CHAPTER 7

1. The discussion on alcohol use in this chapter will focus on !xari, or homebrew, which is, practically speaking, the only alcohol available to the Juǀ'hoansi. It is also referred to as "beer."

2. There is also the important interpretation of alcoholism as a disease that needs to be healed, a viewpoint central to the approach of Alcoholics Anonymous (AA). The AA approach, often in context with traditional treatments, has been very successful in bringing sobriety to many Indigenous communities, especially in North America.

3. The Alkali Lake Band in northern British Columbia, Canada, offers one striking example of an Indigenous community's effective struggle toward sobriety. Drawing strength from a revitalized traditional spirituality to encourage their efforts at community organization and development, the band moved from nearly 90 percent alchohol abuse to nearly 90 percent sobriety. Their journey is documented in the powerful, community-generated film *The Honor of All* (distributed by Four Worlds) and is described in a chapter in York (1989); in Guillory, Willie, and Duran (1988); and in Ben (1991).

CHAPTER 8

1. This chant was recorded and translated by Richard Lee in 1973. He calls it the "Haba-utwe Oration." We use it with his kind permission. The chant was published in Biesele 1993, p. 78, and our discussion of the chant is based on a personal communication with Lee, April 1996, and on Biesele 1993, pp. 78–79.

2. Learning to "drink nǀom"—to know and regulate nǀom for healing, especially in the initial stages such as Kxao ≠Oah recounts here—is a highly social process. New learners are instructed, watched over, and cared for by an

older person who has previously been initiated into nǀom's use. Kxao ≠Oah refers to this person as his "protector."

3. Quoted, with some adaptations, from Biesele 1993, pp. 70–72.
4. The section discussing "seeing properly" is adapted from Katz 1982a, pp. 105–6.
5. Quote appears in Katz 1982a, p. 42.
6. Quote appears in Katz 1982a, p. 105.
7. Quote appears in Katz 1982a, p. 105.
8. Quote appears in Katz 1982a, p. 106.
9. Quote appears in Katz 1982a, p. 98.

CHAPTER 9

1. The drum dance is also known as gǃxoa for an herbal drink used by women initiates when they begin to learn the dance.
2. Quote appears in Katz 1982a, p. 176.
3. Quote appears in Katz 1982a, p. 176.
4. Quote appears in Katz 1982a, p. 127.
5. Marshall 1969, pp. 347–49.
6. As we explored the relationships of giraffe and drum dances to Julʼhoan gender roles in the late 1960s and 1970s, the dances seemed to raise questions about the effects of economic change and sedentism on sexual and political egalitarianism. We took our lead from anthropological work on male and female ceremonies among Australian Aboriginal groups in which questions of class control and power manipulation between male and female sectors in society became central to a number of inquiries. Also, the anthropologist Patricia Draper, our colleague in the Kalahari, had looked into the status of Julʼhoan women and had shown that in transitional contexts of the 1960s and 1970s male and female role conflict was indeed rising (1975, pp. 108–9). We felt it was possible to regard "newer" dances, if in fact the drum dance was such, as possible strategies for expressing or coping with new gender alignments.

Polly Wiessner, another anthropologist who has worked at ǀKaeǀkae, suggested that women's power was being eroded by new forms of economy that excluded them, such as stock-keeping and working for pastoralists. Women also were being marginalized in educational, cultural, and linguistic contexts beyond the degree to which Julʼhoan men themselves were being marginalized. We began to ask whether a newer dance form like the drum dance was expressing emerging subthemes of Julʼhoan culture. Was the drum dance, for example, becoming an arena where women reasserted their power in face of their recently increasing marginalization? Or was the drum dance part of a dynamic that may have been going on between Julʼhoan men and women and between Julʼhoansi and their neighbors for a long time?

7. Drum dances centered around the availability of a drum in a particular camp or the camp of a close relative. The carver and owner of the drum was often the one who also played it for the dance during which it was being used.
8. Though there are other Julʼhoan dances that do have sexual exclusivity—such as puberty dances and several dance games—both the giraffe and drum dances comfortably include both sexes as dancers and singers.
9. It may be that in the traditional hunting-gathering context, sex disparities among the Julʼhoansi were not great enough to generate much need for an alternative dance for women. The giraffe healing dance may have been a complete outlet for most of them, and the healer role was available to be taken up fully by those women, especially among those past childbearing age, who found a need to fulfill themselves in this way. We believe that, to use the phrase of Rohrlich-Leavitt et al. (1975, p. 144), Julʼhoan ceremonial life "reflected the total social organization that the women and men have evolved in their struggle to adapt to a precarious environment." The constraints upon personal aggrandizement and the emphasis on sharing, made necessary by their ecological and technological situation, are also key factors in establishing their relative sexual equality in that situation.

We see the increasing popularity of the drum dance as a response to stress rather than as an expression of a pre-existing equality. In a sense women's healing was there, but its outward form was "potentiated" by the need for a new female outlet and some strategy to cope with the new social alignments of sedentism and economically changed circumstances. This change parallels one recorded by Bogoras around the turn of the century in Siberia (1907, p. 414) where female shamans, traditionally concerned with spirits of foreign origin, saw an upsurge in their numbers and power that was apparently caused by great social upheaval involving external influences, including Christianity.

10. To evaluate this line of thinking, we take a look at formulations about the relationship of environment and means of production to egalitarianism in Julʼhoan social

relations. Summing up her data on male and female work in the more traditional hunting-gathering Jul'hoan relationship to environment, Pat Draper writes that "sexual egalitarianism is a logical outcome given the realities of !Kung [Jul'hoan] life" (1975, p. 105). Extending this argument, Elizabeth Cashdan points out that the egalitarianism of the well-studied western Kalahari (Jul'hoan) hunter-gatherers results from stringent economic constraints and that it cannot be regarded as "a natural condition that represents the absence of stratification" (1980, p. 116). She found that these same constraints do not operate in the eastern Kalahari area she studied. The addition of some food production and storage there supports the existence of greater wealth disparities and differential distribution of political influence among the ǁGana Bushmen. Further, we may expect the work patterns and sedentism accompanying this agriculture, husbandry, and storage, according to Pat Draper (1975, p. 105), to be correlated with greater role differentiation between the sexes and a loss of status for women.

11. Perhaps the most pervasive changes shown by Jul'hoan communities such as ǀKaeǀkae are due to the establishment of some degree of sedentism as opposed to an earlier semi- or water-tethered nomadism. It is tempting to pinpoint this recent sedentism as a watershed between what might have been a more traditional (giraffe) dance form and drum as an incoming form.

Some of the changes accompanying sedentism—identified by Draper (1975), Draper and Cashdan (1988), and Hitchcock (1978)—would indeed seem to be reflected in drum and other newer dances. Because sedentism implies a major shift in the pattern of work, it also implies major shifts in sex roles and the socialization of both male and female children. For instance, the number of female maintenance tasks increases with the greater need for storage and storage-oriented food processing; work roles and tools become sex typed; children are brought into the workforce; female mobility is reduced and female importance diminishes; and children's play groups tend to become single-sex. Woodburn (1980, p. 98) states that the sedentary way of life seems to involve not only a measure of property accumulation and storage but some division of fixed resources among members of the community. Draper (1975, p. 106) describes the change in camp layout from the nomadic to the sedentary context: the close circle of simple huts becomes a loose semicircle of more substantial, Tswana-

or Herero-style houses with less communication between them and more nuclear-family privacy. She draws conclusions from this form (1975, pp. 1080–89) for the privatization of women, for the possibility of greater violence being inflicted on women that cannot be defused by others in the camp, and for reduced female autonomy in using social networks outside their marriages in general.

The single-sex and segregated-task aspects of sedentism, as well as the reduced female mobility accompanied by relative male absenteeism resulting from distant wage labor, appear to be reflected in the women's drum dance, especially in the 1970s. At least provisionally, then, we can say that changes in the dance forms at that time may be connected to introduced economic realities and to sedentism.

12. *San* is a generic term for a fragrant powder usually made by women from dried herbs, and used to perfume clothing and bodies, welcome travelers, and praise healers during a dance. Though ingredients may vary according to preference and availability, its main ingredient, for which it is named, is a plant called *Hemizygia bracteosa*, which grows on the peripheries of water pans.

CHAPTER 10

1. Quote appears in Marshall 1969, p. 366.
2. See Goulet 1985, Schmookler 1984, Trainer 1989.
3. See Katz 1993; Katz, Seth, Nuñez-Molina in press; Lerner 1994; Walsh and Vaughan 1993.
4. See Katz, Seth, Nuñez-Molina in press; Katz and St. Denis 1991. Huxley (1970) identified a core of spiritually based values that run through and guide what he considered the most exemplary spiritual traditions and practices. He called this core the "perennial wisdom," and it is related to what animates the renewed tradition.
5. Rappaport 1978.
6. The following discussion of synergy is adapted from Katz 1982a, chapter 11; Katz 1993.
7. The concept of synergy draws on the seminal work of Buckminster Fuller (e.g., Fuller 1963), Ruth Benedict (Maslow and Honigmann 1970), and the subsequent thinking of Abraham Maslow (Maslow 1971).
8. Katz 1983/84.
9. Quote appears in Katz 1982a, pp. 200–201.
10. Katz 1983/84.
11. Katz 1983/84.
12. Quote appears in Katz 1982a, p. 184.

13. Quote appears in Katz 1982a, p. 64.

14. Quote appears in Katz 1982a, p. 127.

15. Jul'hoan people use the word *xabasi,* which is derived from *dikgaba* in the Tswana language, to refer to the power of ill will or unresolved feelings between people to cause damage or sickness. They visualize xabasi (pl.) as emanations from the angry or jealous heart of one person that may fly forth and injure another.

16. This discussion of life paths is adapted from Katz 1993.

17. Katz 1993.

18. Beck, Walters, and Francisco 1992.

19. Merton 1970.

20. Lame Deer and Erdoes 1972, Neihardt 1972.

21. Musqua 1991.

CHAPTER 11

1. See Bodley 1990.

2. King 1989, pp. 2–3.

CHAPTER 12

1. Quote appears in Katz 1982a, p. 194.

APPENDIX C

1. See Bernard 1980, Wilford 1991.

GLOSSARY

To facilitate the process of looking up unfamiliar words, we have *not* alphabetized the words in this glossary according to standard Jul'hoan orthography. Thus, readers will find words with clicks alphabetized as if they were English words. Also note that *Tsw* refers to a word with a Tswana language origin, and *pl* refers to the plural form of the word. Earlier spellings of a word are enclosed in brackets.

GENERAL VOCABULARY

Afrikaans: Language of Afrikaners.

Afrikaner: White settlers of Dutch descent who arrived in what is now Botswana in 1897 from the South African Cape Colony.

!aia [!kia]: An enhanced state of consciousness that makes healing possible; to enter a healing trance.

BaSarwa: A word used in Botswana by Tswana to denote Bushmen.

Boer: The Afrikaans word for *farmer.*

borehole: A mechanically drilled well; water is brought to the surface through a deep, narrow pipeline.

djo [zho]: Black; a word used by Jul'hoansi to refer to Herero and Tswana people, whose skin is generally darker than their own.

Dobe area: The area in the northwestern Kalahari that includes the traditional water holes of |Kae|kae, Dobe, !Aoan, and G!oci and the villages and settlements that have grown up around them.

g!aeha [!geiha]: Most expert healer or master of n|om.

g!ukxao: Part of core kin group traditionally using a water source; literally, "water steward."

Herero, Hereros (pl): A pastoral ethnic group driven out of South West Africa (now Namibia) into Bechuanaland (now Botswana) in 1904 by the German colonial government; they speak one of the Bantu languages.

≠hoe [≠twe, |hwe]: To heal; literally, "to pull out," meaning (in the context of the dance) "to pull out sickness."

Jul'hoan, Jul'hoansi (pl) [Julwa, Julwasi (pl) or Zhu|twa, Zhu|twasi (pl)]: One language group of Bushmen in Botswana and Namibia. Their name means "real," "genuine," or "ordinary" people.

kgotla (Tsw): A traditional Tswana council and court held outdoors, usually under a prominent shade tree.

kowhedili [kowhidili]: The intense and dramatic cry of healing; the cry expresses the pain and difficulty of the healing work.

!Kung: A linguists' appellation for Jul'hoan Bushmen.

kxao, kxaosi (pl) [kao, k"au, k"ausi (pl)]: A steward, owner, master, or expert.

mafisa (Tsw): A system of farming out cattle for poorer people to care for in exchange for one beast a year for the poor person's own herd.

mokoma [makoma] (Tsw): Literally, a "dance of blood"; some form of healing dance.

mprofiti (Tsw): Evangelists.

n!a'an [n!a]: Old; big; great.

Nama: Sheepherding pastoralists of southern Namibia and western South Africa pejoratively called "Hottentots" by Dutch colonists.

Nharo [Naron]: A Bushman language group from western Botswana—the Ghanzi area—and southeast Namibia.

n|om [n|um]: Spiritual energy or power; spiritual healing energy or power.

n|omkxao, n|omkxaosi (pl) [n|um k"au, n|um k"ausi (pl)]: A healer; literally, "steward of n|om" or "master of n|om."

n!ore, n!oresi (pl): The traditional hunting and gathering territory of a Jul'hoan band.

pan: A shallow depression in the Kalahari that holds water during the rainy season.

SeTswana (Tsw): The language of the Tswana.

tara: Another word for experiences of !aia during drum dance; shaking and quivering during the altered state of !aia; usually used in reference to women.

Tswana: Agricultural/pastoral majority ethnic group of Botswana; they speak one of the Bantu languages.

|Uihaba [|Wihabe, |Wihaba]: Drotsky's Caves; a tourist attraction in the |Kae|kae area.

Vasekela: The Bushman language group from northern Namibia and Angola.

!xari [!khadi]: Beer, alcohol, or homebrew.

xaro [hxaro]: To give, as a gift.

!Xu: One of the names for the great God. Gǂkao Nǃa'an [ǂGao Nǃa] is another name.

BUSH FOODS

ca: Wild sweet potato; *Vigna lobatifolia.*

dcaa: Gemsbok cucumber; *Acanthosicyos naudiniana.*

dshin: Morama (Tsw) bean; *Tylosema esculenta.*

gǁkaa [gǁaa]: Mongongo (Tsw) nut, *Ricinodendron rautanenii.*

gǃoan: Kalahari raisin bush; *Grewia retinervis.*

gǀoq'o [gǀo'o]: An unidentified root food plant.

gǁu'ia [gǁuia, guia]: A leafy food plant; *Talinum esculentum.*

gǃxoa [gǃoah]: Water root; *Fockea angustifolia.*

kaq'amakoq [komako]: Two-color raisin bush; *Grewia bicolor.*

marula (Tsw): Nut tree; *Sclerocarya caffra.*

mongongo, mongongoes (pl) (Tsw): See gǁ*kaa* above.

morama (Tsw): See *dshin* above.

nǂah: Buffalo thorn berry; *Zizyphus mucronata.*

nǀang: Wild currant bush; *Grewia flava.*

nǃoh: Kalahari "orange"; *Strychnos cocculoides.*

ǂ'o: Grove (of nut trees).

ǀore: Rough-leafed raisin bush; *Grewia flavescens.*

ǂube: An unidentified food plant.

BIBLIOGRAPHY

Abrahamson, E. M., and A. W. Pezet. 1951. *Body, mind and sugar.* New York: Avon Books.

Arbousset, T. 1846. *Narrative of an exploratory tour of the northeast Cape of Good Hope.* Cape Town: Robertson.

Barnard, A. 1979. Nharo Bushman medicine and medicine men. *Africa,* 49(1).

———. 1992. *Hunters and herders of southern Africa.* Cambridge: Cambridge University Press.

Beck, P., A. Walters, and N. Francisco. 1992. *The sacred: Ways of knowledge, sources of life.* Tsaile, Ariz.: Navajo Community College Press.

Ben, L. W. 1991. Wellness circles: The Alkali Lake model in community recovery processes. Doctoral dissertation, Northern Arizona University. Ann Arbor, Mich.: University Microfilms International.

Bernard, H. 1980. Orthography for whom? *International Journal of American Linguistics* 46:133–36.

Biesele, M. 1974. A note on the beliefs of modern Bushmen concerning Tsodilo Hills. *Newsletter of the South West Africa Scientific Society* 15(3).

———. 1975a. Folklore and ritual of !Kung hunter-gatherers. Doctoral dissertation, Department of Anthropology, Harvard University, Cambridge, Mass.

———.1975b. Song texts by the Master of Tricks: Kalahari San thumb piano music. *Botswana Notes and Records* 7:171–88.

———. 1975c. Aspects of !Kung folklore. In *Kalahari hunter-gatherers,* edited by R. B. Lee and I. DeVore. Cambridge, Mass.: Harvard University Press.

———. 1983. Interpretation in rock art and folklore: Communication systems in evolutionary perspective. *South African Archaeological Bulletin* 4, June.

———. 1986. "Anyone with sense would know": Tradition and creativity in !Kung narrative and song. In *Contemporary studies in Khoisan,* edited by R. Vossen and K. Keuthmann. Hamburg, Germany: Helmut Buske Verlag.

———. 1988. The Peabody Museum and "The Culture of Imagery." Review of *From Site to Sight: Anthropology, Photography, and the Power of Imagery,* by C. Hinsley and M. Banta. *Exposure* 26(1):5–15.

———. 1992. Integrated environmental development in Namibia: The case of the Ju/'hoan Bushmen. Paper presented at the ninety-first annual meeting of the American Anthropological Association, San Francisco, December.

———. 1993. *Women like meat: The folklore and foraging ideology of the Kalahari Ju/'hoan.* Johannesburg: University of Witwatersrand Press; and Bloomington: Ind.: Indiana University Press.

———. 1995. Human rights and democratization in Namibia: Some grassroots political perspectives. *African Rural and Urban Studies.* 1(2):49–72.

———, ed. 1987. *The past and future of !Kung ethnography: Critical reflections and symbolic perspectives. Essays in honor of Lorna Marshall.* Hamburg, Germany: Helmut Buske Verlag.

Biesele, M., and P. Weinberg. 1990. *Shaken roots: The Bushmen of Namibia.* Marshalltown, South Africa: Environmental and Development Agency.

Bodley, J. 1990. *Victims of progress.* 3rd ed. Mountain View, Calif.: Mayfield Publishing Company.

Borgoras, W. 1907. *The Jesup North Pacific Expedition,* vol. 2 *(The Chukchee).* Leiden.

Burgos-Debray, E., ed. 1984. *I, Rigoberta Menchu: An Indian woman in Guatemala.* London: New Left Books.

Campbell, M. 1973. *Half-breed.* Toronto: McClelland and Stewart.

Cashdan, E. 1980. Egalitarianism among hunters and gatherers: Reports and comments. *American Anthropologist* 82:116–20.

Churchill, W., ed. 1989. *Critical issues in native North America.* Copenhagen: International Work Group for Indigenous Affairs.

Clifford, J., and G. F. Marcus, eds. 1986. *Writing culture: The poetics and politics of ethnography.* Berkeley: University of California Press.

Comaroff, J. 1986. Christianity and colonialism in South Africa. *American Ethnologist,* 13(1):1–22.

Davis-Floyd, R. 1992. *Birth as an American rite of passage.* Berkeley: University of California Press.

Dickens, P. 1991. Ju/'hoan orthography in practice. *South African Journal of African Languages* 11(1):99–104.

———. 1994. *English-Ju/'hoan, Ju/'hoan-English dictionary.* Cologne: Ruediger Koeppe Verlag.

———. 1995. Why anthropologists need linguists: The case of the !Kung. *African Studies* 54(1).

———. In press. *Ju/'hoan grammar.* Cologne: Ruediger Koeppe Verlag.

Dickens, P., and the Ju/'hoan Peoples Literacy Committee. 1990. *Ju/'hoan-English dictionary.* Windhoek, Namibia:

Nyae Nyae Development Foundation of Namibia.

Draper, P. 1975. !Kung women: Contrasts in sexual egalitarianism in the foraging and sedentary contexts. In *Toward an
anthropology of women*, edited by R. Reiter. New York:
Monthly Review Press.

Draper, P., and E. Cashdan. 1988. Technological change and
child behavior among the !Kung. *Ethnology* 27(4):339–65.

Duffy, W. 1975. *Sugar blues.* New York: Warner Books.

Ebert, J. 1976. Hunting in Botswana's past and its role in a
developing Botswana. *UNM Report* (No. 13). Alberquerque:
University of New Mexico.

Eliade, M. 1965. *Rites and symbols of initiation.* New York:
Harper and Row.

England, N. 1992. *Music among the Ju/'hoansi and related
peoples of Namibia, Botswana, and Angola.* New York:
Garland.

Fanon, F. 1963. *The wretched of the earth.* New York: Grove.

Four Worlds and Phil Lukas. 1985. *The honor of all.*
Lethbridge, Alberta, Canada: Four Worlds International
Institute for Human and Community Development. Film.

Freire, P. 1968. *The pedagogy of the oppressed.* New York: Seabury.

Fuller, B. 1963. *Ideas and integrities.* New York: Macmillan.

Gordon, R. J. 1992. *The Bushman myth: The making of a
Namibian underclass.* Boulder, Colo.: Westview Press.

Goulet, D. 1985. *The cruel choice: A new concept in the theory of
development.* Washington, D.C.: University Press of America.

Guenther, M. G. 1973. *Farm Bushmen and mission Bushmen:
Sociocultural change in a setting of conflicts and pluralism of
the San of the Ghanzi District, Republic of Botswana.*
Doctoral dissertation, University of Toronto.

———. 1986. *The Nharo Bushmen of Botswana: Tradition and
change.* Hamburg, Germany: Helmut Buske Verlag.

Guillory, B., E. Willie, and E. Duran. 1988. Analysis of a community organizing case study: Alkali Lake. *Journal of Rural
Community Psychology* 9(1).

Hamilton, A. 1978. Dual social systems: Technology, labour,
and women's secret rites in the eastern Western Desert of
Australia. Paper presented at the International Conference
on Hunter-Gatherers, Paris.

Hermans, J. 1977. Official policy toward the Bushmen of
Botswana. *Botswana Notes & Records* 9:55–67.

Hitchcock, R. 1978. Patterns of sedentism among the hunters
and gatherers in eastern Botswana. Paper presented at the
first international conference on hunting and gathering
societies, Paris.

———. 1988. *Monitoring research and development in
the remote areas of Botswana.* Gaborone, Botswana:
Government Printer.

———. 1992. *Communities and consensus: An evaluation of
the activities of the Nyae Nyae Farmers' Cooperative and the
Nyae Nyae Development Foundation in northeastern
Namibia: A report to the Ford Foundation and the Nyae Nyae
Development Foundation of Namibia.* New York: Ford
Foundation.

———. 1992. The ecology of sustainable and non-sustainable
development in southern Africa. Paper presented at the
91st annual meeting of the American Anthropological
Association, San Francisco.

Hitchcock, R., and J. D. Holm. 1993. Bureaucratic domination
of hunter-gatherer societies: A study of the San in
Botswana. *Development and Change* 24:305–38.

Hitchcock, R. and W. Jeffers. 1982. *Land use planning in the
communal areas.* Report of the Rural Development Unit
and Rural Sociology Unit, Ministry of Finance and
Development Planning and Ministry of Agriculture,
Gaborone, Botswana.

Hitchcock, R., U. Kann, and N. Mbere. 1990. *Let them talk: A
review of the Accelerated Remote Area Development Program.*
Gaborone, Botswana: Ministry of Local Government and
Lands; and Oslo, Norway: Norwegian Agency for
International Development and Ministry of Development
Cooperation.

Hobsbawm, E., and T. Ranger, 1984. *The invention of tradition.*
Cambridge: Cambridge University Press.

Hoch-Smith, J., and A. Spring, eds. 1978. *Women in ritual and
symbolic roles.* New York: Plenum.

Howell, N. 1979. *Demography of the Dobe !Kung.* New York:
Academic Press.

Hurlich, S., and R. B. Lee 1979. Colonialism, apartheid, and
liberation: A Namibian example. In *Challenging anthropology,* edited by D. Turner and G. Smith. Toronto: McGraw-
Hill Ryerson.

Huxley, A. 1970. *The perennial philosophy.* New York:
HarperCollins.

Katz, R. 1981. Education as transformation: Becoming a healer
among the !Kung and Fijians. *Harvard Educational Review*
51(1):57–78.

———. 1982a. *Boiling energy: Community healing among the
Kalahari Kung.* Cambridge: Harvard University Press.

———. 1982b. Commentary on education as transformation.
Harvard Educational Review 52(1):63–66.

———. 1982c. Utilizing traditional healing systems. *American
Psychologist* 37(6):115–16.

———. 1982d. Accepting boiling energy. *Ethos* 10(4):344–68.

———. 1983/84. Empowerment and synergy: Expanding
community healing resources. *Prevention in Human Services*
3(2/3):201–26.

————. 1986. Healing and transformation: Perspectives on development, education, and community. In *The cultural transition: Social transformation in the Third World and Japan,* edited by M. White and S. Pollak. London: Routledge and Kegan Paul.

————. 1993. *The straight path: A story of healing and transformation in Fiji.* Reading, Mass.: Addison-Wesley.

Katz, R., and M. Biesele. 1987. Male and female approaches to healing among the !Kung. In *The past and future of !Kung ethnography: Critical reflections and symbolic perspectives,* edited by M. Biesele. Hamburg, Germany: Helmut Buske Verlag.

Katz, R., and M. Biesele, and M. Shostak. 1982. *Healing music of the Kalahari San.* Folkways Records, New York.

Katz, R., and E. Rolde. 1981. Community alternatives to psychotherapy. *Psychotherapy Theory, Research and Practice* 18(3):365–74.

Katz, R., and N. Seth. 1986. Synergy and healing: A perspective on Western health care. *Prevention in Human Services* 5(1):109–36.

Katz, R., N. Seth, and M. Nuñez-Molina, eds. In press. *Synergy and healing: Multicultural perspectives on transformation and social change.* London: Zed Books.

Katz, R., and V. St. Denis. 1991. Teacher as healer: A renewing tradition. *Journal of Indigenous Studies* (2):23–36.

Kelly, R. L. 1995. *The foraging spectrum: Diversity in hunter-gatherer lifeways.* Washington, D.C.: Smithsonian Institute Press.

King, C. 1989. Here come the anthros. Paper delivered at the eighty-eighth annual meeting of the American Anthropological Society, Washington, D.C.

Kreisberg, S. 1992. *Transforming power: Domination, empowerment, and education.* Albany: State University of New York Press.

Lame Deer, J., and R. Erdoes. 1972. *Lame Deer: Seeker of visions.* New York: Simon and Schuster.

Leacock, E., and R. B. Lee, eds. 1982. *Politics and history in band societies.* Cambridge: Cambridge University Press.

Lee, R. B. 1967. Trance cure of the !Kung Bushmen. *Natural History* (November):30–37.

————. 1979. *The !Kung San: Men, women, and work in a foraging society.* Cambridge: Cambridge University Press.

————. 1985. Foragers and the state: Government policies toward the San in Namibia and Botswana. *Cultural Survival: Occasional Papers* 18:37–46.

————. 1993. *The Dobe Jul'hoansi.* 2nd ed. Fort Worth: Harcourt Brace College Publishers.

————. In press. The public, the private and the world system: The Jul'hoansi-!Kung today. In *Working Papers in the Humanities* series, edied by R. Halford. Windsor, Ontario: University of Windsor.

Lee, R. B. and M. Biesele. In press. From foragers to First Nation: Dependency or self-reliance among the Jul'hoansi-!Kung. *Development and Change.*

Lee, R. B., M. Biesele, and R. Hitchcock. 1996. Thirty years of ethnographic research among the Jul'hoansi of northwestern Botswana: 1963–1993. *Botswana notes and records,* vol. 28, May.

Lee, R. B. and I. DeVore, eds. 1968. *Man the hunter.* Chicago: Aldine.

————. 1976. *Kalahari hunter-gatherers: Studies of the !Kung San and their neighbors.* Cambridge: Harvard University Press.

Lee, R. B., and M. Guenther. 1991. Oxen or onions: The search for trade (and truth) in the Kalahari. *Current Anthropology* 32(5):592–601.

Lerner, M. 1994. *Jewish renewal: A path to healing and transformation.* New York: Putnam.

Lewis-Williams, J. D. 1981. *Believing and seeing: Symbolic meanings in southern San rock paintings.* New York: Academic Press.

Lewis-Williams, J. D., and T. A. Dowson. 1989. *Images of power: Understanding Bushman rock art.* Johannesburg: Southern Book Publishers.

Little Bear, L., M. Boldt, and J. Long. 1984. *Pathways to self-determination: Canadian Indians and the Canadian state.* Toronto: University of Toronto Press.

Marcus, G. E., and M. J. Fisher. 1986. *Anthropology as cultural critique: An experimental moment in the human sciences.* Chicago: University of Chicago Press.

Marshall, J. 1965. *N/um Tchai: The ceremonial dance of the !Kung Bushmen.* Watertown, Mass.: Documentary Educational Resources. Film.

————. 1980. *N!ai: The story of a !Kung woman.* Watertown, Mass.: Documentary Educational Resources. Film.

Marshall, L. 1961. Sharing, talking, and giving: Relief of social tensions among !Kung Bushmen. *Africa* 31(3):231–49.

————. 1969. The medicine dance of the !Kung Bushmen. *Africa* 39(4):347–81.

————. 1976. *The !Kung of Nyae Nyae.* Cambridge: Harvard University Press.

————. Forthcoming. *Beliefs and rites of the Nyae Nyae !Kung.*

Maslow, A. 1971. *The further reaches of human nature.* New York: Viking.

Maslow, A., and J. Honigmann. 1970. Synergy: Some notes of Ruth Benedict. *American Anthropologist* 72(2):320–33.

McGuire, M. 1983. Words of power: Personal empowerment and healing. *Culture, Medicine, and Psychiatry,* 7:221–40.

Memmi, A. 1965. *Colonizer and colonized.* Boston: Beacon.

Merton, T. 1977. *The wisdom of the desert.* New York: New Directions.

Mintz, S. 1986. *Sweetness and power: The place of sugar in modern history.* New York: Penguin Books.

Moody, R., ed. 1988. *The indigenous voice: Visions and realities.* Vol. 2. London: Zed.

Moraga, C., and G. Anzaldua, eds. 1983. *This bridge called my back: Writings by radical women of color.* New York: Kitchen Table Women of Color Press.

Musqua, D. 1991. Traditional Saulteaux human growth and development. Lecture delivered at the Saskatchewan Indian Federated College (March).

Navarro, V. 1976. *Medicine under capitalism.* New York: Prodist.

Neihardt, J. 1972. *Black Elk speaks.* New York: Pocket Books.

Ngugi, W. T. 1986. *Decolonizing the mind.* London: Currey.

Nunez-Molina, M. 1987. "Desarollo del Medium": The process of becoming a healer in Puerto Rican "espiritismo." Doctoral dissertation, Harvard University.

Peacock, J. 1987. *Rites of modernization: Symbols and social aspects of Indonesian proletarian drama.* Chicago: University of Chicago Press.

Rappaport, R. 1978. Adaptation and the structure of ritual. In *Human behavior and adaptation,* edited by N. Blurton-Jones and V. Reynolds. New York: Halsted.

Ritchie, C. 1987. *The political economy of resource tenure in the Kalahari.* Master's thesis, Department of Anthropology, Boston University.

Rohrlich-Leavitt, P., B. Sykes, and E. Weatherford. 1975. Aboriginal women: Male and female anthropological perspectives. In *Toward an anthropology of women,* edited by R. Reiter. New York: Monthly Review Press.

Rosaldo, R. 1993. *Culture and truth: The remaking of social analysis.* 2nd ed. Boston: Beacon Press.

Said, E. 1993. *Culture and imperialism.* New York: Alfred A. Knopf.

Schmookler, A. 1984. *The parable of the tribes: The problem of power in social evolution.* Berkeley: University of California Press.

Shostak, M. 1983. Nisa: *The life and words of a !Kung woman.* New York: Vintage Books.

Silberbauer, G. 1965. *Report to the government of Bechuanaland on the Bushman Survey.* Gaborone, Bechuanaland: Bechuanaland Government Printer.

Singer, M. 1986. Toward a political economy of alcoholism: The missing link in the anthropology of drinking. *Social Science and Medicine* 23(2):113–30.

Snyman, J. W. 1975. Zul'hoasi fonologie en woordeboek (Communication No. 37 of the University of Cape Town, School of African Studies). Cape Town and Rotterdam: A. A. Bakema.

Solway, J., and R. B. Lee. 1990. Foragers, genuine or spurious?: Situating the Kalahari San in history. *Current Anthropology* 32:106–46.

St. Denis, V. 1989. A process of community-based participatory research: A case study. Master's thesis, University of Alaska, Fairbanks.

———. 1992. Community-based participatory research: Aspects of the concept relevant for practice. *Native Studies Review* 8(2):51–74.

Tanaka, J. 1980. *The San, hunter-gatherers of the Kalahari: A study in ecological anthropology.* Tokyo: University of Tokyo Press.

Taussig, M. 1987. *Shamanism, colonialism, and the wild man: A study in terror and healing.* Chicago: University of Chicago Press.

Thomas, E. M. 1989. *The harmless people.* Rev. ed. New York: Vintage.

———. 1990. The old way: Lions and Bushmen of the Kalahari. *The New Yorker,* October 15.

Traill, A., R. Vossen, and M. Biesele, eds. 1995. *The complete linguist: Papers in the memory of Patrick J. Dickens.* Cologne: Ruediger Koeppe Verlag.

Trainer, T. 1989. *Developed to death: Rethinking Third World development.* London: Merlin.

Tsing, A. L. 1993. *In the realm of the diamond queen: Marginality in an out-of-the-way place.* Princeton: Princeton University Press.

Volkman, T. A. 1982. The San in transition: A guide to "N!ai: The Story of a !Kung Woman." Cambridge: Documentary Educational Resources and Cultural Survival.

Walsh, R., and F. Vaughan, eds. 1993. *Paths beyond ego: The transpersonal vision.* New York: G. P. Putnam.

Warnock, J. W. 1987. *The politics of hunger: The global food system.* New York: Methuen.

Wiessner, P. 1982. Risk, reciprocity and social influence on !Kung San economics. In *Politics and History in Band Societies,* edited by E. Leacock and R. Lee. Cambridge, England: Cambridge University Press.

Wilford, J. N. 1991. In a publishing coup: Books in "unwritten languages. *New York Times,* December 31.

Wilmsen, E. 1989. *Land filled with flies: A political economy of the Kalahari.* Chicago: University of Chicago Press.

Woodburn, J. 1980. Hunters and gatherers today and reconstruction of the past. In *Soviet and Western anthropology,* edited by A. Gellner. London: Duckworth.

York, G. 1989. *The dispossessed: Life and death in Native Canada.* Toronto: Lester and Orpen Dennys.

INDEX

Note: notes are indexed by page, chapter, and note number thus: 199n 9.7

advocacy. *See* development work; "paper people"
Afrikaners, 195n 5
agriculturalism, 12. *See also* pastoralists
!aia. *See also* tara
 described, 19
 dying and, 2
|Ai!ae |Aice, 72
|Ai!ae N!a'an, 124
 on dance play, 121
alcohol, use and abuse of, 39, 95–100, 165, 174, 197n 2.8
Alcoholics Anonymous, 198n 7.2
alcoholism, 100, 165, 198n 7.2, 198n 7.3
Alkali Lake Band, 198n 7.3
|Am, on tara, 115–16
|'Angn!ao, 50
animals
 hunted by Jul'hoansi, 16
 transformation into, 24–25
!Aoan, 39
arguing with the gods, during healing work, 24
authors (of this book). *See also individual authors*
 as "paper people," 7–8
 potential influence of, 147–51
 reflections on project, 177–82
 role as cultural translators, 155–61

Beh, origination of healing songs, 131–32
BaSarwa, as term, 186
BaSarwa Development Office, 192
Bechuanaland. *See also* Botswana
 early history of, 36–38
beer brewing. *See* alcohol
Biesele, Megan
 development work, 190–94
biomedical model. *See* clinic

Boiling Energy: Community Healing among the Kalahari Kung (Katz), 2, 196n 3 Prologue
border fence, 39
borehole syndicates, 42, 197n 2.10
Botswana. *See also* Bechuanaland
 effect of independence on Jul'hoansi, 32–35
British Protectorate of Bechuanaland, early history of, 36–38
bush foods, 16. *See also* wild foods
 sharing of, 17
Bushman, as term, xi, 166, 186, 195n 2
Bushman Development Program, 41
Bushmen. *See* Jul'hoansi

caregiving, role men play, 196n 1.1
Cashdan, Elizabeth, 199–200n 9.10
cash economy, effect on Jul'hoansi, 67
cattle, effect on Jul'hoan lifestyle, 34–35, 37, 197n 2.1
cattle care, by Jul'hoansi, 36–37
cattle ownership, Jul'hoansi and, 191
chant, during healing dance, 106
Christianity, among Jul'hoansi, 43–44
chronology, of Jul'hoan history, 187–89
church (Christian) services, 43–44
climbing threads to God's village, 80–81, 108–9
 in joint healing effort, 113
clinic
 healing collaboration and, 92–93
 and Jul'hoan healing, 85–93
 as source of treatment, 61
communication, importance to Jul'hoansi, 155
conflict, healing dance and, 17, 18, 105–6
court system (kgotla), 38, 43
creative process, community and, 132–33

cultural traditions, xiii, 195n 6. *See also* Jul'hoan culture; social change
 government influence on, 67–69
cultural translation, 154–61

Dabe, 59
development work, on behalf of Indigenous peoples, 190–94
DeVore, Irven, 27
Dickens, Patrick, 185
Dillxao (dancer), on dancing, 129
Dillxao ≠Oma, on government, 161
djxani tcxai (to dance a song), 196n 1.12
Dobe area, map, x, 33
Dowson, Thomas, 54–55
Draper, Patricia, 197n 2.4, 199n 9.6, 199–200n 9.10
drum dance, 115, 199n 9.1
 contrasted with giraffe dance, 119–24
 gender roles and, 199n 9.6
drums, for dancing, 121, 199n 9.7
dying, Jul'hoan understanding of, 2, 111

education. *See also* schooling
 conflict with Jul'hoan tradition, 72–74
 employment opportunities and, 72, 74–76
 of healers, 59–61
 value of, 71–72
education programs, for Jul'hoansi, 185–86, 193
educators, attitude to healing dance, 72–73, 80
egalitarianism, among Jul'hoansi, 13–14, 124, 199–200n 9.10
 sedentism and, 200n 9.11
employment opportunities, education and, 72, 74–76
European medicine. *See* clinic

Kinachau, 4
    effects of boiling nǀom, 110
    on the healing dance, 1
    seeing properly, 109
    on women and nǀom, 118
King, Cecil, 149
Koba (ǃXu's wife), 197n 1.18
Koba (young mother)
    nǀom and pregnancy, 125
    tara and, 123
Kodinyau, 29, 166
    on schooling, 74–75, 77
Kommtsa (from Mahopa), on govern-
    ment treatment, 43
Kommtsa Nǃa'an
    on alcohol use, 96
    receiving nǀom, 161
kowhedili, 111, 196n 1.15
Kxao ǂOah
    on European medicine, 89
    on fear of dying, 2, 111
    on nǀom, 19
    "seeing" in the healing dance, 23
    spiritual journey of, 106–8
Kxao ǀOǀOo, 174–75, 183–84
    about, xix
    education and, 72, 76
    effect of alcohol use, 96–97
    on healing collaboration, 93
    schooling and healing, 80–83
kxaosi ("owners"), 16
    sharing and, 17
Kxao Tjimburu, 183, 184
    about, xviii–xix
    on alcohol use, 99–100
    climbing threads to God's village, 108
    on nǀom of women and men, 117
    on schooling, 75, 77
    and transformation to lion,
        24–25
    wife's role when he dances, 126
Kxaru Nǃa'an, 32
    about, xix
    and the clinic, 89
    nǀom and pregnancy, 125
    on wells, 42

land allocation, 42–43, 44–45. See also
    nǀore system

land boards, Juǀ'hoansi and, 42
language. See Juǀ'hoan language
language groups, 195n 3
leaving the body, healers and, 24–25
Lee, Richard, 27, 147, 198n 8.1
Lewis-Williams, David, 54–55
lion, transformation into, 24–25

mafisa (cattle keeping), 36–37
maps, Dobe area, x, 33
Marshall, John, 49, 195
Marshall, Laurence, 38
Marshall, Lorna, 24, 38, 51, 119, 131–32
marula nuts, 196n 1.6
Mathlare, Leonard, 192
meat, sharing of, 17
men
    caregiving role of, 196n 1.1
    roles in healing dance(s) , 21–23,
        117–24, 126–29
missionaries, influence of, 43
Molebatsi, Florence, 183

Nǃae
    gathering wild foods, 49–50
    on singing and ǃaia, 118
Nǂaisa (wife of Kxao Tjimburu), 20, 116,
    183
    about, xix
    importance of heart, 141
    role during healing dance, 126
Nǂaisa Nǃa'an, 183
    about, xx
    on government, 32
    role of healer's wife, 126–27
    on schooling, 75
names. See also Juǀ'hoan names
    importance of, 166
Namibia. See also South West Africa
    effect of independence on Juǀ'hoansi,
        32
Nǃhunkxa, tara and, 123
nǀom
    benefits of, 47–48
    boiling, 26, 110–11
    description of, 18–19
    Dick Katz and, 6–7
    dying and, 2, 111
    Kommtsa Nǃa'an and, 161

learning to "drink," 198–99n 8.2
ǂOma Djo and, 56–59
power of, 104–5
relation to reproductive status, 120,
    124–26
seekers of, 59–61
sources of, 56
synergy of, 137–39
women and, 117–18
young people and, 60–61
nomenclature, 186
nǀore system, 16, 50
nurse (at ǀKaeǀkae clinic), relation to
    Juǀ'hoan healing, 86–88, 90
nurse (regional), relation to Juǀ'hoan
    healing, 87–88
Nyae Nyae Development Foundation of
    Namibia (NNDFN), 193
Nyae Nyae Farmers' Cooperative, 30, 32,
    45, 113, 185, 195n 9
Nyae Nyae Residents' Council, xvii, 195n
    9

Odendaal Commission, 38
ǂOma Djo, 7, 65, 183, 184
    about, xx
    on alcohol use, 95, 96, 97–98, 99, 100
    climbing threads to God's village,
        108–9
    on the clinic, 89
    concern for future healers, 60–61
    death of, 171–72
    drum and giraffe dancing, 123–24
    on effect of cattle, 34–35
    on food scarcity, 32
    on government, 32
    on government food programs, 67
    on the healing dance, 1, 23
    on heart, 139–41, 142
    hoarding of nǀom, 138
    how he received nǀom, 56–57
    hunting-gathering life of, 11, 14–15
    joint healing effort, 112–13
    leaving his body, 24–25
    on nǀom, 47, 55–56, 62, 131
    on nǀom of women and men, 117
    on origination of healing songs, 132
    power as a healer, 58–59
    on purpose of dancing, 133–34

relation to Jul'hoansi, 12, 34–35
Tswana headmen, 197n 2.7

‖Uce N!a'an, 183
  on n‖om, 118
|Ui
  on healing, 25–26
  importance of heart, 141
  on n‖om, 137, 138
  on seeing properly, 109–10
|Uihaba Dancers, 77–80
|Ukxa, 183, 184
  about, xxi
  education and, 71–72, 75–76
  schooling and healing, 81
Utugile, Isak, 38
!U'u N!a'an, on abundance, 161

vegetable foods. *See* bush foods; wild
  foods
Village Development Committees, 43
Village Schools Project, 83

water rights. *See* borehole syndicates;
  g!ukxao; wells
wells, difficulty in obtaining, 42
Westerman, Floyd, 149
Wiessner, Polly, 197n 2.8, 199n 9.6
wild foods. *See also* bush foods
  gathering, 49–50
  use of, 39–40
women
  and n‖om, 117–18
  roles in healing dance, 23, 117–24,
    126–29, 199n 9.9
writing. *See also* Jul'hoan language
  importance to Jul'hoansi, 7

xabasi (ill-will sickness), 141, 201n
  10.15
‖xabe (to open the heart), 141, 161
Xam, 29
  aspirations of, 174
!xari (homebrew), 95–100
xaro (gift-giving), 17

|Xoan (wife of Tshao N!a'an), 183
  on alcohol use, 96
  marriage to a healer, 127–28
  on |Uihaba Dancers, 79
|Xoan N!a'an, 92
  on healing collaboration, 92–93
!Xu (God), 24, 43, 197n 1.18
!Xuma (from Bate), on gift-giving, 17
!Xuma (from Dobe)
  on goverment meetings, 42
  on importance of heart, 142
Xumi N!a'an
  about, xxi
  on alcohol use, 95–96, 98–99, 99–100
  death of, 171
  on First Nations peoples, 164, 165–66
  on government meetings, 7
  on land, 42, 153
  on n‖om of women and men, 117–18
  on |Uihaba Dancers, 77, 79, 80

Committed to the respectful exchange of healing knowledge across cultures, **RICHARD KATZ** began work nearly thirty years ago with Indigenous healers and traditional community healing systems, first in the Kalahari Desert, then in Fiji, Alaska, and several First Nations communities in North America. After receiving his Ph.D. in Clinical Psychology from Harvard, he taught there over a twenty-year period. Currently a Professor at the Saskatchewan Indian Federated College in Saskatoon, Saskatchewan, he works with First Nations elders to create healing environments that draw upon both Indigenous and Western knowledge. In addition to *Boiling Energy: Community Healing Among the Kalahari Kung* (Harvard University Press), an earlier study of Ju/'hoan healing, Katz has written *The Straight Path: A Story of Healing and Transformation in Fiji* (Addison-Wesley); and co-edited *Synergy and Healing: Multicultural Perspectives on Transformation and Social Change* (Zed Books).

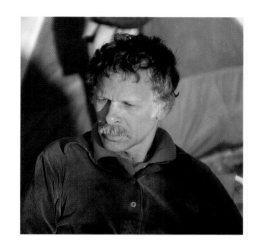

VERNA ST. DENIS, a Cree/Metis from Saskatchewan and a member of Beardy's and Okemasis Band, has a long-term commitment to improving education for Aboriginal people. An Assistant Professor in the Indian and Northern Education Program at the University of Saskatchewan, in Saskatoon, she is currently a Ph.D. student in Anthropology and Education at Stanford University. Her thesis will focus on constructions of cultural identity among Canadian Aboriginal educators. St. Denis also has an interest in community-based research. Her article entitled "Community-based Participatory Research: Aspects of the Concept Relevant for Practice" was recently published in the *Native Studies Review.*

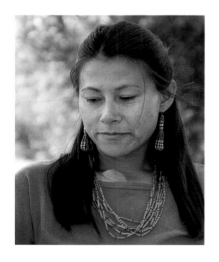

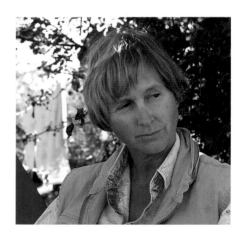

MEGAN BIESELE is an anthropologist who has worked in the Kalahari since 1970. She helped establish and run development and advocacy organizations with the Jul'hoan people in Botswana and Namibia since 1973 and remains active there as a consultant in the area of Indigenous education. Her fields of interest, research, and publication include Jul'hoan folklore and religion, development studies, hunter-gatherer studies, and rock art interpretation. Currently she teaches at the University of Texas. Biesele is the author of *Women Like Meat: The Folklore and Foraging Ideology of the Kalahari Ju/'hoan* (Witwatersrand University Press and Indiana University Press) and *Shaken Roots: The Bushmen of Namibia* (EDA Publications), which includes photography by Paul Weinberg.

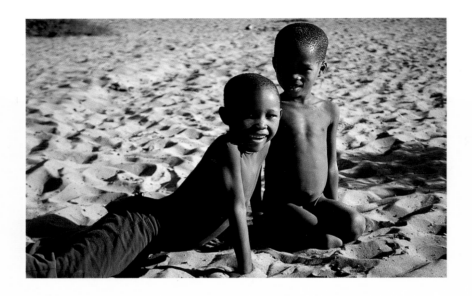

A FUND FOR THE JUǀ'HOANSI

The royalties we receive as authors from this book will be contributed to a fund for the Juǀ'hoansi, and they will decide how to use this money to further their own development. Inner Traditions International, the publisher of this book, is also donating a part of its profits to this cause. We invite you the reader to join in this effort.

The Juǀ'hoansi fund will be administered by The Kalahari Peoples' Fund. Contributions, which are tax deductible, can be sent directly to this fund at:

P.O. Box 7855
University Station
Austin, Texas 78713-7855
U.S.A.

Checks should be made out to The Kalahari Peoples' Fund, earmarked "For the Juǀ'hoansi." For further information, we can be reached in care of the publisher. We look forward to enlarging and enlivening the network of real help.